# MKSAP® for Students 2

## Medical Knowledge Self-Assessment Program®

D1297863

Developed by
American College of Physicians
Clerkship Directors in Internal Medicine

## Publisher's Information

American College of Physicians
190 N. Independence Mall West
Philadelphia, PA 19106-1572
215-351-2600

ISBN: 1-930513-44-5

Library of Congress Card Number: 2002112095

Printed in the United States of America

# Acknowledgements

## MKSAP for Students 2 Development Team

**Eric J. Alper, MD**
Assistant Professor of Medicine
Internal Medicine Clerkship Director
University of Massachusetts Medical School
Worcester, Massachusetts

**Alpesh N. Amin, MD**
Associate Clinical Professor
Medicine Clerkship Director, Associate Program Director,
Internal Medicine Residency
University of California
Irvine, California

**Kimberly Baker-Genaw, MD**
Associate Program Director
Clerkship Coordinator for Year 3 and 4 Medical Student
Programs
Department of Internal Medicine, Henry Ford Hospital
Detroit, Michigan

**Erica Friedman, MD**
Associate Professor of Medicine
Director of Medicine Clerkships, Director of Evaluation
Department of Medicine
The Mount Sinai Hospital
Mount Sinai School of Medicine
New York, New York

**Robert Hirschtick, MD**
Assistant Professor of Medicine
Division of General Internal Medicine
Northwestern University, Feinberg School of Medicine
Chicago, Illinois

**Christopher A. Klipstein, MD**
Assistant Professor
Internal Medicine Clerkship Director
University of North Carolina School of Medicine
Chapel Hill, North Carolina

**Patricia Kutz MD**
Associate Professor of Clinical Medicine
Co-Director, Internal Medicine Clerkship
The University of Chicago Hospitals
Chicago, Illinois

**David R. Lambert, MD**
Associate Professor of Medicine
Associate Dean, Undergraduate Medical Education
University of Rochester School of Medicine and Dentistry
Rochester, New York

**John N. Langenberg, MD**
Associate Professor of Medicine
Associate Medical Clerkship Director
State University of New York, Upstate Medical University
Syracuse, New York

**David Neely, MD**
Assistant Professor
Director, Undergraduate Education, Department of Medicine
Northwestern University, Feinberg School of Medicine
Chicago, Illinois

**Shalini Reddy, MD**
Assistant Professor of Clinical Medicine
Co-Director, Internal Medicine Clerkship
The University of Chicago, Pritzker School of Medicine
Chicago, Illinois

**Steven F. Reichert, MD**
Clinical Assistant Professor
The Mount Sinai Hospital
Mount Sinai School of Medicine
New York, New York

**Rainier Patrick Soriano, MD**
Assistant Professor, Medicine & Geriatrics
Co-Director, Integrated Medicine-Geriatrics Clerkship
Associate Director for Medical Education
Brookdale Department of Geriatrics & Adult Development
Mount Sinai School of Medicine
New York, New York

*Editor-in-Chief (ACP Staff)*
**Patrick C. Alguire, MD, FACP**
Director, Education and Career Development
American College of Physicians
Philadelphia, Pennsylvania

The American College of Physicians gratefully acknowledges the special contributions to MKSAP for Students 2 of Michael Ripca (graphic designer), Francine Martin (administrator), Sheila O'Steen (content production), Lisa Rockey and Heather Cline (manuscript support). All systems and applications were developed by Steven Spadt, Sean O'Donnell, John McKnight, and Adam Schuman of the College's Electronic Product Development group. The College also wishes to acknowledge that many other persons, too numerous to mention, have contributed to the production of this product. Without their dedicated efforts, the publication would not have been possible.

# Foreword

Dear Student:

An essential part of the practice of medicine is the science and art of problem solving. The enormous body of factual material that must be mastered will, in the final analysis, be of value only if intelligently applied to the care of patients.

As a consequence, medical educators have sought to ensure that problem-solving skills are learned and retained throughout the long professional lifetime of the practicing physician.

More than 30 years ago, the American College of Physicians launched a new program to enable practicing internists to measure how well they have kept abreast of new information and how well they are applying it to the care of patients. *The Medical Knowledge Self-Assessment Program* (*MKSAP*) was an instant success, and the current 12th edition has almost 40,000 subscribers who are glowing in their feedback about the impact that the program has had on their professional lives.

Several years ago, the leadership of the College and the Clerkship Directors in Internal Medicine launched a self-assessment product focused on the needs of medical students during their third and fourth years. Modeled after *MKSAP* for internal medicine physicians, the student *MKSAP* was designed to include case-based multiple-choice questions for self-assessment. Each question has a critique, providing information about the topic of the question and why the various options are either correct or incorrect. The first edition was popular and well received. However, with the passage of time come changes in the science and practice of medicine. These are reflected in this second edition of *MKSAP* for Students.

We hope that this program will be a valuable adjunct to your studies and your clerkship experience. If the experiences of hundreds of thousands of internists are a guide, this product will reinforce your learning and help ensure that it is applied in a fashion that will make you the best physician you can be, for your patients deserve no less!

Good luck in your studies and in your future career.

Sincerely,

**Herbert S. Waxman, MD, FACP**
*Senior Vice President, Medical Knowledge and Education*
American College of Physicians

The American College of Physicians wishes to acknowledge the vision and leadership of Herbert S. Waxman, MD, FACP, in the creation of *MKSAP for Students 2*. No individual has contributed more to the realization of the College's commitment to excellence and professionalism in the practice of medicine. He will be dearly missed.

# Preface

The goal of *MKSAP for Students* is to help define and assess mastery of the core knowledge base requisite to internal medicine education in medical school. This study aid is intended primarily for third-year students participating in their required internal medicine clerkship. Other audiences include fourth-year students on an advanced medicine clerkship; second-year students involved in pathophysiology, clinical problem solving, and problem-based learning; and physician assistant students. In creating this product, we have chosen to model it after the highly successful *Medical Knowledge Self-Assessment Program* (*MKSAP*) for internal medicine physicians. We are proud that the first edition of MKSAP for Students was awarded the 2002 Education Development Award from the Clerkship Directors in Internal Medicine.

*MKSAP for Students* consists of a printed and electronic collection of patient-centered self-assessment questions and their answers. The questions begin with a clinical vignette, and the vignettes are organized into 28 different categories that correspond to the *Core Medicine Clerkship Curriculum Guide's* "Training Problems." *The Clerkship Curriculum Guide* is a nationally recognized curriculum for the required third-year internal medicine clerkship created and published by the Clerkship Directors in Internal Medicine (CDIM) and the Society for General Internal Medicine (SGIM). It defines the competencies, knowledge, attitudes, and skills that medical students are expected to master by the end of the clerkship. The "Training Problems" categorize the learning content in the areas of health maintenance and disease screening, disease manifestations, specific diseases, abnormal laboratory findings, and risky lifestyles or behaviors.

Each question has been specifically edited by a group of clerkship directors to meet the learning needs of students participating in the medicine clerkship. Each question comes with an answer critique that supplies the correct answer, an explanation of why that answer is correct and the incorrect options are not, and a short bibliography. We recommend that students read the clinical vignette, select an answer, and then read the associated answer critique.

We would like to emphasize that *MKSAP for Students* is not to be used as a formal evaluation of students. The questions reflect the many real management dilemmas faced daily by internal medicine physicians and when coupled with the answer critiques, provide a focused, concise review of important content. In short, *MKSAP for Students* is a learning text, not an evaluation instrument.

The second edition of *MKSAP for Students* would have been impossible without the valuable and entirely voluntary contributions of many people, some of whom are named in the Acknowledgments section. Others, not specifically named, were representatives of a wide spectrum of constituencies and organizations, such as the Executive Committee of the Clerkship Directors in Internal Medicine and various committees within the American College of Physicians, including the Education Committee, The Counsel of Associates, The Counsel of Student Members, and the Board of Governors.

We need to know if we have accomplished our goal of helping students learn internal medicine content. When finished with this program, please take a few minutes to fill out the electronic evaluation on the CD-ROM and return it to ACP. We value your feedback.

Patrick C. Alguire, MD, FACP
*Editor-in-Chief*

# Contents

# MKSAP for Students 2 User Survey

**Please complete the following electronically by placing the MKSAP for Students 2 CD into the appropriate drive. On the opening page of the CD locate and click on the "User Survey." You must be able to connect to the Internet in order to submit this survey electronically. To thank you for participating in this survey, 20 randomly-selected respondents will receive a complimentary textbook published by the American College of Physicians.**

1. Please indicate whether or not you are using MKSAP for Students to achieve the following learning objectives:

|  | yes | no |
|---|---|---|
| Assess medical knowledge | ☐ | ☐ |
| Enhance clinical knowledge | ☐ | ☐ |
| Enhance clinical problem-solving skills | ☐ | ☐ |
| Improve patient management | ☐ | ☐ |
| Prepare for clerkship examination | ☐ | ☐ |
| Prepare for licensing examination | ☐ | ☐ |

2. How useful is MKSAP for Students in meeting each of your objectives?

|  | not useful | a little useful | useful | very useful | extremely useful | not sure |
|---|---|---|---|---|---|---|
| Assess medical knowledge | ☐ | ☐ | ☐ | ☐ | ☐ | ☐ |
| Enhance clinical knowledge | ☐ | ☐ | ☐ | ☐ | ☐ | ☐ |
| Enhance clinical problem-solving skills | ☐ | ☐ | ☐ | ☐ | ☐ | ☐ |
| Improve patient management | ☐ | ☐ | ☐ | ☐ | ☐ | ☐ |
| Prepare for clerkship examination | ☐ | ☐ | ☐ | ☐ | ☐ | ☐ |
| Prepare for licensing examination | ☐ | ☐ | ☐ | ☐ | ☐ | ☐ |

3. Please rate the Multiple-Choice Questions included with MKSAP for Students on the following:

|  | poor | fair | neutral | good | excellent |
|---|---|---|---|---|---|
| Quality of Questions | ☐ | ☐ | ☐ | ☐ | ☐ |
| Relevance of content to practice | ☐ | ☐ | ☐ | ☐ | ☐ |
| Value as a Board-preparation tool | ☐ | ☐ | ☐ | ☐ | ☐ |

4. Please rate the Critiques included with MKSAP for Students on the following:

|  | poor | fair | neutral | good | excellent |
|---|---|---|---|---|---|
| Quality of Critiques | ☐ | ☐ | ☐ | ☐ | ☐ |
| Source of additional useful information | ☐ | ☐ | ☐ | ☐ | ☐ |
| Explanation for answers | ☐ | ☐ | ☐ | ☐ | ☐ |
| Value as an examination-preparation tool | ☐ | ☐ | ☐ | ☐ | ☐ |

5. Rate the overall quality of MKSAP for Students:

| poor | fair | neutral | good | excellent |
|---|---|---|---|---|
| ☐ | ☐ | ☐ | ☐ | ☐ |

6. Would you recommend MKSAP for Students to a colleague?

| yes | no | not sure |
|---|---|---|
| ☐ | ☐ | ☐ |

*continued on next page...*

7. Did you have any technical difficulty when using the MKSAP for Students CD-ROM?

|  | yes | no |
|---|---|---|
|  | ☐ | ☐ |

(If yes) Did you access the MKSAP technical support site for assistance?

|  | yes | no |
|---|---|---|
|  | ☐ | ☐ |

(If yes) Was it helpful?

|  | yes | no |
|---|---|---|
|  | ☐ | ☐ |

8. Please describe one specific change you plan to make or have recently made in your patient care as a result of something new you learned while working through *MKSAP for Students*:

Your E-mail: _____

(to be used *only* to notify winners of the ACP textbook random drawing)

# Questions

# Cough

## Cough Question 1

A 42-year-old man presents with a 3-month history of a persistent nonproductive cough. The cough occasionally awakens him at night. He has had no wheezing, dyspnea, heartburn, or chest pain.

On physical examination, he appears healthy. His temperature is 36.6 °C (98 °F), pulse rate is 80/min, respiration rate is 16/min, and blood pressure is 122/78 mm Hg. He has mild, nasal, mucosal congestion. Examinations of the heart and lungs are normal; results of chest radiography are normal.

Which of the following is the most likely diagnosis?

(A) Postnasal drip
(B) Gastroesophageal reflux
(C) Sinusitis
(D) Variant asthma
(E) Pneumonia

## Cough Question 2

A 65-year-old man has mild left ventricular dilatation with an estimated ejection fraction of 40% as documented by echocardiography. He also has hypertension. For the past 4 years, he has been taking lisinopril, digoxin, and hydrochlorothiazide. He had done well until several months ago, when he developed paroxysmal coughing that is unrelated to recumbency and can occur at any time of the day or night. The cough is nonproductive but has become debilitating and is not relieved by over-the-counter cough drops.

On physical examination, his pulse rate is 72/min and blood pressure is 120/72 mm Hg. There are no signs of an upper respiratory tract infection, but his pharynx is slightly erythematous. The chest is clear. An $S_4$ is audible. There is no edema. The serum creatinine level is normal.

In addition to a chest radiograph, which one of the following should be done next?

(A) Echocardiography
(B) CT of the chest
(C) Pulmonary function tests
(D) Bronchoscopy

## Cough Question 3

A 54-year-old woman is evaluated because of a dry cough. She is a nonsmoker and noticed the onset of cough about 2 years previously. The cough is not associated with time of day, position, season, or any environmental exposures. The patient has noticed no postnasal drip, frequent clearing of her throat, or nasal discharge, and she has no dyspnea, wheezing, sputum production, or cardiac or gastrointestinal complaints.

Physical examination, chest radiograph, and pulmonary function tests (including spirometry, diffusing capacity, rest and exercise oximetry) are within normal limits. Blood chemistries, liver function tests, and complete blood count are also within normal limits.

Which of the following tests is the next most appropriate option?

(A) Computed tomographic (CT) scan of the sinuses
(B) Bronchoprovocation challenge
(C) Chest CT scan
(D) 24-hour esophageal pH probe monitoring
(E) Fiberoptic bronchoscopy

## Cough Question 4

A 65-year-old male retired teacher is evaluated because of a dry cough and dyspnea on exertion that began 15 months ago and has gradually progressed to the point that he is unable to perform his usual activities. He has never smoked and has had no known exposure to environmental respiratory hazards. Pulmonary function testing shows a restrictive pattern with a forced vital capacity (FVC) 52% of predicted and a carbon monoxide diffusing capacity (DLco) 42% of predicted. He has clubbing, mild cyanosis, and fine basal inspiratory crackles. A chest radiograph shows diffuse linear opacities with basal predominance.

Which of the following disorders is most likely?

(A) Bacterial pneumonia
(B) Idiopathic pulmonary fibrosis
(C) Congestive heart failure
(D) Pulmonary embolism
(E) Asbestosis

**Cough Question 5**

A 45-year-old man is evaluated because of a persistent cough. He is a lifelong nonsmoker without a history of lung disease. He has had a cough productive of clear sputum for approximately 6 months. The cough is particularly troublesome at night and toward the end of the workweek. The patient works in an automobile repair shop spray-painting cars. He has worked in his present job for 2 years. He denies a history of allergies, and there is no family history of asthma or allergies. The chest examination shows a few expiratory wheezes. Spirometry shows moderate airflow obstruction and substantial improvement after inhalation of a bronchodilator.

Which of the following is the best management option for this patient?

(A) Measure carbon monoxide diffusing capacity
(B) Advise him to change jobs
(C) Prescribe an inhaled bronchodilator
(D) Measure IgE antibody to anhydrides

**Cough Question 6**

A 55-year-old man states that he has had persistent coughing for 4 months since he had an upper respiratory infection. He was treated with ciprofloxacin at the time. The cough is intermittent but is worse at night. It is productive of thick, yellow sputum, particularly in the morning. He reports chest pressure and coughing after exertion. He has never been a smoker and has no allergies. The examination findings are normal except for scattered wheezing with forced expiration. Pulmonary function testing shows mild obstruction with normal lung volumes and a normal carbon monoxide diffusing capacity ($DL_{CO}$). The chest radiographic findings and sputum culture are normal.

Which of the following treatments is most likely to be the effective?

(A) Atenolol plus enalapril
(B) Azithromycin
(C) Dextromethorphan plus glyceryl guaiacolate
(D) Budesonide

# Dyspnea

## Dyspnea Question 1

A 55-year-old woman is hospitalized because of new-onset dyspnea on exertion and peripheral edema. She denies chest pain. On physical examination, her pulse rate is 96/min and regular, and her blood pressure is 110/75 mm Hg. The jugular venous pressure is estimated to be 14 cm $H_2O$. There are a few crackles in the right lung field. A prominent $S_4$ and a soft $S_3$ are audible. There is peripheral ankle edema. An electrocardiogram shows left bundle branch block. Echocardiography is performed and the ejection fraction is estimated to be 25%, and the mitral and aortic valves appear normal. Enalapril and furosemide are begun. The patient loses 3.2 kg (7 lb), and her symptoms improve.

Which of the following is the most likely diagnosis?

(A) Myocarditis
(B) Mitral valve stenosis
(C) Chronic obstructive pulmonary disease
(D) Coronary artery disease
(E) Cardiac amyloidosis

## Dyspnea Question 2

A 37-year-old male injection drug user comes to the emergency department because of shortness of breath and fever for 6 days. On physical examination, his temperature is 38.5 °C (101.3 °F), pulse rate is 118/min and regular, respiratory rate is 32/min, and blood pressure is 110/60 mm Hg. Carotid upstrokes are normal, and crackles are heard half way up both lung fields. Cardiac auscultation shows a soft $S_1$, an $S_3$, and a grade 2/6 early diastolic murmur at the left sternal border. An echocardiogram is ordered, blood culture specimens are obtained, and intravenous antibiotics are started.

Which of the following is the most likely diagnosis?

(A) Myocarditis
(B) Pericarditis
(C) Aortic value insufficiency
(D) Septic pulmonary emboli
(E) Staphylococcal aortitis

## Dyspnea Question 3

A 49-year-old man with type 1 diabetes mellitus is evaluated because of exertional dyspnea for the past 2 months. The dyspnea becomes worse after walking two or three blocks. He denies chest, throat, jaw, or arm discomfort with exertion or at rest. In addition to insulin, his other medications include aspirin and atorvastatin. On physical examination, his blood pressure is 160/90 mm Hg. The remainder of the examination and resting electrocardiogram are normal.

Which one of the following is the most likely diagnosis?

(A) Chronic obstructive pulmonary disease
(B) Dilated cardiomyopathy
(C) Coronary artery disease
(D) Aortic stenosis
(E) Pulmonary fibrosis

## Dyspnea Question 4

A 55-year-old woman is evaluated in the emergency department because of severe shortness of breath, which has progressively worsened since midnight the previous evening. She is severely dyspneic and cannot complete a full sentence. Her vital signs are stable except for a pulse rate of 116/min and respiration rate of 40/min. She has diffuse bilateral crackles on posterior lung examination. Chest radiograph shows diffuse airspace disease.

Which one of the following would help to distinguish the acute respiratory distress syndrome from congestive heart failure in this patient?

(A) Subacute to gradual onset
(B) $PaO_2/FiO_2$ ratio $\geq 200$
(C) Bilateral pulmonary infiltrates and a pulmonary capillary wedge pressure $\leq 18$ mm Hg
(D) Response to positive end-expiratory pressure

## Dyspnea Question 5

A 72-year-old man is evaluated because of increasing dyspnea and lower-extremity edema over the past 4 weeks. His history is remarkable for drinking approximately four beers a day and he has smoked 1½ packs of cigarettes daily for 45 years. There is no history of hypertension, diabetes mellitus, or coronary artery disease.

Physical examination reveals a pulse rate of 80/min, respiration rate of 24/min, and blood pressure of 160/80 mm Hg. The lungs are hyperresonant, and no rales are detected. The cardiac impulse is in the sub-xiphoid area. $S_1$ and $S_2$ are distant. A 2/6 midsystolic murmur and an $S_3$ are noted at the lower left sternal border, and both increase slightly on inspiration. The liver span is 16 cm, ascites is present, and there is 3+ to 4+ pitting edema to the knees bilaterally.

The chest radiograph shows hyperinflated lung fields, centrally prominent pulmonary vasculature, and a normal cardiac silhouette.

Which of the following is the most likely diagnosis?

(A) Metastatic carcinoma to the liver and the peritoneum
(B) Alcoholic cirrhosis
(C) Cor pulmonale and right heart failure
(D) Aortic stenosis
(E) Coronary artery disease

## Dyspnea Question 6

A previously healthy 30-year-old man who is a lifelong non-smoker notes the sudden onset of right-sided chest pain and shortness of breath while shoveling snow. He is taken to the emergency department where the chest radiograph shown is obtained.

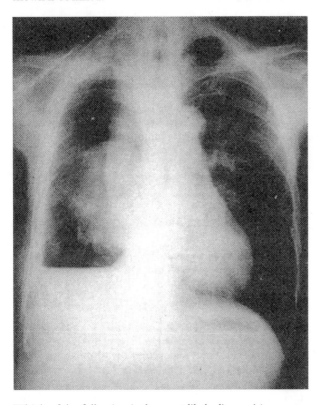

Which of the following is the most likely diagnosis?

(A) Adenocarcinoma
(B) Congestive heart failure
(C) Pneumonia
(D) Pneumothorax

## Dyspnea Question 7

A 38-year-old farmer has acute onset of severe, progressive dyspnea associated with cough and weakness. These symptoms occurred 1 hour he had worked in a silo that had been filled with fresh corn silage the previous day.

Which of the following is most likely to have caused his acute pulmonary decompensation?

(A) Viral pneumonia
(B) Pneumothorax
(C) Nitrogen dioxide pneumonitis
(D) Allergic bronchopulmonary aspergillosis
(E) Hypersensitivity pneumonitis

## Dyspnea Question 8

A 39-year-old woman is seen in the emergency department with an acute attack of asthma that did not respond to self-care at home. She has been using long-term inhaled beclomethasone (with spacer), albuterol as needed, and a single dose of sustained-release theophylline in the evening.

In the emergency department, she is treated with nebulized albuterol every half hour; intravenous methylprednisolone, and oxygen. She improves significantly enough to be discharged home.

Which one of the following changes should be made to her medication program at the time of discharge?

(A) Increase the beclomethasone
(B) Increase the beclomethasone and albuterol
(C) Increase the albuterol
(D) Increase the beclomethasone and begin a prednisone taper
(E) No changes

## Dyspnea Question 9

A 60-year-old man with asthma is evaluated in the emergency department because of the acute onset of chest pain while lifting a heavy object. The pain is sharp and accentuated by deep breathing and by movement of the upper extremities. It is located over the left precordium.

The physical examination and chest x-ray are normal. A ventilation-perfusion lung scan shows matched areas of perfusion and ventilation.

Which one of the following is the correct interpretation of the ventilation-perfusion lung scan?

(A) Normal
(B) Low probability
(C) Indeterminate
(D) High probability

**Dyspnea Question 10**
A 35-year-old woman is evaluated because of worsening dyspnea. She had been well until 6 months ago, when she noted the gradual onset of shortness of breath, worst during exercise but also waking her from sleep at night. There has been no associated chest pain, cough, sputum production, or leg edema. She has a normal physical examination, chest radiograph, and spirometry test. Arterial blood gas studies reveal a $PaO_2$ of 90 mm Hg and a normal $PaCO_2$ and pH.

Which one of the following studies is most likely to yield the cause of the patient's dyspnea?

(A)  High-resolution computed tomography of the chest
(B)  Flow-volume loop
(C)  Bronchoprovocation challenge test
(D)  Echocardiography
(E)  Single-breath $DL_{CO}$

**Dyspnea Question 11**
A 58-year-old man is evaluated because of daytime sleepiness, which has become troublesome over the past 2 years. He did not seek medical attention until an automobile accident resulted from his falling asleep while driving. He is a lifetime nonsmoker and is otherwise healthy.

On examination, he is not obese. There are no obvious abnormalities of his oropharynx. Chest and cardiac examinations are normal. There is no peripheral edema.

Chest radiograph and electrocardiogram are normal. Overnight polysomnography for 6 hours of sleep shows approximately 200 episodes of apnea (cessation of airflow for more than 10 seconds) accompanied by frequent oxygen desaturation below 85%. There is evidence of rib cage and abdominal motion during the apneic periods.

Which of the following is the most appropriate therapy for this patient?

(A)  Nasal continuous positive airway pressure
(B)  Uvulopalatopharyngoplasty
(C)  Progesterone
(D)  Protriptyline
(E)  Nocturnal supplemental oxygen by nasal cannula

**Dyspnea Question 12**
A 22-year-old man with asthma has been treated with inhaled albuterol as needed. He had been using the inhaler fewer than three times per week until the past 6 weeks, when he found he needed the inhaler three or four times each day. He is taking no other medications.

On physical examination, his respiration rate is 16/min, and he is in no respiratory distress. The chest examination has mild wheezing on forced expiration. Spirometry shows a forced expiratory volume in 1 second ($FEV_1$) of 3.1 L (77% predicted) and a forced vital capacity (FVC) of 4.8 L (96% predicted). Chest radiograph is normal.

Which of the following is the most appropriate therapy at this time?

(A)  Continued albuterol as a single agent, used as needed
(B)  Regular albuterol every 4 hours, used as a single agent
(C)  Addition of inhaled ipratropium bromide four times a day
(D)  Addition of oral albuterol
(E)  Addition of an inhaled corticosteroid

**Dyspnea Question 13**
A 30-year-old woman with a history of asthma is evaluated in the emergency department because of severe shortness of breath. She has been using inhaled beta-agonists by metered-dose inhaler (MDI) with increasing frequency, up to every hour, without relief of symptoms.

In the emergency department, she has received continuous beta-agonist by nebulizer for the past hour and 125 mg of intravenous methylprednisolone.

On physical examination, she is using accessory muscles of respiration. Temperature is 37 °C (98.6 °F), pulse rate is 120/min, respiration rate is 32/min, and blood pressure is 130/80 mm Hg. Peak flow is 150 mL/min. Pulsus paradoxus is 18 mm Hg. Cardiac examination reveals tachycardia with distant heart sounds. Lung examination reveals inspiratory and expiratory wheezes in all lung fields. A chest radiograph shows no infiltrates. The leukocyte count is normal. The results of arterial blood gas studies on 60% oxygen by face mask are as follows: $PaO_2$, 150 mm Hg; $PaCO_2$, 48 mm Hg; and pH, 7.28.

Which of the following is the most appropriate management option for this patient?

(A)  Intubation and mechanical ventilation
(B)  Intravenous methylprednisolone
(C)  Nebulized ipratropium bromide solution
(D)  Administration of heliox (helium and oxygen mixture)

**Dyspnea Question 14**
A 42-year-old nurse is evaluated because of coughing, wheezing, and shortness of breath for the past 2 months. The patient relates the onset of her illness to a heavy exposure during an accidental spill of glacial acetic acid at work. At the time of exposure, she experienced dyspnea, as well as irritation of her eyes and nose. Since exposure, she has frequent paroxysms of cough, chest tightness, and awakening at night with shortness of breath. Her physical examination is normal, and her spirometry reveals mild obstructive ventilatory impairment that is partially reversible following the inhalation of bronchodilator.

Which of the following is the most likely diagnosis?

(A)  Reactive airways dysfunction syndrome
(B)  Atopic asthma
(C)  Allergic occupational asthma
(D)  Chronic bronchitis

**Dyspnea Question 15**

A 35-year-old man is evaluted because of shortness of breath and fatigue with exercise. He has been well most of his life but has never been able to participate in sports due to lack of energy.

On physical examination, his vital signs are normal except for a pulse rate of 100/min. Head and neck examination is normal. Lungs are clear to percussion and auscultation. Cardiac examination reveals a widely fixed, split-second sound in the pulmonic area, with the second component louder. A soft grade 2/6 systolic murmur is heard over the left sternal border.

A pulmonary arteriogram reveals a pulmonary artery pressure of 60/30 mm Hg with a mean of 42 mm Hg and a normal wedge pressure.

Which of the following is the most likely diagnosis?

(A) Primary pulmonary hypertension
(B) Mitral valve stenosis
(C) Multiple pulmonary emboli
(D) Atrial septal defect

**Dyspnea Question 16**

A 20-year-old woman has had increased symptoms of asthma for the past 3 months. She has had asthma since early childhood. She has mild eczema on her hands and neck and seasonal conjunctivitis and rhinitis (hay fever), particularly in the late summer. The asthma is worsened by exposure to dust, cats, and dogs. Several years ago the patient had positive skin test reactions to house dust mite, cat, and dog antigens.

Four months ago (in early September) the patient returned to college. She lives in an old and rather dusty dormitory building. She has a large area rug in her bedroom. She has no pets and has not seen mice or cockroaches in the dormitory. She takes most of her meals in the school cafeteria.

Which one of the following is the best initial intervention for this patient?

(A) Allergic immunotherapy (desensitization injections) for dust, cats, and dogs
(B) Allergy skin testing to assess for food sensitivities
(C) Removal of the rug and any carpeting from the bedroom and use of allergy-proof, plastic wraps for the mattress, pillows, and box spring
(D) Use of a room humidifier for the winter months

**Dyspnea Question 17**

A 42-year-old man with asthma has low-grade fevers, productive coughing, and mild exertional dyspnea. He denies chest pain or hemoptysis. Six weeks ago a persistent cough had developed with sputum production. His temperature had been as high as 38.2 °C (100.6 °F), and he had expectorated thick brown cords in the phlegm. The patient was given a diagnosis of pneumonia and received a course of azithromycin without benefit.

The patient has had asthma since childhood. His only medications are inhaled fluticasone 440 µg a day and albuterol as needed. He does not smoke cigarettes but he does smoke marijuana.

The peripheral leukocyte count is 11,200/µL with 35% eosinophils. The chest radiograph shows diffuse pulmonary infiltrates.

What is the most likely diagnosis?

(A) Mycoplasma pneumonia
(B) Pneumococcal pneumonia
(C) Allergic bronchopulmonary aspirgillosis
(D) Tuberculosis
(E) Psittacosis

**Dyspnea Question 18**

A 40-year-old woman is evaluated because she has had exertional breathlessness for the past 3 months and a recent episode of near syncope. She has a history of migraines, but has no cough or snoring. She does not smoke. She takes no medicines, including diet pills.

She is 157 cm (62 in) tall and weighs 52 kg (115 lb), for a body mass index of 21. The pulse rate is 90/min and regular, respiration rate is 18/min, and blood pressure is 95/60 mm Hg. Pulse oximetry shows the oxygen saturation is 95% at rest. Chest examination is normal. The cardiovascular examination reveals a parasternal heave, widely split pulmonic component of $S_2$, and a jugular venous pulse of 10 cm above the sternal angle. The remainder of the examination is normal.

Which if the following is the most likely diagnosis?

(A) Constrictive pericarditis
(B) Coarctation of the aorta
(C) Hypertrophic cardiomyopathy
(D) Pulmonary hypertension
(E) Cor pulmonale secondary to end-stage lung disease

**Dyspnea Question 19**

A 68-year-old woman is evaluated because of exertional breathlessness and lower extremity edema that has progressed over 6 weeks. She has smoked 1 pack of cigarettes a day for 40 years and has a history of hypertension.

The patient is 173 cm (68 in) tall and weighs 104 kg (230 lb), for a body mass index of 35. The respiratory rate is 20/min. Jugular venous pressure is present 5 cm above the sternal angle. A parasternal heave is present, the pulmonic component of $S_2$ is increased in intensity and widely split. No murmurs are audible. Chest examination is normal. There is bilateral 3+ pitting edema to the midcalf level. The hemoglobin 18 g/dL. The arterial blood gas measurements are as follows:

| | |
|---|---|
| $PaO_2$ | 55 mm Hg |
| $PaCO_2$ | 48 mm Hg |
| pH | 7.37 |
| Oxygen saturation | 88% |

Spriometric results are as follows:

| | |
|---|---|
| Forced vital capacity (FVC) | 2.66 L (81% of predicted) |
| Forced expiratory volume in 1 sec ($FEV_1$) | 1.75 L (70% of predicted) |
| Ratio of $FEV_1$ to FVC | 0.66 (83% of predicted) |

Echocardiography shows normal left ventricular size and function, right ventricular hypertrophy and chamber enlargement with diminished right ventricular ejection fraction, an estimated pulmonary arterial systolic pressure of 50 mm Hg above right atrial pressure, 3+ tricuspid regurgitation, and no other valvular lesions.

Which of the following is the most likely immediate cause of her dyspnea and edema?

(A) Right heart failure secondary to pulmonary hypertension
(B) Left heart failure
(C) Atrial septal defect
(D) Chronic obstructive pulmonary disease

# Pneumonia

## Pneumonia Question 1

A 55-year-old man is evaluated because of shaking chills, cough, and dyspnea. The patient is a smoker with a history of chronic obstructive pulmonary disease. On physical examination, his temperature is 39 °C (102.2 °F), pulse is 90/min, respiration rate is 36/min, and blood pressure is 120/70 mm Hg. Examination of the chest reveals diminished breath sounds throughout both lung fields and faint crackles in both bases.

Chest radiograph reveals bibasilar patchy areas of consolidation. A sputum Gram stain is positive for many gram-positive cocci in chains, many large gram-negative rods, a few slender pleomorphic gram-negative rods, a moderate number of polymorphonuclear leukocytes, and a moderate number of epithelial cells. He is begun on antibiotics. Two days later his sputum culture grows *Candida* species, and blood culture grows *Streptococcus pneumoniae*. His physical examination and chest x-ray are unchanged.

Which of the following test results should be used to guide this patient's antimicrobial therapy?

(A) Chest radiograph
(B) Sputum Gram stain
(C) Sputum culture
(D) Blood culture

## Pneumonia Question 2

A 72-year-old man is hospitalized because of fever, chills, and cough that have persisted for the past week. His medical history includes congestive heart failure, chronic bronchitis, and diabetes mellitus.

On physical examination, he is alert and in moderate respiratory distress. His temperature is 39 °C (102.2 °F), pulse rate is 120/min, respiration rate is 36/min, and blood pressure is 100/60 mm Hg. The physical examination reveals crackles in both lung fields at the bases. The jugular venous wave is noted 12 cm above the right atrium, and a soft $S_3$ gallop is present on auscultation.

The leukocyte count is 21,000/µL, serum sodium is 124 meq/L, and serum creatinine is 2.4 mg/dL. Chest x-ray shows infiltrates in the right upper, left upper, and left lower lobes. Bronchiectactic changes are seen throughout the lower lung fields bilaterally. Measurement of arterial blood gases obtained on room air shows the following: pH, 7.38; $PaCO_2$, 32 mm Hg; and $PaO_2$, 58 mm Hg.

Which one of the following antibiotic regimens is the most appropriate for this patient?

(A) Doxycycline
(B) Azithromycin
(C) Ceftriaxone
(D) Ciprofloxacin
(E) Piperacillin-tazobactam and levofloxacin

## Pneumonia Question 3

An 84-year-old man with chronic obstructive pulmonary disease is taken to the emergency department from his nursing home because of fever and increased shortness of breath. On physical examination, he is confused. His temperature is 39.4 °C (103 °F), pulse rate is 110/min, respiration rate is 32/min, and blood pressure is 110/60 mm Hg. His mucous membranes are dry, and his neck is supple. Lung examination reveals only distant breath sounds. The remainder of the examination is normal. The leukocyte count is 14,000/µL with a left shift. Oxygen saturation is 85% by pulse oximetry. Chest radiograph shows changes of emphysema and right lower lobe and right middle lobe infiltrates. The patient is unable to produce sputum.

Which of the following intravenous antibiotics is most appropriate?

(A) Ceftriaxone
(B) Ceftriaxone plus azithromycin
(C) Ciprofloxacin
(D) Azithromycin
(E) Imipenem

## Pneumonia Question 4

A 78-year-old man is evaluated because of a 4-day history of fever and cough productive of thick sputum. He has never smoked. Clarithromycin, given for the past 8 days, has been ineffective. A blood culture drawn in the office 2 days ago is reported to be growing gram-positive cocci in pairs, most likely *S. pneumoniae*. Chest radiograph shows an infiltrate in the right lower lobe. The patient is unable to produce sputum for examination.

Which of the following antibiotics, administered intravenously, is the most appropriate initial therapy?

(A) Azithromycin
(B) Levofloxicin
(C) Ceftazidime
(D) Trimethoprim-sulfamethoxazole

## Pneumonia Question 5

A 55-year-old woman who has chronic obstructive pulmonary disease is hospitalized because of progressive dyspnea. While in the hospital, she develops fever, increased cough, and sputum production. A gram-stained sputum specimen (see Figure 4 in the color plates) is shown.

What is the microscopic diagnosis?

(A) *Neisseria gonorrhoea*
(B) *Neisseria meningitidis*
(C) *Moraxella catarrhalis*
(D) *Haemophilus influenzae*

## Pneumonia Question 6

A 35-year-old man, who is hospitalized and requires mechanical ventilation, develops fever and increased sputum production. A gram-stained sputum specimen (see Figure 2 in the color plates) is shown.

What is most likely etiological cause of the pneumonia?

(A) *Staphylococcus aureus*
(B) *Streptococcus pneumoniae*
(C) *Hemophilus influenzae*
(D) *Escherichia coli*

## Pneumonia Question 7

A 55-year-old man develops fever, cough productive of purulent sputum, and crackles in the right base. A gram-stained smear of sputum (see Figure 3 in the color plates) is shown.

What is the most likely etiological agent causing the pneumonia?

(A) *Staphylococcus aureus*
(B) *Streptococcus pneumoniae*
(C) *Hemophilus influenzae*
(D) *Klebsiella pneumoniae*

## Pneumonia Question 8

A 29-year-old woman with HIV infection and a CD4 cell count of 633/µL has had 3 days of fever, chills, productive cough, and chest pain. Physical examination shows signs of consolidation in the left lower lung fields. Her leukocyte count is 8600/µL, and chest radiograph shows a left lower lobe infiltrate.

Which of the following organisms is most likely present in her sputum?

(A) *Mycoplasma pneumoniae*
(B) *Streptococcus pneumoniae*
(C) *Legionella pneumophila*
(D) *Pseudomonas aeruginosa*
(E) *Pneumocystis carinii*

## Pneumonia Question 9

A 46-year-old hospital janitor develops fevers, sweats, cough, and hemoptysis. He had been in generally good health, although he feels he may have lost about 6 pounds over the previous month. Six months earlier, his annual tuberculin skin test was negative. A chest radiograph now reveals a right upper lobe infiltrate with a small cavity.

Which of the following is the most appropriate management option?

(A) Repeat the PPD skin test (5 tuberculin units)
(B) Gastric fluid stains for acid fast bacilli
(C) Perform a second strength PPD skin test (250 tuberculin units)
(D) Bronchoscopy
(E) Sputum stains for acid fast bacilli

## Pneumonia Question 10

A 48-year-old man with alcoholism and a long history of cigarette smoking is admitted to the hospital with pneumonia. The chest radiograph shows a right lower lobe infiltrate with blunting of the right costophrenic angle. The leukocyte count is 16,100/µL with 82% neutrophils and 10% band forms. Sputum specimen reveals gram-negative coccobacilli. Antibiotic therapy is begun.

Twenty-four hours later, the patient's temperature is 40 °C (104 °F), and breath sounds are diminished over the right base. The leukocyte count is 20,300/µL, and the chest radiograph shows significantly increased haziness and complete loss of the costophrenic angle at the right base.

Which of the following is the most appropriate management option?

(A) A chest CT scan
(B) Inhaled β-agonist
(C) Decubitus radiographs of the chest
(D) Postural drainage and percussion
(E) Endotracheal intubation

## Pneumonia Question 11

A 62-year-old, previously healthy man is taken to the emergency room after 36 hours of cough with slight sputum production, temperature to 39.4 °C (103 °F), and increasing shortness of breath. The patient does not smoke or drink alcohol.

On physical examination, the patient is normotensive. He has a pulse rate of 110/min and a respiration rate of 32/min. Signs of consolidation are noted in the right lower lobe, a finding that is confirmed by chest radiograph. The leukocyte count is 22,000/µL with a left shift, and a sputum Gram stain shows mixed flora and many squamous epithelial cells.

Which of the following is the best empiric therapy for this patient?

(A) Erythromycin

(B) Penicillin

(C) Trimethoprim-sulfamethoxazole

(D) Ceftriaxone and azithromycin

(E) Cephalexin

## Pneumonia Question 12

A 28-year-old woman with a history of HIV is evaluated because of a 2-day history of fever, coughing, shortness of breath, and right-sided pleuritic chest pain. The cough produces yellowish-green phlegm. HIV infection was diagnosed 5 years ago when she was hospitalized with *Pneumocystis carinii* pneumonia. She has not had any other complications. The most recent CD4 cell count, obtained 1 month ago, was 190/µL. She is taking effective anti-retroviral therapy.

The temperature is 38.5 °C (101.3 °F). The pulse rate is 125/min, respiratory rate is 25/min, and blood pressure is 110/70 mm Hg. Examination of the chest shows dullness to percussion and decreased breath sounds at the right base with bronchial breath sounds and egophony just above the region of dullness. A chest radiograph shows consolidation of the right lower lobe and a large, right pleural effusion.

What is the next step in the care of this patient?

(A) Empiric antimicrobial therapy

(B) Diagnostic thoracentesis

(C) Chemotherapy for tuberculosis

(D) Bronchoscopy

(E) Induce sputum for *Pneumocystis carnii*

## Pneumonia Question 13

A 61-year-old man is evaluated because of 2 days of fever, cough with yellow phlegm, and shortness of breath. His medical history includes well-compensated ischemic cardiomyopathy. The patient appears comfortable. The temperature is 38.5 °C (101.3 °F). The pulse rate is 110/min with a regular rhythm, respiratory rate is 28/min, and blood pressure is 90/70 mm Hg. The chest examination reveals dullness and decreased breath sounds at the right base. Cardiac examination reveals an $S_3$ gallop and a 2/6 holosystolic murmur at the apex radiating to the axilla. Oxygen saturation is 93%. The chest radiograph shows a right lower lobe infiltrate and blunting of the ipsilateral costophrenic angle. A radiograph obtained in the lateral decubitus position shows pleural effusion with 5 mm of layering.

Which of the following would be most useful in determining the need for hospitalization?

(A) Thoracentesis

(B) Sputum Gram stain

(C) Serum electrolytes and a complete blood cell count

(D) Exercise oximetry

## Pneumonia Question 14

A 29-year-old woman has had shortness of breath, coughing, and arthralgia for several days. She has had no previous illnesses. She has never smoked cigarettes and has had no exposures to irritant fumes or chemicals. She is working a summer job in a pet shop that specialized in birds. The examination findings include bilateral fine crackles. The $Pao_2$ is 59 mm Hg at rest. A chest radiograph shows reticular nodular opacities at the lung bases and a patchy infiltrate at lower right and left mid lung.

Which of the following steps is most appropriate?

(A) A lung biopsy

(B) Eliminate exposure to the birds

(C) Sputum for culture and sensitivity

(D) Measure the level of angiotensin-converting enzyme

## Pneumonia Question 15

A 42-year-old woman is evaluated because of 2 days of coughing of yellowish phlegm, pleuritic chest pain, and fevers. The patient reports smoking 5 cigarettes a day for 15 years.

The patient appears mildly ill but in no distress. Her dentition is good. The temperature is 38.5 °C (101.3 °F). The pulse rate is 100/min, respiration rate is 24/min, and blood pressure is 110/60 mm Hg. The chest examination shows dullness to percussion, bronchial breath sounds, and coarse crackles at the left base. The findings of the cardiac, abdominal, and extremity examinations are unremarkable. The leukocyte count is 11,300/µL with 20% bands. Oxygen saturation is 96% while the patient is breathing room air. A chest radiograph shows left lower lobe consolidation.

Concern about which of the following pathogens will most directly affect the selection of empiric antibiotics for this patient?

(A) *Pseudomonas aeruginosa*

(B) Methicillin-resistant *Staphylococcus aureus*

(C) Penicillin-resistant *Streptococcus pneumoniae*

(D) *Haemophilus influenzae*

(E) *Legionella pneumophila*

# Chronic Obstructive Pulmonary Disease

**Chronic Obstructive Pulmonary Disease Question 1**

A 77-year-old man is hospitalized with his fourth exacerbation of chronic obstructive pulmonary disease in the past year. His medical history also includes cor pulmonale and depression. After 1 week of therapy with ipratropium, albuterol, broad-spectrum antibiotics, and glucocorticoids, he is discharged to home on supplemental oxygen. At an office visit 4 weeks after discharge, he reports that he has been doing well and no longer complains of dyspnea. Oxygen saturation on room air is 88%.

Which of the following treatments can be expected to have the greatest impact on his long-term survival?

(A) Angiotensin-converting enzyme (ACE) inhibitors
(B) Inhaled bronchodilators
(C) Inhaled glucocorticoids
(D) Chronic suppressive antibiotics
(E) Home oxygen

**Chronic Obstructive Pulmonary Disease Question 2**

A 64-year-old man is ready for discharge from the hospital after a 4-day stay due to an exacerbation of chronic obstructive pulmonary disease. He has been receiving intravenous methylprednisolone, 60 mg every 6 hours, while in the hospital. This is his first hospitalization for chronic obstructive pulmonary disease. Before being admitted, he was taking only ipratropium.

In addition to stopping methyprednisolone and restarting ipratropium, which one of the following is the most appropriate regimen for this patient?

(A) Inhaled glucocorticoids
(B) Prednisone, tapering over 2 weeks
(C) Inhaled N-acetylcysteine
(D) Inhaled albuterol

**Chronic Obstructive Pulmonary Disease Question 3**

A 67-year-old woman with chronic obstructive pulmonary disease and repeated episodes of bronchitis seeks advice about precautions to be taken during a trip from New York City to Hong Kong in January. She asks specifically about antibiotics during the airplane ride to prevent acquisition of bronchitis or pneumonia.

Which of the following agents is most likely to provide prophylactic benefit to this patient?

(A) Antibiotics
(B) Antiviral agents
(C) Immunizations
(D) Zinc lozenges

**Chronic Obstructive Pulmonary Disease Question 4**

A 56-year-old man with chronic obstructive pulmonary disease is evaluated because of disrupted, unrefreshing sleep, daytime fatigue, and morning headaches. He denies paroxysmal nocturnal dyspnea, orthopnea, and chest discomfort but reports development of pedal edema over the preceding several months. He has stable dyspnea on exertion, and there is no history of snoring or observed apnea during sleep.

Physical examination reveals a pulse rate of 96/min, respiration rate of 18/min, and blood pressure of 130/76 mm Hg. Examination of the chest reveals diminished breath sounds bilaterally. Cardiac examination reveals only diminished heart sounds. Extremities demonstrate 2+ ankle edema.

His hematocrit is 42%. Arterial blood gases studies reveals: pH 7.37; $PaO_2$ 63 mm Hg; $PaCO_2$ 46 mm Hg.

A chest radiograph shows pulmonary hyperinflation, and an electrocardiogram shows sinus tachycardia with peaked P waves.

Which of the following is the most appropriate next step for this patient?

(A) An inhaled bronchodilator
(B) A complete sleep study (polysomnogram)
(C) A benzodiazepine
(D) Two consecutive nights of oximetry in the home

**Chronic Obstructive Pulmonary Disease Question 5**

A 68-year-old man has a 10-year history of chronic obstructive pulmonary disease treated with maintenance corticosteroids (10 mg/day) is evaluated because of a 2-day history of increasing dyspnea at rest, cough productive of green-yellow sputum, increased amounts of sputum compared with his baseline, and a low-grade fever of 37.2 °C (99 °F). In the past year, he has had four other similar episodes, each treated with antibiotics, and his last course of antibiotic therapy was with amoxicillin 5 weeks ago. In the office his oxygen saturation is 92% on room air, and a chest radiograph is clear.

Which of the following organisms is likely to be present in the sputum of this patient?

(A) Penicillin-sensitive pneumococcus
(B) Beta-lactamase-negative *Haemophilus influenzae*
(C) Beta-lactamase-negative *Moraxella catarrhalis*
(D) *Pseudomonas aeruginosa*

## Chronic Obstructive Pulmonary Disease Question 6

A 54-year-old man is admitted to the hospital because of cyanosis, ankle swelling, severe shortness of breath, and confusion. He has smoked for 35 years. Physical examination reveals a pulse rate of 120/min, respiration rate is 30/min, and blood pressure of 150/90 mm Hg. The neck veins are distended to the angle of the jaw. Chest examination reveals hyperinflation, prolonged expiration with wheezing, and a few rales at each base posteriorly. The heart's point of maximal impulse is in the epigastrium. Pulmonic second sound is loud, and there is a summation gallop. No murmurs or rubs are heard. The abdominal examination shows an enlarged and tender liver edge felt 2 cm below the costal margin at the mid-clavicular line. Ascites is present, as is ankle edema.

Laboratory studies show a hematocrit of 57%, a leukocyte count of 8000/µL. Serum creatinine, electrolytes, and creatine kinase are normal. Arterial blood gas studies reveal a $PaO_2$ of 50 mm Hg, $PaCO_2$ of 50 mm Hg, and pH of 7.30. A chest radiograph shows hyperinflated lung fields, an enlarged heart with biventricular enlargement, and no infiltrates. A V/Q lung scan shows multiple matched filling defects that are not segmental. Doppler venography of the leg veins is normal.

Which of the following is the single best therapy for this patient?

(A) A calcium-channel blocker
(B) Full-dose heparin
(C) Intravenous methylprednisolone
(D) Oxygen
(E) Phlebotomy

## Chronic Obstructive Pulmonary Disease Question 7

A 75-year-old man with a history of smoking 2 packs of cigarettes per day for 60 years is evaluated because of dyspnea. He reports dyspnea that has been slowly progressive over the last 3 to 4 years, accompanied by a 10-lb (4.5 kg) weight loss. On physical examination, he is using accessory muscles of respiration, and his respiration rate is 24/min at rest. Examination of the heart shows a regular rate and rhythm of 88/min with a right-sided $S_3$, but no murmurs. The lungs show symmetric expansion bilaterally, with reduced air entry and expiratory prolongation. The extremities show 1+ pretibial edema bilaterally.

Oxygen saturation on room air is 88% at rest and decreases to 84% after walking for 1 minute. Other laboratory data are normal, except for a hematocrit of 54%.

Which of the following is the best oxygen therapy option for this patient?

(A) Do not use oxygen
(B) Use only at night when sleeping
(C) Use continuously
(D) Use only with exercise
(E) Use only when short of breath

## Chronic Obstructive Pulmonary Disease Question 8

A 62-year-old woman arrives for a general medical evaluation because she seems to be "slowing down" this past year. She has smoked 1.5 packs of cigarettes a day for 40 years. She has a cough productive of white sputum each morning. She has no history of asthma or pneumonia. The physical examination shows a prolonged expiratory phase and scattered expiratory rhonchi on chest auscultation that clear with coughing. Spirometry gives the following results:

| | |
|---|---|
| Forced vital capacity (FVC) | 3.13 L (92% of expected) |
| Forced expiratory volume in 1 sec ($FEV_1$) | 1.08 L (40% of expected) |
| Ratio of $FEV_1$ to FVC | 0.35 (46% of expected) |

Which of the following interventions is most likely to preserve the patient's lung function over the next 5 years?

(A) Inhaled β-adrenergic agonists
(B) Inhaled cholinergic antagonist
(C) Inhaled glucocorticoids
(D) Pulmonary rehabilitation
(E) Smoking cessation

## Chronic Obstructive Pulmonary Disease Question 9

Which one of the following statements regarding inhaled glucocorticoids is accurate?

(A) Inhaled glucocorticoids are contraindicated during pregnancy.
(B) Inhaled glucocorticoids are useful immediately before exercise in preventing exercise-induced bronchoconstriction.
(C) Inhaled glucocorticoids are best taken twice a day.
(D) Inhaled glucocorticoids are not associated with systemic absorption.

## Chronic Obstructive Pulmonary Disease Question 10

A 47-year-old man has exertional dyspnea. He does not smoke. He has no history of asthma or allergic diseases. He has only an occasional cough that is nonproductive. He has no history of heart disease. His brother, father, and two cousins all developed emphysema before 50 years of age. The physical examination findings are normal. Pulmonary function tests show moderate airflow obstruction without change after administration of a bronchodilator. Resting oxygen saturation measured with a pulse oximeter is 97%. The chest radiograph findings are normal.

Which of the following is the best study to confirm the diagnosis in this patient?

(A) CT of the chest
(B) Carbon monoxide diffusing capacity ($DL_{CO}$)
(C) Exercise pulse oximetry
(D) Measurement of $\alpha_1$-antitrypsin
(E) Genetic testing of the patient and family members

# Deep Venous Thrombosis

## Deep Venous Thrombosis Question 1

A 63-year-old woman is scheduled to undergo a total knee replacement and needs prophylaxis for deep venous thrombosis. She has no previous history of increased bleeding or of a hypercoagulable state. She takes aspirin, 325 mg/d, for primary prevention of cardiovascular disease and wants to continue taking it; she does not want subcutaneous injections.

Which one of the following would you recommend for prophylaxis?

(A) Aspirin
(B) Full-dose intravenous heparin
(C) Intermittent pneumatic compression
(D) Warfarin
(E) Elastic stockings

## Deep Venous Thrombosis Question 2

A 76-year-old woman with metastatic breast cancer is evaluated because of a 3-day history of swelling of her right leg and pleuritic chest pain. Ultrasonography shows an occlusive thrombus in the femoral vein. Results of a ventilation-perfusion scan are normal, and therapy with continuous intravenous heparin is begun. On the fourth day of heparin therapy and after oral warfarin has been started, the activated partial thromboplastin time is therapeutically prolonged, but the prothrombin time has not yet reached the therapeutic range; at this time, the patient develops dyspnea.

On physical examination, her blood pressure is 140/90 mm Hg; she is tachypneic and tachycardic, but the remainder of her cardiopulmonary examination is normal. Chest radiograph shows no abnormalities. Measurement of arterial blood gases reveals new hypoxemia on room air. Ventilation-perfusion scan shows perfusion defects in the entire right lower lobe and the inferior subsegment of the lingula.

Which one of the following should be part of this patient's management at this time?

(A) Continued observation until warfarin dosing is therapeutic
(B) Placement of an inferior vena caval filter
(C) Readminister heparin bolus and increase the rate of the continuous infusion
(D) Administer an increased dose of warfarin

## Deep Venous Thrombosis Question 3

A 45-year-old woman is evaluated in the emergency department because of the sudden onset of shortness of breath and chest tightness earlier this afternoon. She has been in excellent health and returned 2 days ago from a trip to Japan. On physical examination, her pulse rate is 116/min and respiration rate is 36/min. Cardiopulmonary examination is otherwise unremarkable, and a chest radiograph shows no infiltrates. Measurement of arterial blood gases on room air shows the following: pH 7.48, $PaCO_2$ 24 mm Hg, and $PaO_2$ 78 mm Hg; oxygen saturation is 96%.

What is the most appropriate immediate next step in this patient's management?

(A) Pulmonary angiogram
(B) Compression ultrasonography of the lower extremities
(C) Therapy with diazepam
(D) Intravenous heparin
(E) Ventilation-perfusion lung scan

## Deep Venous Thrombosis Question 4

A 75-year-old man comes to the emergency department because of a 2-day history of a swollen and tender left calf following a 10-hour automobile trip. Ultrasonography confirms the presence of a deep venous thrombosis of the left calf extending to the popliteal region. The patient has an extensive smoking history, but his medical history is otherwise unremarkable. Physical examination is normal, and a stool specimen is negative for occult blood. The complete blood count, prothrombin time, activated partial thromboplastin time, and routine serum chemistry studies are normal.

In addition to a thorough physical examination, which one of the following should be included in the evaluation of this patient?

(A) Chest radiograph
(B) Abdominal CT scan
(C) Prostate-specific antigen and cystoscopy
(D) Serum carcinoembryonic antigen level

## Deep Venous Thrombosis Question 5

A 38-year-old man is receiving warfarin therapy for treatment of a deep venous thrombosis of the left leg that he developed 3 weeks ago. He comes for his scheduled prothrombin time INR determination. He denies gingival bleeding, hematuria, nosebleeds, or gastrointestinal disorders but reports a sore throat and fever that started about 1 week ago. He has not been able to swallow and has consequently been on a mostly clear liquid diet for the last week.

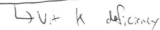 → V.t K deficiency

On physical examination, his temperature is 38.0 °C (100.4 °F). His posterior pharynx is erythematous but without exudate. There are several scattered ecchymoses on the forearms and legs. The remainder of the examination is normal.

The laboratory evaluation reveals a hematocrit of 41%; activated partial thromboplastin time of 37 s; and a prothrombin time INR of 6.0.

Which of the following is most appropriate for initial management of this patient's elevated INR?

(A) Transfuse two to four units of fresh frozen plasma

(B) Stop warfarin; give vitamin K, orally

(C) Stop warfarin; give vitamin K, intravenously

(D) Stop warfarin; give vitamin K, intramuscularly

(E) Stop warfarin

### Deep Venous Thrombosis Question 6

A 58-year-old man is admitted for elective cholecystectomy. Five days after surgery, he acutely develops moderate dyspnea with a systemic blood pressure that dropped from an immediate postoperative value of 135/85 mm Hg to 95/55 mm Hg. He is afebrile and has no complaints of cough or chest pain, and on physical examination, breath sounds are clear. A chest radiograph shows no infiltrates. The arterial oxygen saturation on room air is 89%, and a ventilation-perfusion scan is ordered, which shows two unmatched lobar defects and two segmental defects. A Doppler study shows a deep venous thrombosis in the femoral vein of the right leg.

Which of the following is the best treatment option for this patient?

(A) Intravenous unfractionated heparin

(B) Subcutaneous low-molecular weight heparin

(C) Intravenous tissue plasminogen activator (t-PA)

(D) Intravenous heparin plus an inferior vena cava filter

(E) Oral warfarin

### Deep Venous Thrombosis Question 7

A 53-year-old man has sudden-onset dyspnea that developed an hour ago. He had undergone total hip arthroplasty 48 hours earlier. He is otherwise healthy except for controlled hypertension. The patient has a minimal dry cough and no wheezing or chest pain. Temperature is 38.5 °C (101.3 °F). The pulse rate is 110/min. Respiration rate is 24/min with increased respiratory effort. Blood pressure is 156/92 mm Hg. The lungs are clear, and the findings of the cardiac examination are normal. Arterial saturation measured with a pulse oximeter is 87% while the patient is breathing oxygen at 3 L/min through a nasal cannula. A ventilation-perfusion scan of the lungs shows large defects over the right upper lobe and the lingula. Ventilation is normal.

Which of the following is the best management option?

(A) A pulmonary angiogram

(B) Measurement of dimerized plasmin fragment D (D-dimer)

(C) Malignancy workup

(D) Unfractionated heparin

(E) Assay for factor V Leiden mutation

### Deep Venous Thrombosis Question 8

A 23-year-old otherwise healthy woman has a pulmonary embolism while hospitalized after a motor vehicle accident. She is 8 weeks pregnant. She has completed 1 day of therapy with unfractionated heparin.

In addition to completing 5 to 7 days of intravenous administration of unfractionated heparin, which of the following is the next management option for this patient?

(A) Unfractionated heparin

(B) Low-molecular-weight heparin

(C) Warfarin

(D) Inferior vena cava filter

(E) Compression stockings

### Deep Venous Thrombosis Question 9

A 24-year-old man is evaluated because of a swollen right calf. The calf has been swollen for 1 day. He had a deep venous thrombosis of the opposite leg when he was 17 years old, for which he took warfarin for 3 months. He has never smoked cigarettes. His father also had a deep venous thrombosis, but he is currently in good health. Physical examination shows a tender, swollen, right calf. Doppler studies confirm a deep venous thrombosis.

Which of the following is the most likely risk factor for hypercoagulability in this patient?

(A) Antiphospholipid antibodies

(B) Occult malignancy

(C) Paroxysmal nocturnal hemoglobinuria

(D) Factor V Leiden mutation

(E) Homocysteinemia

## Deep Venous Thrombosis Question 10

A 56-year-old man with a 15-year history of active rheumatoid arthritis is evaluated because of left lower leg pain that began suddenly while he was climbing stairs 2 days ago. In recent years, his arthritis has been reasonably well controlled with a combination of disease-modifying agents. His principal symptom has been continual swelling in his knees, for which arthrocentesis has been done twice in the last year on the left knee with concurrent injection of glucocorticosteroids. The last injection was done 2 weeks ago.

On physical examination, he has a temperature of 37.5 °C (99.5 °F). Fluid is palpable in both knees, but more so in the right than the left, with fullness in both popliteal fossae. The left calf is tender, and at 25 cm below the patella the circumference is 3 cm greater than on the right. Dorsiflexion of his left foot with the knee extended elicits sharp calf pain.

What step should be taken next in managing this patient?

(A) Venography of the left leg
(B) Ultrasonography of the left thigh, knee, and calf
(C) Arthrocentesis of both knees
(D) Anticoagulation
(E) Inject triamcinolone hexacetonide into the left knee

# Nosocomial Infection

### Nosocomial Infection Question 1
A 23-year-old woman on the rehabilitation service develops a temperature of 38.8 °C (102.0 °F). She is quadriplegic secondary to a diving accident that occurred 1 month ago. The patient has had a peripheral intravenous catheter in place for the past 7 days; the original catheter has not been changed. She also has had a urinary catheter for the past month; the urine is now cloudy, and Gram stain of an unspun specimen reveals gram-negative rods. After a thorough investigation, there is no other apparent source of the patient's temperature elevation.

What is the most likely route of bacterial access to the patient's urinary system?

(A) Hematogenous spread from the intravascular device
(B) Migration from the distal urethra along the external catheter surface
(C) Direct inoculation of organisms into the bladder at the time of catheterization
(D) Contamination of the urine collection bag
(E) Pre-existing asymptomatic colonization of the bladder from before the injury

### Nosocomial Infection Question 2
Which one of the following recommendations should be included in a hand washing protocol to decrease the rate of nosocomial infections?

(A) A minimum hand washing time of 5 seconds
(B) Antimicrobial hand washing solutions in all patient care areas
(C) The requirement to wash hands even after the use of sterile gloves
(D) Targeting only the nursing staff

### Nosocomial Infection Question 3
Which one of the following statements is true regarding the risk of a catheter infection?

(A) A lower extremity site has a higher risk of infection than an upper extremity site.
(B) An internal jugular line has a lower risk of infection than a subclavian line.
(C) A venous catheter inserted in the wrist has a lower risk of infection than one inserted in the dorsum of the hand.
(D) A triple-lumen catheter has the same rate of infection as a single-lumen catheter.

### Nosocomial Infection Question 4
A 28-year-old woman with ulcerative colitis was admitted to the medical service 1 week ago with abdominal pain and hematochezia. She has been treated with high-dose glucocorticoids with slow improvement; however, last night she developed fever, leukocytosis, and respiratory distress and required intubation. Chest radiograph shows multilobar infiltrates.

Which of the following is the most appropriate treatment regimen for this patient?

(A) An antipseudomonal penicillin
(B) An aminoglycoside plus trimethoprim-sulfamethoxazole
(C) A fluoroquinolone
(D) A fluoroquinolone plus imipenem
(E) A fluoroquinolone plus clindamycin

### Nosocomial Infection Question 5
A 32-year-old man in the intensive care unit develops a new fever with a temperature to 40 °C (104 °F), shivering, and a decrease in blood pressure to 90/40 mm Hg on the fifth postoperative day following neurosurgery for a cerebral aneurysm. The postoperative course was complicated by a persistent coma.

On physical examination, the patient has orotracheal and nasogastric tubes, an internal jugular central venous catheter, and a urinary catheter, all of which have been in place since admission. The catheter sites are clean without adjacent erythema. Auscultation reveals rhonchi over both lungs and no cardiac murmur. The abdomen is quiet but soft. Neurologic examination is unchanged from previous findings. The remainder of the examination is normal. Leukocyte count is 15,000/μL with 95% polymorphonuclear neutrophils, 3% band forms, and 2% lymphocytes. Blood chemistries are normal. Urinalysis shows 2 to 3 erythrocytes and 2 to 3 leukocytes per high-power field. Lumbar puncture is performed and the findings are normal except for 900/μL red blood cells and xanthochromia. Sputum suctioned from the orotracheal tube shows moderate polymorphonuclear neutrophils and small numbers of gram-positive and gram-negative bacteria. Oxygen saturation on room air is 96% by pulse oximetry. Chest radiograph shows only subsegmental atelectasis at the right base. Results of blood, urine, sputum, and cerebrospinal fluid cultures are pending.

Which of the following is the most likely cause of his fever?

(A) Pneumonia
(B) Meningitis
(C) Pulmonary embolism
(D) Cystitis
(E) Central venous catheter

## Nosocomial Infection Question 6

A 36-year-old woman is intubated and admitted to the medical intensive care unit because of respiratory depression following a barbiturate overdose.

Which one of the following will diminish her risk of developing a nosocomial infection?

(A) Ventilator tube changes every 12 hours
(B) Elevation of the head of the patient's bed to 45 degrees
(C) Intravenous ceftriaxone
(D) Spraying of the oropharynx with a polymyxin B solution every 8 hours

## Nosocomial Infection Question 7

An 80-year-old woman is admitted from a rehabilitation center with sudden shortness of breath and hypoxia of 3-hours duration. She had a stroke 3-weeks ago resulting in right hemiparesis and she is receiving feeding through a gastrostomy tube. Her pulse oximetry is 83% on room air and temperature is 38.3 °C (101.1 °F). The patient is edentulous. There is diffuse wheezing and rhonchi over all lung fields. Chest x-ray reveals bilateral lower lobe infiltrates.

Which of the following is the best initial therapy?

(A) Furosemide
(B) Levofloxacin
(C) Levofloxacin and clindamycin
(D) Deep tracheal suction

# Myocardial Infarction

## Myocardial Infarction Question 1

A 65-year-old man is evaluated in the emergency department because of a 2-hour history of precordial discomfort radiating to his left arm. On physical examination, his pulse rate is 80/min and regular, and blood pressure is 120/75 mm Hg. There are crackles at the right base, and an $S_4$ is present at the apex. An electrocardiogram shows 2-mm ST-segment elevation in leads $V_3$ through $V_6$. Chest x-ray reveals mild congestive heart failure. The patient is treated with chewable aspirin and a thrombolytic agent, following which his symptoms resolve and the ST segments return to normal.

He is started on atenolol. Aspirin is continued. He receives furosemide and is started on heparin. Laboratory studies 12 hours after admission show a markedly elevated troponin I level (50 ng/mL). An echocardiogram reveals a large anterior wall motion abnormality and an estimated ejection fraction of 30%.

In addition to the medications listed above, which one of the following should you prescribe?

(A) A calcium-channel blocker
(B) Quinidine
(C) An angiotensin-converting enzyme inhibitor
(D) An angiotensin II antagonist

## Myocardial Infarction Question 2

A 54-year-old man with angina pectoris comes to the emergency department because of increasingly severe and frequent chest discomfort on exertion. His physician had previously prescribed aspirin, isosorbide mononitrate, simvastatin, and atenolol. The chest discomfort is usually relieved by sublingual nitroglycerin, but last night it lasted for 30 minutes and required two sublingual nitroglycerin tablets for relief. On admission to the emergency department, his pulse rate is 58/min and regular, and blood pressure is 110/80 mm Hg. Chest and cardiac examinations are normal. The electrocardiogram shows new ST-segment depression in leads $V_4$ through $V_6$, which resolve over several hours. The QRS complexes are normal. An initial troponin I determination is normal, but a value obtained 6 hours later is elevated at 4 ng/mL (normal < 0.05).

Which of the following diagnostic tests should be done next?

(A) Coronary angiography
(B) Stress echocardiography
(C) Exercise electrocardiography
(D) Stress scintigraphy (thallium or sestamibi)
(E) No testing necessary; start thrombolytics and heparin

## Myocardial Infarction Question 3

A 54-year-old postmenopausal woman with type 2 diabetes mellitus is brought to an outlying urgent care center because of the sudden onset of severe substernal burning pain 3 hours ago. She has taken four sublingual nitroglycerin and had a syncopal spell after taking the last tablet.

An electrocardiogram shows ST elevation in leads II, III, and aVF, and there is an R wave and ST depression in lead $V_1$. Aspirin and an intravenous thrombolytic agent are administered. During the admission physical examination, her bedside monitor shows the abrupt onset of ventricular tachycardia. Electrical cardioversion is performed, and her arrhythmia is converted to sinus rhythm. Her peak troponin levels are 28 (normal < 0.05), but the remainder of her 5-day hospital course is uneventful.

In addition to aspirin and a β-blocker, which of the following is most appropriate for treatment of ventricular tachycardia at hospital discharge?

(A) Amiodarone
(B) Sotalol
(C) Diltiazem
(D) Add nothing
(E) Insert an automatic implantable cardiac defibrillator (AICD)

## Myocardial Infarction Question 4

A 62-year-old man is evaluated in the emergency department because of retrosternal chest pain and shortness of breath of 2 hours duration. He has no prior history of acute myocardial infarction or coronary artery disease but has a history of hypertension and type 2 diabetes mellitus. The patient is admitted to the hospital with the diagnosis of "rule out myocardial infarction."

Which information upon hospital admission would be most predictive of an uncomplicated hospital course?

(A) Normal chest radiograph
(B) Normal admission electrocardiogram
(C) Normal serum creatine kinase concentration
(D) Normal serum troponin I
(E) Pulse within normal limits

**Myocardial Infarction Question 5**
A 65-year-old man with a history of smoking and partially controlled hypertension is evaluated in the emergency department because of a 2-hour history of acute chest pain, worsened hypertension, and an electrocardiogram indicative of a large anterior myocardial infarction. The patient had gastrointestinal bleeding 4 weeks ago requiring hospitalization and transfusion therapy.

Which of the following is the most appropriate treatment?

(A)  Thrombolytic therapy
(B)  Percutaneous coronary angioplasty with stenting
(C)  Heparin
(D)  Aspirin

**Myocardial Infarction Question 6**
A previously healthy 49-year-old man has had severe chest pain for 2 hours. Heart rate is 74/min, blood pressure is 110/70 mm Hg, and the estimated jugular venous pressure is 9 cm $H_2O$; lungs are clear to auscultation. Cardiac examination reveals a normal $S_1$ and $S_2$, an $S_4$ gallop, and no murmur. Electrocardiography reveals sinus rhythm, ST-segment elevation in leads II, III and aVF, and a small Q wave in lead III.

Because of persistent chest pain, nitroglycerin ointment is applied topically. Fifteen minutes later the patient is confused, diaphoretic, and agitated. Systolic blood pressure is 64 mm Hg. Heart sounds are less audible, but there is no other change in the cardiac or pulmonary examination. The electrocardiographic monitor reveals sinus rhythm at 120/min.

Which of the following is the most likely cause of this patient's hypotension?

(A)  A ruptured anterior papillary muscle
(B)  A ruptured interventricular septum
(C)  Inadequate right ventricular filling pressure
(D)  Anaphylactic reaction to nitroglycerin
(E)  Left ventricular failure

**Myocardial Infarction Question 7**
A 44-year-old man had sudden onset of severe, crushing, retrosternal chest pain.

On physical examination, the patient had a pulse rate of 150/min, respiratory rate of 28/min with moderately labored respirations, and a blood pressure of 80/50 mm Hg. He appeared diaphoretic and ashen and was apprehensive. Jugular venous pressure was not clearly seen, carotid pulsation was thready, and examination of the lungs revealed inspiratory crackles bilaterally throughout the lower lung fields. Cardiac examination revealed a soft first and second heart sound, a third heart sound, but no murmur. A chest radiograph showed pulmonary edema. The ECG reveals ST elevations in $V_3$-$V_6$, and aVL. He received thrombolytic therapy in the emergency department 5 hours after the onset of pain, with incomplete relief.

This patient is most likely experiencing which of the following complications?

(A)  Cardiogenic shock
(B)  Pericarditis
(C)  Papillary muscle rupture
(D)  Ventricular septal rupture

**Myocardial Infarction Question 8**
A 52-year-old man is admitted with an acute anteroseptal infarction. His pulse rate is 115/min and blood pressure is 88/60 mm Hg; his urine flow is only 15 mL/h. His skin is cool, and he is confused. Bedside right-heart catheterization reveals the following: mean right atrial pressure, 0 mm Hg (normal 0-8); right ventricular pressure, 29/0 mm Hg (normal 25-30/0-8 mm Hg); pulmonary artery pressure, 20/10 mm Hg (normal 15-30 / 6-12 mm Hg); and mean pulmonary artery occlusive (wedge) pressure, 5 mm Hg (normal 4-12 mm Hg). Cardiac index is 2.2 L/min/m² (normal 2.5-4.2 L/min/m²).

The most important next step in the initial management of this patient is intravenous administration of which of the following?

(A)  Cardiac glycosides
(B)  A β-adrenergic blocking agent
(C)  Normal saline
(D)  Dopamine
(E)  Isoproterenol

**Myocardial Infarction Question 9**
A 54-year-old man is evaluated in the emergency department because of 2.5 hours of chest discomfort. He is hemodynamically stable, and an electrocardiogram shows an acute inferolateral myocardial infarction. The patient is treated with aspirin, intravenous β-blockers, and thrombolytics. Serial cardiac enzymes confirm an infarction, with a peak creatine kinase of 900 U/L (normal is less than 250 U/L). Five days later the electrocardiogram shows T-wave inversion in the inferolateral leads but no Q waves. A predischarge exercise test reveals no angina or ECG changes. He is discharged on an angiotensin-converting enzyme (ACE) inhibitor.

What additional medication should be added at the time of hospital discharge?

(A)  Aspirin
(B)  β-blocker
(C)  Warfarin
(D)  Oral nitrate

**Myocardial Infarction Question 10**

An active, 80-year-old woman is evaluated in a small community hospital because of severe crushing chest pain of approximately 5-hours duration. She has no history of a previous stroke, transient ischemic attack, or bleeding propensity. Her initial pulse rate is 80/min and blood pressure is 165/95 mm Hg. She has no signs of peripheral hypoperfusion, and the lungs fields are clear. Initial electrocardiogram reveals 4 mm of ST-segment elevation in the $V_2$-$V_6$. The hospital is nearly 2 hours from the nearest cardiac catheterization laboratory.

In addition to aspirin, which of the following is the most appropriate initial therapy?

(A) Warfarin
(B) Streptokinase
(C) IV heparin
(D) Nitrates

**Myocardial Infarction Question 11**

Which of the following constitutes an absolute contraindication to the use of intravenous β-blockers in acute myocardial infarction?

(A) Type 1 diabetes mellitus
(B) History of stable bronchospastic disease
(C) Inferior infarction
(D) Sinus bradycardia without hypotension
(E) None of the above

# Chest Pain

## Chest Pain Question 1

A 37-year-old man is evaluated because of a 2-week history of substernal chest "burning" that occurs mostly with meals or with exertion after a meal. The symptoms last 30 to 40 minutes, are not immediately relieved by rest, and do not radiate. He was awakened one night with similar symptoms, which were relieved when he drank some milk. Physical examination is normal.

Which of the following is the most cost-effective next step in this patient's management?

(A) Antacids as needed
(B) Proton pump inhibitor therapy
(C) Esophagogastroduodenoscopy
(D) Treadmill stress electrocardiogram
(E) Trial of nitroglycerin at time of symptoms

## Chest Pain Question 2

A 52-year-old woman is evaluated because of a 6-week history of substernal chest pressure that occurs with exercise, especially in the mornings, lasts 10 to 15 minutes, and resolves with rest. The pressure radiates to her shoulders but is not accompanied by shortness of breath, lightheadedness, diaphoresis, nausea, or vomiting. The episodes occur every 3 to 4 days and have caused her to reduce her activity level.

On physical examination, her pulse rate is 80/min and regular, and blood pressure is 120/80 mm Hg. The lungs, heart, abdomen, and peripheral pulses are normal. Hemoglobin level is 12 g/dL. The resting electrocardiogram is normal.

What is the best next diagnostic step in this patient?

(A) Stress electrocardiogram
(B) Stress electrocardiogram with thallium imaging
(C) Dipyridamole stress test with thallium imaging
(D) Coronary angiography
(E) Dobutamine stress echocardiogram

## Chest Pain Question 3

Which of the following patients with no acute ECG changes is the best candidate for evaluation in an emergency department chest pain center?

(A) A 64-year-old man with a prior history of coronary artery bypass grafting 7 years ago, stent placement 8 months ago, and a prolonged episode of typical substernal chest pain that awakened him from sleep

(B) A 44-year-old man with a single 40-minute episode of sharp left anterior chest pressure earlier today after exercise, which resolved spontaneously by the time he made it to the emergency department

(C) A 32-year-old woman with sharp left anterior chest pain, which came on during exertion and persisted as a "sore" sensation for about 1.5 hours before her arrival in the emergency department

(D) A 52-year-old man with diabetes mellitus and onset of persistent substernal chest pain that has lasted for 45 minutes and is continuing during the patient's initial evaluation in the emergency department

(E) An 80-year-old woman with known aortic stenosis who developed substernal chest discomfort, increasing shortness of breath, and diaphoresis and whose symptoms improved with oxygen and furosemide administration by paramedics

## Chest Pain Question 4

A 68-year-old woman comes to the emergency department because of precordial discomfort of 30 minutes' duration. She has a history of hypertension, type 2 diabetes mellitus, and stable angina pectoris. Her electrocardiogram shows 3-mm ST-segment elevation in leads $V_2$ through $V_6$.

Which of the following therapies is the most appropriate for this patient?

(A) Angioplasty
(B) Thrombolysis
(C) Thrombolysis or angioplasty
(D) Neither thrombolysis nor angioplasty

## Chest Pain Question 5

A 55-year-old postmenopausal woman with a history of breast cancer and type 2 diabetes mellitus is evaluated because of exertional chest discomfort. She had a non Q-wave myocardial infarction documented by cardiac enzyme elevation 1 year ago. She is currently taking sublingual nitroglycerin as needed, daily aspirin, an oral hypoglycemic agent, and a lipid-lowering drug. Her resting blood pressure is 155/90 mm Hg, and her low-density lipoprotein cholesterol is 106 mg/dL. A treadmill exercise test shows 2-mm ST-segment depression after 5 minutes of exercise using the Bruce protocol. Thallium scintigraphy reveals a mild reversible anterior defect. Coronary arteriography shows mild diffuse coronary artery disease with no discrete obstructions greater than 50%.

Which of the following is the most appropriate additional medication for this patient?

(A) A long-acting β-blocker
(B) A long-acting calcium-channel blocker
(C) A long-acting nitrate
(D) An α-blocker
(E) Estrogen replacement therapy

### Chest Pain Question 6

A 62-year-old man with known coronary artery disease was admitted to the emergency department because of a 4-hour history of chest discomfort the previous night. The discomfort awoke him from sleep and finally subsided after he took several sublingual nitroglycerin tablets. His medications include atenolol, lisinopril, aspirin, and simvastatin.

On physical examination, his pulse rate was 58/min and regular, and blood pressure was 115/70 mm Hg. There was no jugular venous distention, and his chest was clear. Cardiac examination revealed an apical $S_4$ with no murmurs. Troponin I levels were normal. He again complained of chest discomfort shortly after transfer to the coronary care unit, and an electrocardiogram taken at that time showed new 3-mm ST-segment depression in leads I, aVL, and $V_4$ through $V_6$.

Which of the following should be given at this time?

(A) Warfarin
(B) Heparin
(C) Heparin plus a platelet glycoprotein IIb/IIIa inhibitor
(D) Clopidogrel

### Chest Pain Question 7

A 69-year-old man is evaluated because of a 2-week history of burning retrosternal discomfort related to exertion. He denies any discomfort at rest. The discomfort subsides with rest and has never lasted more than a few minutes. He does not have any other cardiac symptoms. He recently discontinued smoking. On physical examination, he is normotensive. The cardiac examination is unremarkable. A resting electrocardiogram is normal.

In addition to prescribing aspirin, sublingual nitroglycerin, and a β-blocker, which of the following should be done next?

(A) Echocardiography
(B) Coronary angiography
(C) Admit the patient to the coronary care unit
(D) Exercise stress test

### Chest Pain Question 8

A 57-year-old man is evaluated because of increasing precordial chest discomfort with progressively milder exertion for the past few months. The patient had an acute anterior myocardial infarction 10 years ago. Daily medications include aspirin, furosemide, isosorbide mononitrate, lisinopril, and long-acting diltiazem. Exertional angina is somewhat relieved by sublingual nitroglycerin.

On physical examination, his pulse rate is 98/min and regular and blood pressure is 125/80 mm Hg. Jugular venous pressure is mildly elevated with a dominant *a* wave. Bibasilar crackles and an $S_3$ is present at the apex without any murmurs. There is 2+ pretibial edema. An electrocardiogram shows sinus rhythm with occasional ventricular premature contractions and evidence of significant Q waves in leads $V_4$ through $V_6$. Electrocardiographic findings are unchanged from those obtained 2 years ago. An echocardiogram shows diffuse anterior wall hypokinesis with an estimated ejection fraction of 25%. A dipyridamole-thallium perfusion study shows no evidence of reversibility of the abnormalities.

Which one of the following should be done at this time?

(A) Increase the dose of diltiazem
(B) Discontinue the diltiazem
(C) Discontinue the diltiazem and add metoprolol
(D) Continue the diltiazem and add metoprolol

### Chest Pain Question 9

A 62-year-old man is evaluated because of the sudden onset of severe substernal chest pain that radiates to his neck and back and has persisted for 45 minutes. He has a 20-year-history of hypertension and a 60-pack-year smoking history but has no prior history of myocardial infarction or congestive heart failure.

Physical examination shows an anxious, diaphoretic man. His pulse rate is 96/min and regular, respiratory rate is 24/min, and blood pressure is 160/90 mm Hg in his right arm. His lungs are clear to percussion and auscultation. Cardiac examination shows a normal $S_1$, a loud $A_2$, and an $S_4$. The electrocardiogram shows left ventricular hypertrophy with abnormal repolarization. A chest radiograph reveals mediastinal widening, mild cardiomegaly, and clear lung fields.

Which of the following is the most likely diagnosis?

(A) Coronary thrombosis
(B) Percarditis
(C) Aortic dissection
(D) Pulmonary embolism
(E) Interventricular rupture

### Chest Pain Question 10

A 65-year-old woman with type 2 diabetes mellitus is evaluated because of precordial exertional discomfort. A treadmill exercise electrocardiogram shows 3-mm ST-segment depression after 2 1/2 minutes of exercise. Coronary arteriography is performed promptly and shows high-grade obstruction (> 80%) in the proximal left anterior descending and right coronary arteries. Both vessels are widely patent distal to the obstructions. Left ventricular function is mildly depressed with an ejection fraction of 45%. Current medications are aspirin, atenolol, isosorbide mononitrate, glyburide, and simvastatin. Her blood pressure is 130/75 mm Hg.

Which one of the following should be done next?

(A) Continue current treatment
(B) Percutaneous transluminal coronary angioplasty with possible stenting
(C) Thrombolysis
(D) Coronary artery bypass surgery

## Chest Pain Question 11

A 72-year-old man is diagnosed with dissection of the midsection of the descending thoracic aorta.

Which of the following is the most appropriate initial management for this patient?

(A) Prompt surgical intervention
(B) A β-blocker
(C) Furosemide
(D) Heparin
(E) A nonsteroidal anti-inflammatory drug

## Chest Pain Question 12

A 40-year-old man is evaluated because of increasing chest pressure and exertional dyspnea. He had been experiencing exertional dyspnea after climbing two flights of stairs. Physical examination disclosed a regular pulse rate of 65/min. His blood pressure was 155/90 mm Hg. The carotid pulse had a brisk upstroke and a bifid contour. There was a grade 4/6 systolic murmur heard best at the left sternal border in the fourth left interspace. The murmur increased with Valsalva maneuver and became louder with standing. An electrocardiogram was done and showed left ventricular hypertrophy. An M-mode echocardiogram showed thickening of the interventricular septum to 2.0 cm.

Which of the following is the most likely diagnosis?

(A) Aortic stenosis
(B) Atrial septal defect
(C) Coarctation of the aorta
(D) Hypertrophic cardiomyopathy
(E) Ventricular septal defect

## Chest Pain Question 13

A 38-year-old woman, who is a nonsmoker, is evaluated in the emergency department at 0330 hours because of severe retrosternal chest pain, graded 10/10. She is diaphoretic and nauseated. She reports that this is the fourth such episode in the last week, the previous episodes having terminated spontaneously. She has no history of exertional pain. She has no risk factors for coronary artery disease but does have a history of migraine headaches.

Her physical examination is notable for a pulse rate of 110/min and a blood pressure of 140/90 mm Hg but is otherwise unremarkable. An electrocardiogram is obtained just prior to the administration of sublingual nitroglycerin. This shows 4-mm ST-segment elevation in leads $V_1$, $V_2$, $V_3$, with reciprocal depression in leads II, III, aVF. The pain resolves within 3 minutes of nitrate administration, and a

repeat electrocardiogram shows complete resolution of the ST-segment changes.

Which one of the following is the most likely diagnosis?

(A) Pericarditis
(B) Myocardial infarction
(C) Unstable angina
(D) Variant (Prinzmetal's) angina
(E) Esophageal spasm

## Chest Pain Question 14

A treadmill electrocardiographic (ECG) exercise test would most likely help diagnose the presence or absence of significant coronary artery disease in which of the following patients?

(A) A 62-year-old man who smokes and has atypical chest pain
(B) A 70-year-old man who is asymptomatic 6 months after coronary angioplasty
(C) A 31-year-old sedentary woman
(D) A 55-year-old man who has rest angina pectoris associated with transient ECG changes
(E) An asymptomatic 69-year-old woman

## Chest Pain Question 15

Which of the following is the best treatment for long-term management of Printzmental's angina?

(A) Captopril
(B) Aspirin
(C) Propranolol
(D) Nifedipine
(E) Percutaneous transluminal coronary angioplasty (PTCA)

## Chest Pain Question 16

A 22-year-old woman is admitted to the hospital because of 3 days of high-grade fever, shaking chills, and precordial chest pain that is made worse by inspiration and relieved by bending forward. On physical examination the neck veins are normal, the lungs are clear, and there is a scratchy, three-component friction rub heard best at the lower left sternal border. The complete blood count is normal. The erythrocyte sedimentation rate is 40 mm/h. Chest radiograph, electrocardiogram, and echocardiogram are all normal.

Which of the following is the most likely diagnosis?

(A) Myocardial infarction
(B) Myocarditis
(C) Multiple pulmonary emboli
(D) Pericarditis

**Chest Pain Question 17**

A 60-year-old man with multiple risk factors for coronary atherosclerosis is evaluated because of a 6-month history of exertional chest tightness and diaphoresis, relieved promptly by rest. During a recent hospital admission, the patient underwent coronary angiography, which revealed single-vessel coronary disease involving a large, obtuse marginal vessel, and a normal left ventricular ejection fraction. β-Blockers, aspirin, and sublingual nitroglycerin were begun. He was discharged on one aspirin tablet daily and sublingual nitroglycerin as needed.

Which of the following chronic nitrate regimens is most likely to provide long-term symptomatic relief of angina in this patient?

(A) Slow-release nitroglycerin, orally every 8 hours
(B) Nitroglycerin patch, every 24 hours
(C) Slow-release isosorbide dinitrate, orally every 12 hours
(D) Nitroglycerin ointment, topically every 6 hours
(E) Slow-release isosorbide mononitrate, orally once daily

**Chest Pain Question 18**

A 39-year-old housewife with systemic lupus erythematosus who has been receiving long-term glucocorticoid therapy is evaluated because of substernal chest pain, which she has had for the past several hours. The pain is not positional or pleuritic. Physical examination does not show chest wall tenderness. Lung fields are clear on auscultation. On cardiac examination, she is tachycardic. Previous laboratory tests have not shown antiphospholipid antibodies. Electrocardiogram shows some T-wave changes in anterior leads.

Initial treatment includes a liquid antacid, which has no effect on her pain.

What test should be done next in this patient?

(A) Creatine kinase MB band and troponin
(B) Ventilation and perfusion lung scan
(C) Echocardiography
(D) Esophageal manometry
(E) High-resolution chest CT

# Congestive Heart Failure

**Congestive Heart Failure Question 1**

A 65-year-old man was hospitalized with symptoms of increasing dyspnea on exertion and at rest, peripheral edema, and a weight gain of 6.8 kg (15 lb). Four years ago, an echocardiogram showed an estimated ejection fraction of 30% and a dilated ventricle. Myocardial scintigraphy, performed 1 year ago, was negative. Admission medications include benazepril, furosemide, and digoxin. Effective diuresis of 2 liters was obtained overnight with intravenous furosemide.

The following day he feels better. On physical examination, his pulse rate is 90/min, and his blood pressure is 110/80 mm Hg. The jugular venous pressure is estimated at 12 cm $H_2O$. The chest is clear. An $S_4$ and an $S_3$ are heard. There is 2+ pedal edema.

In addition to measuring serum electrolytes, which of the following diagnostic procedures should be done next?

(A) Ultrafast CT of the chest
(B) Repeat echocardiography
(C) Chest radiograph
(D) Serum digoxin level

**Congestive Heart Failure Question 2**

A 52-year-old man is being treated for dilated cardiomyopathy and heart failure. He is receiving a maximal dose of enalapril and is considered to be New York Heart Class II. On physical examination, his pulse rate is 70/min, and his blood pressure is 110/72 mm Hg. The jugular venous pressure is estimated at 8 cm $H_2O$.

β-Blocker therapy with metoprolol, 6.25 mg twice daily, is begun. One week later, the patient feels well, and he is instructed to increase the dose of metoprolol to 12.5 mg twice daily. The patient returns 1 week later, complaining of fatigue and increasing dyspnea. On physical examination, pulse rate is 80/min, blood pressure is 100/72 mm Hg, and estimated jugular venous pressure is 12 cm $H_2O$. He has gained 2.4 kg (5 lb). His chest is clear, and there is no peripheral edema.

Which one of the following should be done now?

(A) Stop the metoprolol
(B) Decrease the dose of metoprolol
(C) Administer furosemide
(D) Decrease the dose of enalapril
(E) Increase the dose of metoprolol

**Congestive Heart Failure Question 3**

A 64-year-old man with heart failure due to coronary artery disease underwent coronary artery bypass surgery 6 years ago. Medical history includes hypertension and hyperlipidemia. His last ejection fraction by echocardiography was 25%. He has occasional orthopnea but can walk up to three blocks without symptoms. He denies chest pain. Current medications include digoxin, lisinopril, furosemide, simvastatin, low-dose aspirin, and potassium.

On physical examination, he is 174 cm (69 in) tall and weighs 86 kg (190 lb). His pulse rate is 84/min and regular, and his blood pressure is 130/80 mm Hg. The jugular venous pressure is estimated at 12 cm $H_2O$. The chest is clear. Heart sounds are distant, but an $S_4$ can be appreciated. There are no cardiac murmurs. The liver is normal in size, and there is no peripheral edema. Blood urea nitrogen is 34 mg/dL, serum creatinine is 1.3 mg/dL, and serum potassium is 4.1 meq/L. An electrocardiogram shows an old inferior wall myocardial infarction.

In addition to weight loss and exercise, which one of the following should be done?

(A) Continue current medications
(B) Discontinue the furosemide
(C) Increase the lisinopril
(D) Increase the lisinopril and furosemide
(E) Increase the furosemide

**Congestive Heart Failure Question 4**

A 24-year-old woman developed heart failure during her first pregnancy 2 years ago and was diagnosed as having peripartum cardiomyopathy. Her heart failure improved after delivery, and a recent echocardiogram showed almost normal left ventricular systolic function with an ejection fraction of 50% and moderate residual mitral regurgitation. The patient is now asymptomatic and is on no cardiac medications. She wishes to conceive again.

On physical examination, she appears well. Her pulse rate is 80/min and regular, and blood pressure is 114/60 mm Hg. Her cardiac examination is normal except for a grade 2/6 holosystolic murmur heard at the apex.

Which one of the following statements is correct?

(A) She is at no increased risk of recurrence of peripartum cardiomyopathy
(B) She is at increased risk of recurrence of peripartum cardiomyopathy
(C) Prophylactic therapy with an angiotensin-converting enzyme inhibitor is indicated
(D) Salt avoidance will reduce the risk of recurrence of peripartum cardiomyopathy

### Congestive Heart Failure Question 5
Which one of the following best explains why the prevalence of heart failure is increasing in the United States?

(A) An increase in the prevalence of hypertension
(B) Improvement in revascularization techniques
(C) An increase in the development of rheumatic valvular disease
(D) An increase in the development of cardiomyopathy

### Congestive Heart Failure Question 6
A 58-year-old postmenopausal woman was evaluated because of symptoms of exertional dyspnea for several months. Stress echocardiography showed anterior wall ischemia, and coronary angiography documented a 90% obstruction in the proximal left anterior descending coronary artery and mild obstruction in the right and first obtuse marginal coronary vessels. The patient was placed on a lipid-lowering diet, a β-blocker, and aspirin and agreed to have an angioplasty procedure. She was treated with the platelet glycoprotein IIb/IIIa inhibitor abciximab before the procedure and underwent uneventful angioplasty and stent placement.

Now, 3 months later, the patient has developed exertional dyspnea after vigorous exercise, which she resumed following the angioplasty procedure. She has no other symptoms. Her physical examination and resting electrocardiogram are normal.

Which of the following is the most likely diagnosis?

(A) Coronary artery stent occlusion
(B) New coronary artery obstruction
(C) Ventricular aneurysm
(D) Gastroesophageal reflux
(E) Pulmonary embolism

### Congestive Heart Failure Question 7
In a patient with heart failure, which one of the following is a poor prognostic indicator?

(A) Pulmonary artery systolic pressure of > 50 mm Hg
(B) Female gender
(C) Serum sodium level of 145 meq/L
(D) Male gender

### Congestive Heart Failure Question 8
A 78-year-old woman with a history of moderately severe asthma is referred for evaluation following three emergency department visits for flash pulmonary edema. The episodes of acute dyspnea are unrelated to physical activity and rapidly respond to intravenous diuretics. She denies chest pain. Medical history includes hypertension treated with a thiazide diuretic. On physical examination, her pulse rate is 90/min and regular, and her blood pressure is 180/90 mm Hg. The chest is clear. There is a prominent $S_4$ and a grade 2/6 holosystolic murmur at the apex radiating to the left axilla. The pulmonic component of $S_2$ is pronounced. There is no peripheral edema. An electrocardiogram shows

left ventricular hypertrophy. Echocardiography shows that the left ventricular end-diastolic dimension is 5 cm and the left atral dimension is 4 cm. The ejection fraction is 60%. There is mild concentric left ventricular hypertrophy.

Which of the following is the most likely cause of her acute episodes of heart failure?

(A) Acute diastolic dysfunction
(B) Coronary artery disease
(C) Mitral regurgitation
(D) Myocarditis
(E) Dietary indiscretion

### Congestive Heart Failure Question 9
Which of the following is the most appropriate therapeutic regimen for the patient in the preceding question?

(A) Stop hydrochlorothiazide, begin furosemide and long-acting diltiazem
(B) Add a β-blocker
(C) Add an angiotensin-converting enzyme inhibitor
(D) Stop hydrochlorothiazide, begin terazosin

### Congestive Heart Failure Question 10
A 70-year-old woman is hospitalized with pulmonary edema. An echocardiogram shows significant left ventricular systolic dysfunction. After 5 days of treatment in the hospital, her symptoms improve and she is discharged to home on digoxin, enalapril, spironolactone, and metoprolol. She is examined in the office 1 week later; although her pulmonary examination and chest radiograph still show crackles and mild congestive heart failure, respectively, her symptoms are markedly improved.

Which one of the following medications can be safely discontinued without compromising patient survival?

(A) Digoxin
(B) Angiotensin-converting enzyme (ACE) inhibitor
(C) Spironolactone
(D) Metoprolol

### Congestive Heart Failure Question 11
Angiotensin II receptor blockers have been shown to have which one of the following benefits in patients with congestive failure?

(A) Significantly greater reductions in long-term clinical events (death and hospitalization) compared with placebo
(B) Significantly greater improvements in symptoms compared with angiointensin-converting enzyme (ACE) inhibitors
(C) Significantly greater improvements in left ventricular function compared with angiointensin-converting enzyme (ACE) inhibitors
(D) Significantly greater reductions in in-hospital mortality compared with placebo

## Congestive Heart Failure Question 12

A 50-year-old man is evaluated because of dyspnea. He has noticed progressive worsening of his exercise tolerance over the previous 8 months and has had two-pillow orthopnea over the previous 6 weeks. His other complaints are nocturia, a decreased sex drive, and hand pain. On physical examination, his pulse rate is 110/min, and his blood pressure is 80/60 mm Hg. His skin appears to be deeply tanned. Examination of the lungs reveals bibasilar crackles. Cardiac examination demonstrates both an $S_4$ and $S_3$ gallop, with a grade 2/6 systolic ejection murmur. There is mild tenderness and bony enlargement of his metacarpophalangeal joints. An electrocardiogram demonstrates sinus rhythm with low voltage and there are nonspecific ST-segment changes. A chest radiograph demonstrates an enlarged heart with interstitial pulmonary edema. A chemistry profile reveals elevated blood glucose and elevated liver function tests.

Which of the following is most likely responsible for all of the patient's findings?

(A) Coronary artery disease
(B) Hemochromatosis
(C) Hypothyroidism
(D) Addison's disease

## Congestive Heart Failure Question 13

A 59-year-old man with long-standing obesity is evaluated because of worsening pedal edema for the last 6 weeks. He has chronic obstructive pulmonary disease with severely limited exercise capacity. He routinely takes hydrochlorothiazide for hypertension and uses albuterol and ipratropium metered-dose inhalers, which provide mild relief of his dyspnea.

On physical examination, his height is 175 cm (68.9 in), and his weight is 110 kg (242 lb). His pulse rate is 92/min, respiration rate is 20/min, and blood pressure is 152/94 mm Hg. He has an elevated jugular venous pressure that decreases significantly with inspiration and shows no "cannon" a waves. Auscultation of the lungs reveals decreased breath sounds and diffuse soft expiratory wheezes. Cardiac examination reveals a soft systolic murmur on the left sternal border and a third heart sound, both of which increase with inspiration. There is obvious pitting edema to the mid-calf. He has a hematocrit of 57% and an oxygen saturation of 87%.

Which of the following is most likely responsible for his symptoms?

(A) Constrictive pericarditis
(B) Cardiac tamponade
(C) Cor pulmonale
(D) Mitral regurgitation
(E) Pulmonic stenosis

## Congestive Heart Failure Question 14

A 24-year-old woman is admitted to the hospital because of the sudden onset of severe shortness of breath and two-pillow orthopnea associated with palpitations. She is 4 months pregnant.

On physical examination, the pulse rate is 125/min and irregular, respiration rate is 20/min, and blood pressure is 90/60 mm Hg. There is marked jugular venous distention with no visible a waves. Bibasilar pulmonary rales are present, as well as a right ventricular lift, a loud $S_1$, a loud $P_2$, an opening snap, and a pandiastolic rumble. The chest radiograph reveals pulmonary venous congestion, right ventricular enlargement, and left atrial enlargement. The electrocardiogram reveals atrial fibrillation and right ventricular hypertrophy.

Which of the following is the most likely diagnosis?

(A) Aortic regurgitation
(B) Atrial septal defect
(C) Mitral valve stenosis
(D) Tricuspid stenosis
(E) Patent ductus arteriosus

## Congestive Heart Failure Question 15

A 58-year-old retired man has had pharyngitis and a nonproductive cough for approximately 4 days. Since that time, he has noted increasing effort dyspnea and orthopnea.

On physical examination, he has an irregular pulse with a rate of 120/min and a blood pressure of 140/90 mm Hg. There are rales at the bases of both lungs. The mean central venous pressure is 15 cm $H_2O$; the left ventricular impulse is in the sixth left interspace 7 cm from the midsternal line. $S_1$ is variable in intensity, and $S_2$ splits normally. There is a grade 2/6 midsystolic murmur at the apex. No $S_3$ is noted. The liver span is 14 cm. The extremities are cool and without edema.

A chest radiograph reveals increased vascular markings and mild cardiomegaly. The electrocardiogram shows atrial fibrillation. An echocardiogram demonstrates only global left ventricular hypokinesis, with an ejection fraction estimated at 30%. The aortic and mitral valves are normal. Laboratory studies show mildly elevated creatine phosphokinase (CPK)-MB and troponin I levels.

What is the most likely cause of this patient's cardiac problem?

(A) Myocardial infarction
(B) Hypertensive heart disease
(C) Myocarditis
(D) Valvular heart disease
(E) Pericardial effusion

**Congestive Heart Failure Question 16**

A 44-year-old woman with a history of morbid obesity is evaluated because of gradually progressive peripheral edema and shortness of breath. Several years ago, she took "phen-fen" in an attempt to lose weight but stopped taking the drugs in 1997. She was diagnosed with obstructive sleep apnea 6 years ago but has been unable to tolerate nasal continuous positive airway pressure (CPAP). The patient has no cardiac history and does not smoke cigarettes. She takes no medications.

On physical examination, she has a body mass index of 36 kg/m$^2$. She has a pulse rate of 78/min, a respiration rate of 14/min, and a blood pressure of 180/110 mm Hg. Examination of the chest reveals decreased breath sounds. Cardiovascular examination reveals a right ventricular heave, a prominent second heart sound, and a murmur of tricuspid regurgitation. Jugular venous pressure cannot be estimated because of the size of her neck. The liver is palpated 4 cm below the costal margin, and 4+ peripheral edema is noted. An arterial blood gas study on room air reveals a $PaO_2$ of 52 mm Hg, $PaCO_2$ of 74 mm Hg, and pH of 7.34.

What is the most likely cause of her right heart failure?

(A) Appetite-suppressant drug-induced valvulopathy
(B) Primary pulmonary hypertension
(C) Obesity-hypoventilation syndrome
(D) Acute pulmonary thromboembolic disease

**Congestive Heart Failure Question 17**

A 65-year-old woman with a history of congestive heart failure is eveluted because she has had shortness of breath for the past 2 weeks. She denies any fever, coughing, history of smoking, weight loss, or pleuritic chest pain.

A chest radiograph shows a small left pleural effusion, a large right pleural effusion, interstitial edema, and cardiomegaly. The patient is sent home with a prescription for an increased dosage of furosemide and captopril and she is told to return in 1 week.

When the patient returns in 1 week, she is less breathless and has less edema, but the right pleural effusion remains large and asymmetric. Diagnostic thoracentesis yields yellow, translucent fluid, and the following findings:

| | |
|---|---|
| Erythrocyte count | 12,400/μL |
| Leukocyte count | 1,800/μL |
| Lymphocytes | 70% |
| Pleural fluid protein | 2.8 g/dL |
| Pleural fluid lactate dehydrogenase | 110 U/L |
| Pleural fluid pH | 7.49 |
| Pleural fluid glucose | 110 mg/dL |
| Pleural fluid cholesterol | 40 mg/dL |

What additional diagnostic tests are needed?

(A) Microscopic examination of the fluid for asbestos bodies
(B) Serum and fluid albumin concentrations
(C) Polymerase chain reaction for *Mycobacterium tuberculosis* in the pleural fluid
(D) Pleural fluid triglyceride concentration

# Lipid Disorders

## Lipid Disorders Question 1
A 50-year-old man is evaluated for cardiovascular risk factors following a recent uncomplicated inferior wall infarction. He is a nonsmoker, is normotensive, and does not have diabetes mellitus. He exercises regularly. His height is 183 cm (72 in), weight is 104 kg (230 lb), and body mass index is 31.3. He is following a Step I fat reduction diet. His current medications are a β-blocker and aspirin. His total cholesterol is 164 mg/dL, low-density lipoprotein cholesterol is 92 mg/dL, high-density lipoprotein cholesterol is 32 mg/dL, and triglycerides are 200 mg/dL.

Which of the following is the most appropriate next step in managing this patient?

(A) Discontinue the β-blocker
(B) Further lower his dietary fat intake (Step II diet)
(C) Begin simvastatin
(D) Begin gemfibrozil

## Lipid Disorders Question 2
A 50-year-old man is evaluated for cardiovascular risk factors because his father had a myocardial infarction at age 52. He is a nonsmoker. His blood pressure is 120/80 mm Hg and his body mass index is 28.

In addition to obtaining a lipoprotein analysis, which of the following is most appropriate for this patient?

(A) Determine the ankle-brachial index
(B) Measure serum lipoprotein(a)
(C) Measure fasting plasma glucose
(D) Measure C-reactive protein
(E) Measure plasma homocysteine

## Lipid Disorders Question 3
A 60-year-old man with diabetes mellitus and peripheral arterial disease (ankle-brachial index of < 0.90) is evaluated because of limited walking capacity. He is otherwise asymptomatic.

In addition to obtaining a standard lipoprotein profile (serum total cholesterol, triglycerides, high-density lipoprotein cholesterol, and low-density lipoprotein cholesterol), which of the following tests is most appropriate for this patient?

(A) Perform glucose tolerance test
(B) Measure hemoglobin $A_{1C}$
(C) Measure lipoprotein(a)
(D) Perform treadmill exercise test

## Lipid Disorders Question 4
A 56-year-old postmenopausal woman is evaluated for cardiovascular risk factors during a routine examination. She smokes one pack of cigarettes per day, and does not have diabetes mellitus. Her family history is negative for coronary artery disease, and she has no symptoms to suggest coronary artery disease. Her blood pressure is 136/88 mm Hg.

| | |
|---|---|
| Plasma glucose (fasting) | 100 mg/dL |
| Plasma total cholesterol | 238 mg/dL |
| Plasma high-density lipoprotein cholesterol | 45 mg/dL |
| Plasma low-density lipoprotein cholesterol | 166 mg/dL |
| Serum triglycerides | 135 mg/dL |
| Serum thyroid-stimulating hormone | Normal |

In addition to advising her to stop smoking and to engage in regular physical activity, which of the following is the most appropriate next step?

(A) Begin a Step I diet
(B) Begin a Step II diet
(C) Begin hormone replacement therapy
(D) Begin a Step I diet plus simvastatin

## Lipid Disorders Question 5
A 47-year-old man seeks advice concerning "staying healthy." His mother underwent coronary artery bypass surgery at age 59 years. He has no personal or family history of diabetes mellitus. He is a nonsmoker and exercises three times weekly for at least 30 minutes each session, and says that he sweats during the exercise bouts. His blood pressure is 146/92 mm Hg, and his body mass index is 28.

Based on the information provided, which of the following lipoprotein test results is most desirable for this patient?

(A) His low-density lipoprotein cholesterol goal should be 130 mg/dL or less
(B) His total cholesterol goal should be 220 mg/dL or less
(C) His high-density lipoprotein cholesterol goal should be 75 mg/dL or greater
(D) His triglyceride goal should be 300 mg/dL or less

**Lipid Disorders Question 6**

A patient has the following laboratory study results:

| | |
|---|---|
| Plasma total cholesterol | 290 mg/dL |
| Plasma high-density lipoprotein cholesterol | 32 mg/dL |
| Plasma low-density lipoprotein cholesterol | 193 mg/dL |
| Serum triglycerides | 325 mg/dL |

Which one of the following lipid-lowering drugs is *contraindicated* in this patient?

(A) Cholestyramine
(B) Niacin
(C) Lovastatin
(D) Gemfibrozil

**Lipid Disorders Question 7**

A 60-year-old man with a 7-year history of type 2 diabetes mellitus is evaluated for cardiovascular risk factors. His only medication is glyburide, 5 mg/d. His physical examination shows: weight, 94 kg (207 lb); height, 175 cm (69 in); blood pressure, 152/96 mm Hg; background retinopathy, and a mild peripheral neuropathy.

| | |
|---|---|
| Hemoglobin $A_{1c}$ | 12.3% |
| Triglycerides (fasting) | 225 mg/dL |
| Total cholesterol | 231 mg/dL |
| HDL cholesterol | 35 mg/dL |
| LDL cholesterol | 152 mg/dL |

What is the most appropriate next step?

(A) Begin a low-sodium, low-saturated fat, reduced-calorie diet
(B) Begin lovastatin
(C) Begin hydrochlorothiazide
(D) Increase the glyburide dosage
(E) Begin insulin

**Lipid Disorders Question 8**

A 68-year-old woman is evaluated because of hypercholesterolemia. She has no family history of premature heart disease and no personal history of hypertension, diabetes, cigarette smoking, peripheral vascular disease, or coronary heart disease. She takes no medications. She follows a strict low-fat, low-cholesterol diet and consumes less than 25% of her calories as fat (less than 7% saturated fat) and less than 200 mg/d of cholesterol. She is close to her ideal body weight. She has previously been treated with cholestyramine but was unable to tolerate the medication owing to bloating, gas, and constipation. She later tried lovastatin, but this was discontinued owing to myalgias, even though her creatine kinase (CK) level was normal.

Results of her laboratory studies (fasting) include: plasma cholesterol (total) 275 mg/dL; HDL cholesterol 75 mg/dL; LDL cholesterol 180 mg/dL; triglycerides 100 mg/dL; glucose, thyroid, renal, liver function tests, and CK level are normal.

What is the most appropriate therapy for this woman?

(A) Refer her to the dietitian
(B) Continue present program
(C) Reinstitute lovastatin
(D) Begin niacin

**Lipid Disorders Question 9**

A 52-year-old woman requests a dietary consultation to decrease the level of fat in her diet.

She initially was seen 8 weeks ago with the following lipid profile: cholesterol, 420 mg/dL; triglycerides, 86 mg/dL; and HDL cholesterol, 40 mg/dL. Her father and two brothers had myocardial infarctions before age 40 years. On physical examination she has several nodular enlargements on her Achilles tendons. She is begun on a low saturated fat and cholesterol diet. After this intervention her HDL cholesterol level decreased to 38 mg/dL.

What is the best therapeutic approach to take now?

(A) Discontinue the low-fat diet
(B) Begin a HMG-CoA reductase inhibitor
(C) Advise moderate alcohol ingestion
(D) Begin gemfibrozil

**Lipid Disorders Question 10**

A 45-year-old woman is evaluated because of an elevated serum cholesterol level. She is otherwise healthy and has no other risk factors for atherosclerotic cardiovascular disease. Her total serum cholesterol after a 12-hour fast is 260 mg/dL.

Which one of the following should be done next?

(A) Repeat total cholesterol measurement
(B) Perform fasting lipoprotein analysis
(C) Dietary modification
(D) Prescribe an exercise program

# Abdominal Pain

**Abdominal Pain Question 1**

A 48-year-old woman (gravida 3, para 3) is evaluated because of right upper quadrant pain. She has had three discrete episodes of moderate to severe right upper quadrant pain that radiates to the right scapula and lasts 4 to 5 hours. The last of these episodes occurred 72 hours ago. These attacks occur 30 minutes to 90 minutes after eating and are associated with nausea, but not vomiting. Her medical history is otherwise unremarkable. Physical examination reveals moderate obesity, and abdominal examination is normal. She takes no medications.

Which of the following is the best test to confirm the diagnosis?

(A) CT scan of abdomen
(B) Ultrasonography
(C) Hepatoiminodiacetic acid (HIDA) scan
(D) Oral cholecystography
(E) Upper endoscopy

**Abdominal Pain Question 2**

A 35-year-old woman is evaluated because of epigastric pain radiating to the back and vomiting. She has no significant medical history, takes no medications, and occasionally has a glass of wine. The physical examination is significant for a temperature of 38 °C (100.4 °F), pulse rate of 104/min, blood pressure of 118/74 mm Hg, anicteric sclerae, normal heart and lungs, absence of bowel sounds, and severe epigastric tenderness with voluntary guarding. Results of laboratory studies include the following: leukocyte count, 14,000/μL; amylase, 2482 U/L; lipase, 18,756 U/L; alkaline phosphatase, 189 U/L; aspartate aminotransferase (AST), 88 U/L; total bilirubin, 1.2 mg/dL; and normal calcium, magnesium, phosphate, and triglyceride levels. An upright chest radiograph is normal.

Which of the following would be the most appropriate next diagnostic study?

(A) Upright and supine abdominal radiographs
(B) Abdominal ultrasonography
(C) CT of the abdomen
(D) Endoscopic retrograde cholangiopancreatography (ERCP)

**Abdominal Pain Question 3**

A 32-year-old man is evaluated because of upper abdominal pain of 2 years' duration. His pain has been intermittent and improves with antacids, eating, and over-the-counter $H_2$-receptor antagonists. His latest episode began 2 weeks ago but resolved when proton pump inhibitor therapy was

initiated at that time. He has not been tested or treated for *Helicobacter pylori* infection in the past.

Considering both cost and accuracy, which of the following is the best screening test to detect *H. pylori* infection?

(A) Urea breath test
(B) Serum or whole-blood antibody test
(C) Endoscopic rapid urease test
(D) Endoscopic biopsy

**Abdominal Pain Question 4**

A 62-year-old asymptomatic woman undergoes abdominal ultrasonography for evaluation for a possible aortic aneurysm. Ultrasonography shows a normal aorta, as well as a normal abdomen and pelvis; however, gallstones are detected. The rest of the biliary tree and liver are normal, without evidence of ductal dilation or gallbladder wall abnormalities.

Which one of the following represents the appropriate management of this patient?

(A) No treatment at this time
(B) Elective cholecystectomy
(C) Dissolution therapy with ursodeoxycholic acid
(D) Stone fragmentation by lithotripsy
(E) Low-fat diet

**Abdominal Pain Question 5**

In which of the following individuals is it appropriate to test for and treat *Helicobacter pylori* infection?

(A) A 50-year-old asymptomatic man
(B) A 42-year-old asymptomatic woman with a family history of gastric cancer
(C) A 38-year-old patient with abdominal pain but without an ulcer (nonulcer dyspepsia)
(D) A 62-year-old patient with gastroesophageal reflux disease
(E) A 45-year-old man with a peptic ulcer

**Abdominal Pain Question 6**

A 34-year-old woman is evaluated because of heartburn. She has tried double-dose, over-the-counter $H_2$-receptor antagonists, with inadequate relief. Her only other medications are birth control pills, calcium, and selenium. She is 162.6 cm (64 in) tall and weighs 47.2 kg (104 lb).

The patient is given a prescription for omeprazole, 20 mg daily. Two weeks later her heartburn is no better. The dosage of omeprazole is increased to 20 mg before breakfast and 20 mg before dinner. One month later her symptoms are no better.

Which of the following is the next best step in managing this patient?

(A) Laparoscopic fundoplication
(B) Increased dose of proton pump inhibitor
(C) Upper endoscopy
(D) 24-hour esophageal pH recording

## Abdominal Pain Question 7

A 48-year-old man is hospitalized with acute pancreatitis, which resolves after 8 days. He has no significant medical history, takes no medications, and has never used alcohol. Results of his evaluation include a normal blood count, normal liver tests, and normal abdominal ultrasonography.

Which of the following diagnostic tests might identify the cause of this patient's pancreatitis?

(A) Fasting serum triglyceride level and a serum calcium level
(B) Serum cholesterol
(C) Glucose tolerance test
(D) Serum CA 19-9

## Abdominal Pain Question 8

A 16-year-old girl returns from a weekend campout with a local youth group complaining of abdominal cramping and malaise. She had two loose, bloody bowel movements. She has always been in good health and has no medical problems. On physical examination, she is in no acute distress. Her temperature is 37.2 °C (99 °F). Other vital signs are normal. Examination is normal except for hyperactive bowel sounds and diffuse, mild abdominal tenderness. The stool on the rectal examination is spotted with red blood.

Ingestion of which of the following is the most likely cause of this patient's findings?

(A) Fried chicken
(B) Untreated water
(C) Aspirin
(D) Hamburgers
(E) Precooked ham

## Abdominal Pain Question 9

A 66-year-old man is evaluated because of severe left lower quadrant pain. This morning he awoke with progressive lower abdominal pain. He described both a steady lower abdominal discomfort as well as waves of pain that came in "spasms."

Physical examination reveals a man in considerable abdominal distress. His temperature is 38.7 °C (101.5 °F), blood pressure is 160/88 mm Hg, and pulse rate is 108/min. He has occasional, high-pitched bowel sounds, and he is quite tender over the left lower quadrant. The remainder of the examination is normal. Laboratory abnormalities include a

hemoglobin of 16 g/dL; leukocyte count of 12,600/μL with 15% band forms and 52% polymorphonuclear cells. A computed tomographic (CT) scan shows several air-filled loops of small intestine. There are multiple diverticula in the left colon, with thickening of wall and an inflammatory mass but no definite abscess.

Which of the following is the most appropriate management?

(A) Laparotomy and colon resection
(B) CT-guided biopsy of the inflammatory mass
(C) Colonoscopy
(D) Nasogastric suction and an antibiotic

## Abdominal Pain Question 10

A 31-year-old female accountant is evaluated because of intermittent epigastric pain, which is relieved by food and antacids. She had similar pain 3 years ago, at which time a duodenal ulcer was diagnosed. She was treated with an $H_2$-receptor antagonist with good relief of her symptoms.

Her medical history is unremarkable. She takes no medications, including aspirin and NSAIDs. Physical examination shows only minor epigastric tenderness. The complete blood count is normal, as is the serum gastrin level.

Upper gastrointestinal endoscopy shows a 0.7-cm ulcer in the duodenal bulb. Scarring is noted in the bulb and pyloric channel, suggesting prior ulcer disease. The remainder of the examination is normal. A biopsy of the gastric antrum demonstrates a superficial chronic active gastritis.

In addition to antisecretory therapy with a proton-pump inhibitor, which of the following is the best therapeutic option?

(A) Magnesium hydroxide antacids
(B) Calcium carbonate antacids
(C) Therapy for *Helicobacter pylori* infection
(D) Sucralfate
(E) Parietal cell vagotomy

## Abdominal Pain Question 11

A 65-year-old man has had sudden onset of left lower abdominal quadrant cramping pain associated with an urge to defecate. Passage of stool fails to relieve his pain, and within 2 hours, the patient passes bright red blood per rectum. After the third bloody bowel movement in 12 hours, he is evaluated in the emergency department.

Physical examination shows normal vital signs, and marked tenderness in the left lower abdominal quadrant associated with guarding and rebound. Leukocyte count is 18,000/μL with a left shift. Sigmoidoscopy is normal to 60 cm.

Which of the following is the most likely diagnosis ?

(A) Acute diverticulitis
(B) Pseudomembranous colitis
(C) Acute colonic ischemia
(D) Polyposis coli
(E) Multiple angiodysplastic lesions

## Abdominal Pain Question 12

A 75-year-old man is evaluated for progressive abdominal symptoms. He has been hospitalized for an exacerbation of chronic congestive heart failure complicated by atrial fibrillation. On the fifth hospital day, he developed progressive midabdominal pain over the prior 12 hours. He vomited once and refused his last meal. His medications include only digoxin and furosemide.

Physical examination reveals an elderly man in abdominal distress. The pulse is 110/min, respiration rate is 24/min, and blood pressure is 160/90 mm Hg. Cardiac examination reveals atrial fibrillation. He has bilateral cervical and femoral bruits. His abdomen is diffusely tender with hypoactive bowel sounds. There is no rebound tenderness or hepatosplenomegaly. Stool in the rectum is positive for occult blood. Laboratory tests from the previous day show normal electrolytes and liver enzymes, but persistent mild chronic renal insufficiency. A stat blood count reveals a leukocyte count of 11,000/μL with a left shift. An abdominal radiograph shows nonspecific gas and no evidence of subdiaphragmatic air.

Which of the following is the most likely diagnosis?

(A) Pancreatitis
(B) Cholelithiasis
(C) Duodenal ulcer
(D) Angiodysplasia
(E) Embolism to the superior mesenteric artery

## Abdominal Pain Question 13

A 28-year-old woman with a 15-year history of heavy alcohol use is evaluated because of severe abdominal pain exacerbated by meals. An abdominal radiograph reveals diffuse calcifications in the pancreas.

Which one of the following is the most likely diagnosis?

(A) Cholelithasis
(B) Nephrolithiasis
(C) Ischemic colitis
(D) Diverticulitis
(E) Acute and chronic pancreatitis

## Abdominal Pain Question 14

A 36-year-old woman is evaluated because of abdominal pain. She has had epigastric distress for the past 10 years. She describes a sense of fullness, bloating, and mild nausea. Her symptoms occur irregularly, approximately two to four times each month, and are not associated with vomiting, anorexia, weight loss, or change in bowel habit. Her symptoms may be more prominent during times of stress. She does take any medications and does not smoke.

On physical examination, her vital signs are normal. There is minimal epigastric tenderness to deep palpation. Stool is negative for occult blood.

Medical records from the previous 6 months show: complete blood count, erythrocyte sedimentation rate, chemistry panel (including amylase and lipase), urinalysis, and abdominal ultrasonography were all normal. An upper gastrointestinal endoscopy was unrevealing.

What is the most appropriate management plan for this patient?

(A) CT scan of the abdomen
(B) Endoscopic retrograde cholangiopancreatography (ERCP)
(C) Omeprazole
(D) Metronidazole, tetracycline, and bismuth subsalicylate
(E) Reassurance

## Abdominal Pain Question 15

A 41-year-old man is evaluated because of intermittent epigastric pain partially relieved by food and antacids. The pain awakens him at night. He had three similar episodes in the past 2 years that were treated empirically with an $H_2$-receptor antagonist for 6 weeks with good relief of his symptoms. He takes no aspirin or NSAIDs.

Physical examination shows epigastric tenderness. Results of a complete blood count are normal, but examination of the stool for occult blood is positive. Upper gastrointestinal endoscopy shows erosive esophagitis. A 1.0-cm, clean-based ulcer is identified in the duodenal bulb; prominent gastric folds are noted, but no other abnormalities are identified. A urease test of an antral mucosal biopsy is negative. Histologic assessment of antral biopsies demonstrates no gastritis and no *Helicobacter pylori*.

Which of the following is the next most appropriate diagnostic test?

(A) Upper gastrointestinal series
(B) *H. pylori* serologies
(C) Fasting serum gastrin level
(D) Colonoscopy

## Abdominal Pain Question 16

A 20-year-old woman is evaluated because of a lower abdominal pain and a heavy, yellowish vaginal discharge 3 weeks after having unprotected intercourse with a new partner. Speculum examination shows a reddened, friable cervix with yellow discharge emanating from the os. A Gram stain of the discharge is obtained. (see Figure 5 in the color plates)

What is the most likely diagnosis?

(A) Chlamydia
(B) Bacterial vaginosis
(C) HIV
(D) Gonorrhea
(E) Syphilis

**Abdominal Pain Question 17**

A 17-year-old woman is evaluated because of left lower quadrant cramping pain, nausea, fever, and increased vaginal discharge. She has been sexually active for more than 2 years with multiple partners. Her last menstrual period was 2 weeks ago and normal.

Physical examination reveals an uncomfortable young woman. Her temperature is 38.5 °C (101.3 °F), pulse rate is 72/min, and blood pressure is 110/80 mm Hg. Abdominal examination reveals diffuse bilateral tenderness to palpation without rebound in the lower quadrants. On pelvic examination, a profuse, frothy, yellow-green vaginal discharge is present. The cervix is tender to manipulation. Bimanual examination reveals tenderness in the right fallopian tube with a 2-cm mass noted. Laboratory data includes a normal urinalysis and a cervical Gram stain showing many leukocytes but no gram-negative intracellular diplococci. Examination of the vaginal fluid shows motile trichomonads but no clue cells. The potassium hydroxide preparation for yeast is negative.

Which of the following is the most appropriate antibiotic regimen for this patient?

(A) Ceftriaxone, intramuscularly, followed by doxycycline, orally

(B) Metronidazole, orally

(C) Gentamicin, intravenously, plus clindamycin, intravenously

(D) Amoxicillin, orally

(E) Cefixime, orally

# Gastrointestinal Bleeding

## Gastrointestinal Bleeding Question 1

A 67-year-old man is evaluated because of bright red blood in his stool 2 weeks ago, which seemed to resolve spontaneously. Rectal examination reveals increased sphincter tone, a small fissure, and a normal prostate gland. Stool is brown and negative for occult blood.

Which of the following is the most appropriate next step in managing this patient?

(A) No further investigation
(B) Three tests of stool for occult blood
(C) Colonoscopy
(D) Barium enema
(E) CT scan of the abdomen

## Gastrointestinal Bleeding Question 2

A 35-year-old man with chronic alcoholism is evaluated because of bright-red hematemesis and syncope. At 11 PM his pulse rate is 100/min and his blood pressure is 100/60 mm Hg, and there is red-tinged irrigant present in the nasogastric tube. The patient has multiple, vascular spider angiomata and a distended abdomen with shifting dullness. He has received 2 L of normal saline solution, and an octreotide drip. His vital signs have stabilized.

What is the optimal management for this patient?

(A) Immediate endoscopy
(B) Endoscopy in the morning
(C) Portocaval shunt surgery
(D) Transjugular intrahepatic portosystemic shunt (TIPS)

## Gastrointestinal Bleeding Question 3

A 64-year-old woman is admitted to the hospital because of bright red blood per rectum and hypotension. She has passed blood per rectum four times in the last 12 hours.

Her general health is good. Her only medication is aspirin, 81 mg/day. She does not smoke or drink alcohol. She has had no abdominal pain, weight loss, or change in bowel habits. On physical examination, her vitals signs and abdominal examination are unremarkable, and she has bright-red blood in her rectum. Nasogastric tube aspiration is clear.

After volume restoration and laboratory assessment, which of the following is the next most important management step?

(A) Visceral angiography
(B) Nuclear medicine scan
(C) Barium enema
(D) Flexible sigmoidoscopy
(E) Colonoscopy

## Gastrointestinal Bleeding Question 4

A 42-year-old woman is evaluated after three episodes of melena. Her only medication is a nonsteroidal anti-inflammatory drug (NSAID) for a long-standing tennis elbow. In the supine position, her pulse rate is 85/min, and her blood pressure is 125/80 mm Hg. Sitting, her pulse rate is 115/min, and her blood pressure is 90/60 mm Hg.

In addition to discontinuing the NSAID, which of the following is the next most important management step?

(A) Vigorous volume replacement
(B) Treatment of *Helicobacter pylori* infection
(C) Upper endoscopy
(D) Intravenous administration of an $H_2$-receptor antagonist

## Gastrointestinal Bleeding Question 5

A 47-year-old man with chronic alcoholism is evaluated because of two episodes of hematemesis over the previous 3 hours. Physical examination demonstrates cutaneous stigmata of cirrhosis, splenomegaly, and ascites. The patient is hemodynamically stable after intravenous administration of 2 L of crystalloid.

Which of the following treatments is appropriate to initiate in the emergency department before transfer to the intensive care unit?

(A) Intravenous octreotide
(B) Intravenous vasopressin
(C) Intravenous nitroglycerin
(D) Balloon tamponade
(E) Transjugular intrahepatic portosystemic shunt (TIPS)

## Gastrointestinal Bleeding Question 6

A 72-year-old woman is evaluated because of lightheadedness and passage of red blood from her rectum. Her pulse rate is 122/min, and her blood pressure is 90/52 mm Hg. Abdominal examination demonstrates no masses, organomegaly, or tenderness. After hemodynamic stabilization, upper endoscopy reveals a nonbleeding visible vessel in a duodenal ulcer.

What is the most appropriate therapy for this patient?

(A) Oral proton-pump inhibitor
(B) Intravenous $H_2$-receptor antagonist
(C) Intravenous vasopressin
(D) Endoscopic injection and/or thermal coagulation therapy

**Gastrointestinal Bleeding Question 7**

A 46-year-old man is evaluated because of melena. He undergoes endoscopy, which demonstrates a nonbleeding, clean-based gastric ulcer. He uses ibuprofen chronically for low back pain. A whole-blood antibody test for *Helicobacter pylori* is positive.

In addition to discontinuing the ibuprofen, which of the following is the most appropriate long-term management of his ulcer disease?

(A) No additional changes
(B) Substitute celecoxib or rofecoxib for ibuprofen
(C) Treat the *H. pylori* infection
(D) Begin misoprostol

**Gastrointestinal Bleeding Question 8**

A 45-year-old man with alcoholic cirrhosis is admitted to the intensive care unit for evaluation of hematemesis. On the morning of admission, he developed nausea and dizziness followed by a liquid, maroon stool. He subsequently vomited "a quart" of bright red blood.

The patient's hemodynamic condition was stabilized. Upper gastrointestinal endoscopy shows large esophageal varices, one of which has adherent clot. No other bleeding site is seen. Sclerotherapy is administered to all visible varices. Twenty-four hours later he suddenly vomits a large volume of bright red blood. His pulse rate is 140/min, respiration rate is 36/min, and blood pressure is 70/40 mm Hg. Despite fluid resuscitation, he continues to be hypotensive and vomit bright red blood.

Which of the following is the most appropriate next step?

(A) Portosystemic shunt procedure
(B) Balloon-tamponade of the bleeding varices
(C) Intravenous vasopressin
(D) Transjugular intrahepatic portosystemic shunt (TIPS) procedure

**Gastrointestinal Bleeding Question 9**

A 74-year-old woman is evaluated because of a second episode of painless, large-volume hematochezia. Three months ago, following her first episode, colonoscopy demonstrated both right- and left-sided diverticula, with a pigmented spot on a right-sided diverticulum. She is now admitted to the hospital for evaluation of a similar bout of painless hematochezia. Physical examination reveals tachycardia with orthostatic blood pressure changes, pale conjunctivae and skin, and mild bilateral abdominal tenderness. Laboratory tests show a hemoglobin of 10 g/dL.

Which of the following is the most likely diagnosis?

(A) Colon cancer
(B) Diverticulosis
(C) Ischemic colitis
(D) Diverticulitis
(E) Ulcerative colitis

**Gastrointestinal Bleeding Question 10**

A 33-year-old man is admitted to the hospital for gastrointestinal bleeding. Several skin lesions were noted. The photograph (see Figure 6 in the color plates) shows examples of the lesions on his thumb. When these lesions are lightly compressed with a glass side, they pulsate, and with increasing the pressure, they blanch.

Which of the following is the most likely etiology of the gastrointestinal bleeding?

(A) Peptic ulcer disease
(B) Hereditary hemorrhagic telangiectasias
(C) Portal hypertension
(D) Thrombocytopenia

# Liver Disorders

## Liver Disorders Question 1

A 46-year-old man with a history of cirrhosis is evaluated because of increasing abdominal girth, swelling of his ankles, and a 30-lb weight gain. Physical examination demonstrates moderate ascites, muscle wasting, cutaneous stigmata of advanced liver disease, and no sign of hepatic encephalopathy. Laboratory studies reveal the following: albumin, 3.0 g/dL; aspartate aminotransferase (AST), 66 U/dL; alanine aminotransferase (ALT), 78 U/dL; total bilirubin, 1.4 mg/dL; international normalized ratio (INR), 1.2; sodium, 132 meq/L; potassium, 3.8 meq/L; serum creatinine, 0.9 mg/dL; and $U_{Na}$, 15 meq/d. Ascitic fluid findings on paracentesis include a leukocyte count of 270/µL (60% polymorphonuclear leukocytes) and an albumin level of 1.3 g/dL.

In addition to a salt-restricted diet, which of the following initial measures is most appropriate to manage this patient's ascites?

(A) Dietary protein and fluid restriction
(B) Serial large-volume paracentesis
(C) A loop diuretic
(D) Spironolactone and a loop diuretic

## Liver Disorders Question 2

A healthy 35-year-old woman is planning to travel to rural Mexico in 2 weeks on a 7-day trip and seeks advice regarding prophylaxis against viral hepatitis. She denies any prior history of liver disease or use of illicit drugs and has a monogamous heterosexual relationship. She is asymptomatic, and her physical examination is normal. Serologic testing for antibody to hepatitis A virus (anti-HAV) (both IgG and IgM) is negative.

Administration of which of the following options is the most appropriate?

(A) Immune serum globulin
(B) Immune serum globulin (ISG) and hepatitis B immune globulin (HBIG)
(C) Hepatitis A vaccine
(D) Hepatitis A and B vaccines

## Liver Disorders Question 3

A 20-year-old male college student is diagnosed with acute hepatitis B. Hepatitis B immune globulin (HBIG) and hepatitis B vaccine should be administered to which of the following?

(A) Members of his swim team
(B) Classmates in his English class
(C) The medical assistant who took his vital signs
(D) His coworkers at a fast-food restaurant
(E) His roommate

## Liver Disorders Question 4

A 50-year-old woman with a remote history of blood transfusions is found on a screening physical examination to have spider angiomas and palpable splenomegaly. She is otherwise healthy. Subsequent evaluation reveals that she is positive for antibody to hepatitis C virus (anti-HCV), and liver biopsy reveals cirrhosis. Screening endoscopy demonstrates large, distal esophageal varices.

Which of the following management options is most appropriate at this time?

(A) Nonselective β-blocker
(B) Band ligation of esophageal varices
(C) Band ligation and sclerotherapy of esophageal varices
(D) Dietary protein restriction
(E) Isosorbide mononitrate

## Liver Disorders Question 5

A 38-year-old woman is evaluated because of jaundice and mental confusion. She admits to drinking 1 quart of vodka per day for the last 3 weeks. On physical examination, she has a temperature of 37.8 °C (100.04 °F), with jaundice, spider telangiectasias, a tender and enlarged liver, a protuberant abdomen with a fluid wave, and asterixis. Her hematocrit is 31%, and her leukocyte count is 17,500/µL with 75% polymorphonuclear leukocytes.

Ultrasonography confirms hepatomegaly and ascites. Paracentesis is performed, and ascitic fluid studies show a leukocyte count of 150/µL (80% polymorphonuclear leukocytes) and an albumin level of 1.3 g/dL.

Which of the following is the most likely diagnosis?

(A) Cholelithiasis
(B) Alcoholic hepatitis
(C) Spontaneous bacterial peritonitis
(D) Pyelonephritis
(E) Alcohol withdrawal

**Liver Disorders Question 6**

A 45-year-old man is evaluated because of a 4-year history of progressive arthritis involving predominantly the joints in his hands. He has a long history of alcoholism and continues to drink four cocktails daily. He has mildly abnormal liver function test results for 10 years, which are attributed to alcohol consumption.

On physical examination, his temperature is 37.6 °C (99.7 °F). His pulse is 66/min, and blood pressure is 130/60 mm Hg. His skin shows a slight bronze pigmentation on sun-exposed areas but is otherwise unremarkable. There is slight swelling and tenderness of the second and third proximal interphalangeal joints bilaterally. Cardiac examination reveals an $S_4$ gallop. Abdominal examination discloses a liver edge that is palpable 6 cm below the right costal margin at the midclavicular line. The remainder of his examination is normal.

| | |
|---|---|
| Hemoglobin | 14.8 g/dL |
| Mean corpuscular volume | 90 fL |
| Serum ferritin | 3255 µg/mL |
| Serum copper | 600 µg/dL |
| Serum ceruloplasmin | 28 mg/dL |
| Plasma glucose (fasting) | 230 mg/dL |
| Serum alkaline phosphatase | 333 U/L |
| Serum aspartate aminotransferase | 77 U/L |
| Serum alanine aminotransferase | 66 U/L |

A liver biopsy shows iron deposited in the periportal areas and in hepatocytes and demonstrates evidence of early cirrhosis. Very little iron is noted in the Kupffer cells. Quantitative studies show 34,000 µg of iron/g dry weight.

Which of the following is the most likely diagnosis?

(A) Thalassemia
(B) Hemochromatosis
(C) Alcohol-induced liver disease
(D) Idiopathic acquired sideroblastic anemia
(E) Wilson's disease

**Liver Disorders Question 7**

A 43-year-old woman is evaluated because of itching that keeps her awake at night. Physical examination is normal, except for the liver, which is felt 7 cm below the right costal margin.

The blood count is normal; the results of selected serum chemistry tests are as follows:

Creatinine 0.8 mg/dL

Bilirubin 0.6 mg/dL

Alanine aminotransferase 78 U/L

Albumin 4.2 g/dL

Alkaline phosphatase 450 U/L

Which of the following is the most likely diagnosis?

(A) Hepatitis A infection
(B) Hepatitis B infection
(C) Primary biliary cirrhosis
(D) Cholelithiasis
(E) Autoimmune hepatitis

**Liver Disorders Question 8**

A 22-year-old woman has had fatigue for 8 months and dark urine, which she first noticed 6 weeks ago. Positive physical findings include scleral icterus, multiple spider telangiectasias over the chest and back, a liver edge palpated 4 cm below the right costal margin, and an enlarged spleen palpated 6 cm below the left costal margin.

Results of complete blood count as well as measurement of serum electrolytes, urea nitrogen, and creatinine are normal. Other laboratory tests show:

| | |
|---|---|
| Alanine aminotransferase | 780 U/L |
| Aspartate aminotransferase | 680 U/L |
| Serum bilirubin | 20.8 mg/dL |
| Direct bilirubin | 8.7 mg/dL |
| Alkaline phosphatase | 145 U/L |
| Serum albumin | 2.8 g/dL |
| Serum globulin | 8.7 g/dL |
| Prothrombin time | 12 sec (international normalized ratio, 1.2) |

Which one of the following diagnostic studies should be performed next?

(A) Endoscopic retrograde cholangiopancreatography (ERCP)
(B) Hepatoiminodiacetic acid (HIDA) scan
(C) Percutaneous liver biopsy
(D) Technetium-99m liver-spleen scan
(E) Magnetic resonance imaging of the abdomen

**Liver Disorders Question 9**

A 22-year-old male graduate student is evaluated because of yellow eyes for 2 weeks. He has a history of ulcerative colitis for 5 years with recurrent flares, requiring steroids for control. He is taking 3 g of sulfasalazine per day, a medication that he has been on for 5 years. His health has otherwise been good, and he has had no abdominal pain, nausea, vomiting, or weight loss. He also denies alcohol intake, known exposure to hepatitis, intravenous drug abuse, or homosexual activity. He denies taking other medications, including acetaminophen.

Physical examination is significant for yellow sclerae; there are no other stigmata of chronic liver disease. His liver has an 8-cm span to percussion in the right midclavicular line and cannot be felt. The remainder of his examination is normal. Laboratory studies reveal a normal blood count and differential, but his bilirubin is 5 mg/dL with a direct fraction of 3; alkaline phosphatase is 400 U/L, aspartate aminotransferase (AST) is 50 U/L, and alanine aminotransferase (ALT) is 60 U/L. Prothrombin time and albumin are normal. A hepatitis panel shows the following: hepatitis B surface antigen (HBsAg), negative; HBs core antibody, negative; hepatitis C antibody, negative; and hepatitis A antibody, negative. Ultrasonography is performed and shows a liver of normal size and density, a gallbladder without stones, and no dilatation of the common bile duct. The pancreas also appears unremarkable.

Which of the following is the most likely diagnosis?

(A) Viral hepatitis
(B) Cholelithiasis
(C) Hemolytic anemia
(D) Sclerosing cholangitis
(E) Cancer of the head of the pancreas

## Liver Disorders Question 10

A 24-year-old male student with severe acute hepatitis B infection is evaluated because of mental status changes. He has had nausea, vomiting, and fatigue for 5 to 7 days and jaundice for 2 to 3 days.

| Prothrombin time | 28 sec (control, 11-13 sec) |
| Total serum bilirubin | 12.6 mg/dL |
| Serum aspartate aminotransferase | 1640 U/L |
| Serum ammonia | 136 µg/dL |

In the last 24 hours, he developed grade II hepatic encephalopathy.

Which of the following is the most appropriate, immediate set of options?

(A) Lactulose
(B) Intravenous glucose
(C) Lactulose, intravenous glucose
(D) Low protein diet, proton-pump inhibitor
(E) Intravenous glucose, proton-pump inhibitor

## Liver Disorders Question 11

A 52-year-old woman has an annual check-up. She has type 2 diabetes mellitus, for which she takes an oral sulfonylurea medication. Her medical history is otherwise unremarkable. She occasionally drinks a glass of wine with dinner. On physical examination, she is 152.4 cm (60 in) tall and weighs 90.7 kg (200 lb). The liver is mildly enlarged and nontender. The remainder of the examination is normal. Results of laboratory studies are as follows: aspartate aminotransferase (AST), 75 U/L; alanine aminotransferase (ALT), 52 U/L; alkaline phosphatase, 110 U/L; albumin, 4.0 g/dL; globulin, 2.5 g/dL; international normalized ratio (INR), 1.1; total bilirubin, 1.0 mg/dL; and glucose level, 254 mg/dL. Further studies were then performed that showed negative serology for hepatitis virus B and C and negative studies for antimitochondrial and anti–smooth

cell antibodies. Ultrasonography showed decreased echogenicity of the liver but no ductal dilatation.

Which of the following is the most likely diagnosis?

(A) Alcoholic steatosis
(B) Nonalcoholic steatohepatitis
(C) Chronic cholecystitis
(D) Biliary cirrhosis
(E) Autoimmune hepatitis

## Liver Disorders Question 12

A 25-year-old man is evaluated because of jaundice. He returned from a trip to Mexico 2 months ago. He denies exposure to individuals with hepatitis or blood transfusions. He is an office worker and denies exposure to toxins. He denies taking any medications. Family history is positive for a brother who died 1 year earlier at age 35 years of "liver disease." Physical examination reveals normal vital signs. Sclerae are jaundiced. The remainder of the examination is normal.

| Complete blood count | Normal |
| Aspartate aminotransferase | 500 U/L |
| Alanine aminotransferase | 450 U/L |
| Lactate dehydrogenase | 1000 U/L |
| Albumin | 2.5 g/dL |
| Uric acid | 3.5 mg/dL |

Testing for all known hepatitis viruses is negative. Antinuclear antibody (ANA) testing is negative. A liver biopsy reveals chronic active hepatitis with some bridging and early fibrosis. Iron stain on the liver biopsy is normal.

Which of the following is the most likely diagnosis?

(A) Wilson's disease
(B) Hemachromatosis
(C) Viral hepatitis
(D) Autoimmune hepatitis
(E) Primary biliary cirrhosis

## Liver Disorders Question 13

A 42-year-old male attorney is evaluated because of recent onset of jaundice. He also has vague epigastric and right upper quadrant discomfort but no severe pain. The patient estimates his daily alcohol intake to be one pint of vodka. He says that he has never used intravenous drugs, been transfused, or had homosexual contact. Recently, he had an upper respiratory illness for which he used acetaminophen several days before hospital admission.

On physical examination, he is alert and oriented but has jaundice. The heart and lungs are normal, but there is hepatomegaly.

| | |
|---|---|
| Prothrombin time | 20 s (control, 11-13 s) |
| Blood urea nitrogen | 38 mg/dL |
| Serum creatinine | 3.0 mg/dL |
| Total serum protein | 7.7 g/dL |
| Serum albumin | 4.8 g/dL |
| Total serum bilirubin | 11.2 mg/dL |
| Serum alkaline phosphatase | 70 U/L |
| Serum aspartate aminotransferase | 14,830 U/L |
| Serum alanine aminotransferase | 6740 U/L |
| Serum ammonia | 96 μg/dL |

Which of the following is the most likely cause of this patient's liver disease?

(A) Alcoholic hepatitis
(B) Acute viral hepatitis
(C) Acetaminophen hepatotoxicity
(D) Reye's syndrome
(E) Hepatic ischemia

## Liver Disorders Question 14

A 63-year-old woman comes to the emergency department because of nausea, vomiting, shaking chills, fever, and abdominal pain of 4 hours' duration. Physical examination reveals a temperature of 39.2 °C (102.5 °F), scleral icterus, and epigastric tenderness.

Ultrasonography of the abdomen reveals gallstones and dilatation of the common bile duct. The liver and pancreas appear to be normal.

Which of the following is the most likely diagnosis?

(A) Viral hepatitis
(B) Ascending cholangitis
(C) Hepatic abscess
(D) Gallstone ileus
(E) Pancreatic pseudocyst

## Liver Disorders Question 15

A 26-year-old woman (G4P3A0) in her thirty-fourth week of pregnancy is evaluated because of a 4-day history of malaise and right upper quadrant pain and a 2-day history of nausea and vomiting. Her pregnancy has been uneventful to this point, and her three previous pregnancies were uneventful. On physical examination, her blood pressure is 140/90 mm Hg, and her other vital signs are normal. No abdominal masses other than an appropriately enlarged uterus are found. Murphy's sign is negative. She has 3+ pitting leg edema. Laboratory studies reveal the following:

| | |
|---|---|
| Hemoglobin | 8 g/dL (normal 1 month previously) |
| Leukocyte count | 12,000/μL, with 80% segmented neutrophils |
| Platelet count | 80,000/μL |
| Blood smear | Helmet cells and erythrocyte fragments |
| Bilirubin | 5.0 mg/dL (direct measurement, 0.4 mg/dL) |
| Aspartate aminotransferase (AST) | 300 U/L |
| Alanine aminotransferase (ALT) | 300 U/L |
| Lactate dehydrogenase (LDH) | 1000 U/L |
| Blood urea nitrogen | 19 mg/dL |
| Uric acid | 6.0 mg/dL |
| Creatinine | 0.8 mg/dL |
| Urinalysis | 4+ proteinuria |

Which of the following is the most probable diagnosis in this patient?

(A) HELLP syndrome (hemolysis, elevated liver enzymes, low platelet count)
(B) Acute fatty liver of pregnancy
(C) Cholestasis of pregnancy
(D) Hemolytic-uremic syndrome
(E) Immune thrombocytopenic purpura

## Liver Disorders Question 16

A 58-year-old woman with cirrhosis is evaluated because of a 1-week history of diffuse abdominal discomfort, feverishness, and night sweats. The patient is taking furosemide and spironolactone. She denies alcohol consumption.

On physical examination, the patient appears unwell, with a temperature of 37.5 °C (99.5 °F), pulse rate of 90/min and regular, and blood pressure of 110/80 mm Hg. There is no jaundice, but mild asterixis is present. The abdomen is soft, with tenderness to palpation in all quadrants. Ascites is present. The liver edge cannot be palpated, but a spleen tip is present just below the left costal margin. Bowel sounds are diminished.

Laboratory studies include a hemoglobin of 11.5 g/dL, leukocyte count of 8500/ml, and serum albumin of 2.6 g/dL.

Diagnostic paracentesis yields ascitic fluid with a neutrophil count of 750/mL and a negative Gram's stain for bacteria. Cultures are pending.

Which of the following would be the most reasonable next step?

(A) Continued observation
(B) Administer lactulose
(C) Perform abdominal ultrasonography
(D) Increase diuretic doses
(E) Prescribe antibiotics

## Liver Disorders Question 17

A 19-year-old female student comes to the university health service with a 6-day history of fever, sore throat, malaise, and right upper quadrant abdominal discomfort. Physical examination reveals an oral temperature of 38.9 °C (102 °F), diffuse pharyngeal infection without exudate, several slightly tender anterior cervical lymph nodes, and a palpable spleen tip 2 cm below the left costal margin.

| | |
|---|---|
| Leukocyte count | 11,700/μL |
| Polymorphonuclear leukocytes | 39% |
| Lymphocytes | 60%, with 20% atypical forms |
| Eosinophils | 1% |
| Serum alkaline phosphatase | 74 U/L |
| Serum aspartate aminotransferase | 122 U/L |
| Heterophil antigen test | Negative |
| Epstein-Barr virus antibody titer | <10 |

Which one of the following infections is the most likely cause of the elevated liver function studies?

(A) Epstein-Barr virus
(B) Adenovirus
(C) *Mycoplasma pneumoniae*
(D) Cytomegalovirus
(E) *Chlamydia pneumoniae* (TWAR)

## Liver Disorders Question 18

A 30-year-old male health care worker comes to your office to be evaluated because one of his coworkers has acute hepatitis B infection. One year ago he was immunized for hepatitis B virus (HBV). The physical examination is normal. Serologic tests reveal that he is positive for antibody to hepatitis B surface antigen (anti-HBs) and negative for hepatitis B surface antigen (HbsAg), IgM anti-HBc (IgM antibodies to the hepatitis B core antigen), anti-hepatitis D virus, anti-hepatitis C virus, and IgM anti-hepatitis A virus.

Which of the following best describes the clinical state of this patient?

(A) Acute HBV infection
(B) Chronic HBV infection
(C) Convalescent HBV infection
(D) Vaccinated for HBV

# Anemia

## Anemia Question 1

An 80-year-old man who had a hemicolectomy for colon cancer is evaluated because of a 4-month history of diarrhea, anorexia, and fatigue. He had a remote history of alcoholism.

On physical examination, he is cachectic and mildly confused. His pulse rate is 70/min, and blood pressure is 140/85 mm Hg. His tongue is smooth. The abdomen is soft; there are no palpable masses or hepatosplenomegaly. A stool specimen is negative for occult blood. Neurologic examination shows loss of position sense in the feet. He has a wide-based gait. The Romberg test is positive. His hemoglobin is 9.4 g/dL, reticulocyte count is 2.5%, mean corpuscular volume is 125 fL, and serum lactate dehydrogenase is 400 U/L.

Which of the following is the most likely cause for his symptoms?

(A) Alcoholic cerebellar degeneration
(B) Vitamin $B_{12}$ deficiency
(C) Brain metastases
(D) Folate deficiency
(E) Liver metastases

## Anemia Question 2

A 22-year-old woman with active systemic lupus erythematosus is evaluated because of a 3-week history of dark stools. For the past 3 months, she has taken large doses of ibuprofen and aspirin for joint pain. She takes no other medications or vitamin supplements.

On physical examination, she is thin and appears chronically ill. She has a prominent "butterfly" facial rash. A stool specimen is strongly positive for occult blood.

| | |
|---|---|
| Hematocrit | 29.2% |
| Mean corpuscular volume | 72 fL |
| Erythrocyte sedimentation rate | 91 mm/h |
| Reticulocyte count | 1.3% |

Which of the following iron indices will most likely be found in this patient?

(A) Serum iron 21 mgldL; serum total iron-binding capacity 490 mgldL; serum ferritin 10 mgldL
(B) Serum iron 24 mgldL; serum total iron-binding capacity 211 mgldL; serum ferritin 440 mgldL
(C) Serum iron 36 mgldL; serum total iron-binding capacity 218 mgldL; serum ferritin 32 mgldL
(D) Serum iron 172 mgldL; serum total iron-binding capacity 328 mgldL; serum ferritin 940 mgldL

## Anemia Question 3

A 26-year-old man is evaluated because of progressive fatigue, dyspnea on exertion, and orthostatic dizziness for the past 2 to 3 weeks. He takes no medications. Physical examination is normal except for pallor.

| | |
|---|---|
| Hematocrit | 13% |
| Leukocyte count | 8300/µL; normal differential |
| Reticulocyte count | 0 |
| Platelet count | 320,000/µL |

A routine biochemical profile, including liver function tests, is normal. A chest radiograph shows normal lung fields and a widened mediastinum, suggestive of an anterior mediastinal mass. Bone marrow biopsy shows absent erythrocyte precursors, normal megakaryocytes, and normal leukocyte numbers and maturation.

Which of the following is the most likely cause of the mediastinal mass and anemia?

(A) Hodgkin's disease
(B) Non-Hodgkin's lymphoma
(C) Thyroid carcinoma
(D) Thymoma
(E) Germ cell carcinoma

## Anemia Question 4

A 36-year-old black man with known sickle cell anemia is evaluated because of a 2-week history of fever, a macular rash on his trunk, and arthralgias. Subsequently, he developed weakness and dyspnea on exertion. Several of his children had febrile illnesses with associated rashes and fatigue over the past month. These illnesses resolved spontaneously without sequelae.

On physical examination, his temperature is 38.8 °C (101.8 °F), pulse rate is 100/min, and blood pressure is 160/70 mm Hg. A maculopapular, truncal rash is noted. There is conjunctival pallor. The remainder of his examination is unremarkable.

| | |
|---|---|
| Hemoglobin | 5.2 g/dL |
| Leukocyte count | 5000/µL |
| Reticulocyte count | 0% |
| Platelet count | 130,000/µL |
| Serum lactate dehydrogenase | 622 U/L |

Which of the following is the most likely diagnosis?

(A) Paroxysmal nocturnal hemoglobinuria
(B) Parvovirus infection
(C) Glucose-6-phosphate dehydrogenase deficiency
(D) Aplastic anemia

## Anemia Question 5

A 43-year-old woman is evaluated for a routine physical examination. She reports progressive mild weakness and fatigue and slight numbness and tingling in her fingers. The patient had previously been treated with levothyroxine for hypothyroidism. She denies having black or tarry stools and has no gastrointestinal complaints. She drinks one cocktail every other evening, as she has for many years. She has been a vegetarian for the past 16 months.

On physical examination, her skin is sallow, and her hair is predominantly gray. She has blue eyes with slight scleral icterus. Temperature is normal. Her pulse rate is 68/min and blood pressure is 140/80 mm Hg. Her tongue is smooth. The remainder of the examination is normal.

| | |
|---|---|
| Hemoglobin | 10.0 g/dL |
| Mean corpuscular volume | 128 fL |
| Leukocyte count | 5600/μL |
| Reticulocyte count | 1.2% |
| Platelet count | 145,000/μL |
| Peripheral smear | Macrocytosis and hypersegmented neutrophils |

Which of the following is the most likely cause of her anemia?

(A) Myelodysplastic syndrome
(B) Pernicious anemia
(C) Hypothyroidism
(D) Alcoholic liver disease
(E) Folate deficiency

## Anemia Question 6

A 31-year-old man with sickle cell disease is hospitalized because of right-sided pleuritic chest pain, a nonproductive cough, fever, and pain in his upper legs and pelvis.

On physical examination, his temperature is 38.6 °C (101.1 °F). His pulse rate is 95/min, respiratory rate is 20/min, and blood pressure is 130/85 mm Hg. Crackles and rhonchi are heard over both lower lung fields. There is no tenderness over the joints or bones. Hemoglobin is 6.7 g/dL, the reticulocyte count is 18%, and the leukocyte count is 17,000/μL with 65% neutrophils. Sputum is clear, and no neutrophils are seen on a sputum smear. A chest radiograph shows a large infiltrate in the right lower lobe. His arterial $PaO_2$ is 60 mm Hg. The patient is started on antibiotics and supplemental oxygen.

Which of the following management options should be performed next?

(A) Red blood cell transfusion
(B) Red blood cell exchange transfusion
(C) Treatment with erythropoietin
(D) Treatment with hydroxyurea

## Anemia Question 7

An 18-year-old woman is found to be anemic during a pre-college screening program. Her older brother is anemic. Physical examination is normal except for an enlarged spleen.

| | |
|---|---|
| Hemoglobin | 8.2 g/dL |
| Mean corpuscular volume | 85 fL |
| Mean corpuscular hemoglobin concentration | 38 g/dL |
| Reticulocyte count | 6% |
| Direct antiglobulin test | Negative |
| Osmotic fragility test | Increased |

Which of the following is the most likely diagnosis?

(A) Iron deficiency anemia
(B) β-Thalassemia minor
(C) Autoimmune hemolytic anemia
(D) Hereditary spherocytosis

## Anemia Question 8

A 27-year-old woman delivers a small-for-gestational-age infant at 33 weeks of pregnancy. Postpartum, she develops nausea, malaise, and epigastric pain, accompanied by a falling hematocrit. Her pulse rate is 88/min, blood pressure is 100/60 mmHg, and she is afebrile.

| | |
|---|---|
| Reticulocyte count | 12% |
| Platelet count | 30,000/μL |
| Prothrombin time | Normal |
| Activated partial thromboplastin time | Normal |
| Plasma fibrinogen | Normal |
| Fibrin degradation products | Markedly elevated |
| Serum creatinine | 0.5 mg/dL |
| Urinalysis | No proteinuria |
| Serum aspartate aminotransferase | 140 U/L |
| Serum alanine aminotransferase | 110 U/L |
| Peripheral blood smear | Numerous schistocytes |

Which of the following is the most likely diagnosis?

(A) Preeclampsia
(B) Postpartum hemolytic uremic syndrome
(C) HELLP syndrome
(D) Acute fatty liver of pregnancy

## Anemia Question 9

A 52-year-old woman is evaluated because of fatigue and easy bruising. The patient had a hysterectomy with unilateral oophorectomy 14 years ago. She received 2 units of packed red blood cells perioperatively. She has well-controlled hypertension and has taken lisinopril for 12 months. She does not use alcohol, tobacco, or illicit drugs.

On physical examination, the patient appears pale. There are a few spider telangiectasias on her upper trunk. The liver measures 7 to 8 cm by percussion, and the spleen tip is palpable 4 cm below the left costal margin. There is no evidence of ascites or jaundice. Scattered ecchymoses without petechiae are present on her lower extremities.

| | |
|---|---|
| Hematocrit | 27% |
| Leukocyte count | 2800/μL; normal differential |
| Reticulocyte count | 5.3% |
| Platelet count | 72,000/μL |
| Serum aspartate aminotransferase | 82 U/L |
| Serum alanine aminotransferase | 108 U/L |
| Serologic studies for hepatitis A, B, and C | Positive for antibodies to hepatitis C (anti-HCV) |

A complete blood count obtained during a routine gynecologic examination 15 months ago showed the following: hemoglobin, 10.5 g/dL; hematocrit, 33%; leukocyte count, 3900/μL; and platelet count, 110,000/μL. A peripheral blood shows normal cell morphology.

Which of the following is the most likely cause of this patient's pancytopenia?

(A) Hepatitis-associated aplastic anemia
(B) HIV-associated bone marrow suppression
(C) Cirrhosis-associated hypersplenism
(D) Lisinopril-induced bone marrow suppression

## Anemia Question 10

A 36-year-old man is evaluated because of fatigue. He has had two episodes of acute gouty arthritis over the past 6 months. He has a 10-year history of significant alcohol use, but he quit drinking 4 months ago. He works in a factory making battery products. A complete blood count obtained prior to elective hernia repair surgery 4 years ago was normal. He takes no medications.

On physical examination, his temperature is 37.3 °C (99.1 °F), pulse is 60/min, and blood pressure is 135/70 mm Hg. His skin is normal. There is slight scleral icterus. There is a blue line at the edge of his gums (see Figure 7 in the color plates).

The remainder of the examination is normal. Stool specimens are negative for blood on three occasions.

| | |
|---|---|
| Hemoglobin | 7.5 g/dL |
| Mean corpuscular volume | 71 fl |
| Leukocyte count | 9400/μL |
| Reticulocyte count | 5.3% |
| Platelet count | 435,000/μL |
| Serum lactate dehydrogenase | 553 U/L |
| Serum uric acid | 11 mg/dL |

A peripheral blood smear (see Figure 8 in the color plates) is shown.

Which of the following diagnostic studies is most useful for determining the cause of this patient's anemia?

(A) Serum iron, total iron-binding capacity, and ferritin levels
(B) Serum lead levels
(C) Direct and indirect antiglobulin tests
(D) Hemoglobin $A_2$ quantitation
(E) Serum ethanol and folic acid levels

## Anemia Question 11

A 64-year-old man has osteoarthritis and needs to undergo hip replacement surgery. He has been a regular blood donor and donates blood every 8 weeks. The patient has no other medical problems. Because he is concerned about receiving blood from an unknown donor, he has donated 4 units of blood preoperatively. During the surgical procedure, all four units of blood were needed. He is re-evaluated on the fourth postoperative day because of anemia.

He feels well and is ambulating without difficulty. On physical examination, he appears pale. His pulse rate is 82/min, and blood pressure is 120/80 mm Hg. Hemoglobin is 8.0 g/dL, with normal indices. The reticulocyte count is 2.0%.

Which of the following should be done regarding treating this patient's anemia?

(A) Transfusion of two units of packed red blood cells
(B) Evaluation for a bleeding disorder
(C) Treatment with oral iron replacement
(D) Treatment with intravenous iron replacement

## Anemia Question 12

A 77-year-old man was found to have a hemoglobin level of 10.0 g/dL as part of a routine physical examination. He had noted easy fatigability for several months but had no symptoms of gastrointestinal blood loss. A stool specimen was negative for occult blood on three separate occasions.

Three months later, repeat hemoglobin was 8.4 g/dL, leukocyte count was 3400/μL, reticulocyte count was 1.7%, and platelet count was 132,000/μL. An upper and lower gastrointestinal endoscopy showed no abnormalities. Vitamin $B_{12}$ and serum folate levels were normal; serum ferritin level was 680 μg/ml.

On physical examination, he is pale. His temperature is normal. His pulse rate is 64/min and regular, respiratory rate is 18/min, and blood pressure is 150/84 mm Hg. The remainder of the examination is normal.

| | |
|---|---|
| Hematocrit | 25% |
| Mean corpuscular volume | 102 fL |
| Leukocyte count | 3100/μL |
| Reticulocyte count | 1.7% |
| Platelet count | 128,000/μL |

A peripheral blood smear shows dimorphic erythrocytes, many macrocytes, no oval macrocytes, and no hypersegmented polymorphonuclear cells. Bone marrow aspirate is hypercellular with marked erythroid hyperplasia and dyserythropoiesis. Megakaryocytes are normal, and there is moderate myelodysplasia. Prussian blue (iron) stain of the bone marrow aspirate shows increased iron with pathologic and ringed sideroblasts.

Which of the following treatments is most likely to improve the anemia?

(A) Pyridoxine
(B) Erythropoietin
(C) Androgen therapy
(D) Red blood cell transfusions

### Anemia Question 13
A 22-year-old man is evaluated in the intensive care unit because of bleeding immediately after scoliosis surgery. During surgery, 12 units of packed red blood cells and 12 units of fresh frozen plasma were transfused. There is no history of a bleeding disorder or of drug administration that could affect platelet function.

On physical examination, the patient is afebrile. His pulse rate is 100/min, and blood pressure is 110/72 mm Hg. Petechiae are present on his arms, and blood is oozing from the drains.

| | |
|---|---|
| Hemoglobin | 9.0 g/dL |
| Platelet count | 43,000/μL |
| Prothrombin time | 12 s |
| Activated partial thromboplastin time | 32 s |
| Plasma fibrinogen | 400 g/dL |
| D-Dimers | Negative |

Which of the following is the most likely cause of the thrombocytopenia and bleeding?

(A) Dilutional thrombocytopenia
(B) Incompatible blood transfusion
(C) Posttransfusion purpura
(D) Septic transfusion reaction

### Anemia Question 14
A 32-year-old man of Italian descent is evaluated during a routine pre-employment physical examination. He has always been healthy and his examination is normal. Laboratory studies reveal a hematocrit of 35%, mean corpuscular volume of 63 fL, leukocyte count of 6800/μL, reticulocyte count of 40,000/μL (0.7%), and a platelet count of 270,000/μL. His stools are negative for occult blood.

Which of the following is the most direct way to confirm the diagnosis?

(A) Peripheral blood smear
(B) Measurement of hemoglobin $A_2$
(C) Glucose-6-phosphate dehydrogenase screen
(D) Measurement of serum iron binding capacity, and serum ferritin level

### Anemia Question 15
A 74-year-old woman is evaluated as part of a screening program in a geriatrics clinic. She has a hemoglobin level of 13.8 g/dL and a mean corpuscular volume of 90 fL. The peripheral blood smear is normal. Serum iron is 70 μg/dL, and serum vitamin $B_{12}$ is 180 pg/mL, with 200 as the lower boundary of the reference range. Serum folate is normal. Her neurologic and Mini-Mental State examinations are normal.

What is the next best step in the management of this patient?

(A) Daily vitamins containing cobalamin
(B) Bone marrow aspirate
(C) Measure erythrocyte folate concentration
(D) Measure serum homocysteine concentration
(E) Measure serum or urine methylmalonic acid concentration

### Anemia Question 16
A 20-year-old male university student of Cambodian descent presents for his college preadmission physical examination. He has no medical problems. His physical examination reveals a grade 2/6 systolic flow murmur and a spleen that is palpable at the left costal margin.

The hematocrit is 33% and the mean corpuscular volume is 66 fL. The neutrophil count, platelet count, and iron studies are normal. Hemoglobin electrophoresis reveals a hemoglobin A of 97%, hemoglobin $A_2$ of 2.5%, and hemoglobin F of 0.5%. Numerous target cells are seen on peripheral blood smear.

Which of the following is the most likely diagnosis?

(A) Thalassemia minor
(B) Sickle cell anemia
(C) Hereditary spherocytosis
(D) Iron deficiency anemia
(E) Anemia of chronic disease

## Anemia Question 17

A 22-year-old nulliparous college student of Greek descent notes that for the past 2 to 3 months she tires easily and has palpitations when playing tennis. She reports no night sweats or weight loss. Family history is negative for anemia.

Physical examination is unremarkable. A blood count shows a hemoglobin of 9.0 g/dL with a hematocrit of 28% and an erythrocyte count of 3.7 million. The MCV is 70 fl and the red cell distribution width is elevated at 17. The neutrophil, lymphocyte, and platelet counts are normal.

Which one of the following would you recommend?

(A) Hemoglobin electrophoresis for $A_2$ and F
(B) Blood counts on her family members
(C) Serum ferritin concentration
(D) Spleen ultrasonography
(E) $\alpha/\beta$ globin chain synthesis rate ratio

## Anemia Question 18

A 52-year-old man is evaluated in the emergency department because of nausea, fever, and malaise. He describes an antecedent watery diarrheal illness for the past 2 days. Two family members suffered a similar illness, and all affected individuals developed symptoms within 24 hours of eating hamburgers at a local fast-food restaurant.

On physical examination, the patient appears pale and in moderate distress. His temperature is 39.9 °C (103.8 °F), the pulse rate is 78/min and regular, respiration rate is 24/min, and supine blood pressure in the right arm is 90/60 mm Hg with no orthostatic changes. There is an extensive petechial rash over the lower extremities.

| | |
|---|---|
| Hematocrit | 22% |
| Leukocyte count | 16,000/µL |
| Reticulocyte count | 100,000/µL |
| Platelet count | 8000/µL |
| Prothrombin time | 11 sec |
| Activated partial thromboplastin time | 32 sec |
| Blood urea nitrogen | 78 mg/dL |
| Direct antiglobulin (Coombs) test | Negative |
| Urinalysis | 3+ blood with gross hematuria |

Blood smear reveals numerous schistocytes.

Which of the following is the most likely diagnosis?

(A) Evans's syndrome (autoimmune hemolytic anemia and thrombocytopenia)
(B) Hemolytic uremic syndrome
(C) Intravascular hemolysis due to *Clostridium* species
(D) Babesiosis

## Anemia Question 19

A 57-year-old woman (gravida 5, para 5) is admitted to the hospital with a bleeding, peptic duodenal ulcer. Her condition stabilizes after she is given 3 units of packed erythrocytes. She is placed on a regimen of antacids and cimetidine and is discharged after 3 days.

Two days later she returns to the hospital because of weakness and increased malaise. Her hematocrit, which was 37% at discharge, is now 26%. She has dark urine, and liver studies reveal a total bilirubin of 6.1 mg/dL with a direct value of 2.3 mg/dL and a lactate dehydrogenase of 467 U/L. Her renal function is normal. Stools are trace-positive for occult blood, and a gastric lavage is negative for blood. Peripheral blood smear shows numerous microspherocytes.

Which of the following is the most appropriate next management step?

(A) Recheck her type and crossmatch
(B) Osmotic fragility test
(C) Infuse immunoglobulin
(D) Surgery

## Anemia Question 20

A previously healthy 65-year-old male corporate executive is evaluated because of easy fatigability. He is found to have pallor and a hemoglobin level of 8.6 g/dL. A peripheral blood smear (see Figure 9 in the color plates) is shown.

Which of the following is the most likely diagnosis?

(A) Iron deficiency anemia
(B) Thalassemia minor
(C) Hereditary spherocytosis
(D) Sickle cell anemia

## Anemia Question 21

An 18-year-old man undergoing evaluation for military service is found to have the peripheral blood smear (see Figure 10 in the color plates) shown. His history and physical examination and the remainder of his diagnostic studies are normal.

Which of the following is the most likely diagnosis?

(A) Iron deficiency anemia
(B) Thalassemia minor
(C) Hereditary spherocytosis
(D) Sickle cell anemia

**Anemia Question 22**
A 12-year-old boy is evaluated because of pallor and easy fatigability. His hemoglobin level is 9.5 g/dL and his mean corpuscular volume is 93 fL. A peripheral blood smear is shown.

Which of the following is the most likely diagnosis?

(A) Iron deficiency anemia
(B) Thalassemia minor
(C) Hereditary spherocytosis
(D) Sickle cell anemia

**Anemia Question 23**
A 13-year-old girl is hospitalized because of the sudden development of left hemiparesis and aphasia. A peripheral blood smear (see Figure 12 in the color plates) is shown.

Which of the following is the most likely diagnosis?

(A) Iron deficiency anemia
(B) Thalassemia minor
(C) Hereditary spherocytosis
(D) Sickle cell anemia

**Anemia Question 24**
A 60-year-old woman is evaluated because of easy fatigability and pallor. Her hemoglobin level is 7.3 g/dL, leukocyte count is 2800/μL, platelet count is 90,000/μL, and mean corpuscular volume is 115 fL. A peripheral blood smear (see Figure 13 in the color plates) is shown.

Which of the following is the most likely diagnosis?

(A) Cirrhosis
(B) Aplastic anemia
(C) Paroxysmal nocturnal hemoglobinuria
(D) Vitamin $B_{12}$ deficiency

# Cancer

## Cancer Question 1

A 59-year-old woman is seen for her annual examination. She has no signs or symptoms of illness. Her medical and family history are negative. She has two children. Her last menstrual period was 3 years ago. She has occasional hot flashes and vaginal dryness.

On physical examination, there is a round, firm, nontender, and mobile mass approximately 1 cm in diameter in the upper outer quadrant of the patient's left breast. A mammogram is negative, and a subsequent ultrasound identifies no cysts.

Which of the following is the best approach to the management of this patient?

(A) Reexamine the breast during a different part of the menstrual cycle.
(B) Needle aspiration of the mass
(C) Reassurance and yearly examinations and mammograms
(D) Mammogram in 3 months
(E) Biopsy of the mass

## Cancer Question 2

A 37-year-old man is evaluated for a melanoma on his upper back. Except for some freckle-like lesions across his shoulders and upper back, his skin does not seem to be photodamaged or weathered. The patient reports that he does not have many outdoor pursuits, other than coaching the boys' soccer team after school. He says he tans if he spends enough time outdoors.

What history would best explain the development of this patient's melanoma?

(A) A series of five tanning booth sessions
(B) Periodic weekend hiking trips
(C) Multiple childhood sunburns
(D) Radiation from indoor fluorescent lighting
(E) A sunburn last summer

## Cancer Question 3

On screening flexible sigmoidoscopy, a 60-year-old man is found to have a 5-mm polyp in the rectum. Histopathologic examination of biopsy specimens demonstrates a hyperplastic morphology. He has no symptoms, family history of colorectal cancer, or significant medical history and takes no medications. A six-window fecal occult blood test is negative.

What is the most appropriate follow-up for this patient?

(A) Repeat sigmoidoscopy in 1 year
(B) Colonoscopy
(C) Barium enema
(D) Yearly fecal occult blood testing and sigmoidoscopy in 3 to 5 years

## Cancer Question 4

A 72-year-old woman was evaluated because of fatigue and exercise intolerance. She has no other symptoms and no significant medical or family history and takes no medications. She has no abdominal discomfort. She has never had screening for colorectal cancer. Her physical examination is unremarkable. Results of laboratory studies include the following: hematocrit, 28%; mean corpuscular volume, 70 fL; ferritin, 2 ng/mL; transferrin saturation, 11%; and normal electrolyte levels and renal and liver tests. A six-window fecal occult blood test is negative. Urinalysis is normal.

What is the most appropriate next recommendation?

(A) Flexible sigmoidoscopy
(B) Barium enema
(C) Colonoscopy
(D) Esophagogastroduodenoscopy (EGD)
(E) CT of the abdomen

## Cancer Question 5

On a six-window fecal occult blood test on appropriate dietary and medication restrictions, a 63-year-old woman has one positive window. She is otherwise healthy, has no family history of colorectal cancer, and takes no medications. Her physical examination and complete blood count are normal.

Which of the following is the most appropriate approach to this patient?

(A) Colonoscopy
(B) Sigmoidoscopy
(C) Barium enema
(D) Repeat fecal occult blood test
(E) Anoscopy

## Cancer Question 6

A 35-year-old man is evaluated for routine health maintenance. He has no complaints and no significant medical history and takes no medications. His family history is significant for colon cancer in his mother at age 52 years, his brother at age 42 years, and his sister at age 40 years. His physical examination is normal.

What is the most appropriate recommendation for this man?

(A) Yearly fecal occult blood testing and sigmoidoscopy every 3 to 5 years beginning at age 50 years
(B) Colonoscopy every 5 years beginning at age 50 years
(C) Colonoscopy now
(D) Barium enema now

## Cancer Question 7

A 68-year-old man underwent resection of an adenocarcinoma of the transverse colon 6 months ago. There was adequate resection and nodal dissection. Neither invasion of other organs nor lymph node metastases were found. The patient feels fit, with no complaints, and he has no significant medical history. The physical examination and complete blood count are normal.

Which of the following should be performed in one year?

(A) Liver tests
(B) CT scan of the abdomen
(C) Fecal occult blood testing and sigmoidoscopy
(D) Colonoscopy

## Cancer Question 8

A 35-year-old otherwise healthy woman comes to the office interested in screening, prevention, and the "breast cancer gene." Both her maternal and paternal grandmothers had breast cancer, one at age 62 years and the other at age 75 years. No one else in her family has breast or ovarian cancer; however, her paternal grandfather had lung cancer and her mother has had a few colonic polyps removed after routine screening. She has two older sisters, both of whom are alive and healthy. Her physical examination is normal. She has multiple densities in both breasts but no dominant masses and no nipple discharge.

Which of the following should be done for this patient at this time?

(A) *BRCA1* and *BRCA2* screening
(B) Mammograms every 6 months
(C) Tamoxifen therapy
(D) No genetic evaluation, screening, or chemoprevention

## Cancer Question 9

A 68-year-old woman evaluated because of a painless enlargement of a mass above her clavicle. She has had hemoptysis in the past 2 weeks but has no shortness of breath, fever, chills, or weight loss. She has smoked one pack of cigarettes per day for 53 years and continues to smoke.

On physical examination, she has a 3-cm hard, nontender mass in the right supraclavicular fossa. Her oral cavity and pharynx show no lesions, and she has no other adenopathy. Her lungs are clear to auscultation and percussion. She has no breast masses or tenderness and no hepatomegaly or abdominal masses. A chest radiograph shows an increased anterior-posterior diameter and a low diaphragm but no parenchymal masses. A biopsy specimen of the supraclavicular lymph node is positive for squamous cell carcinoma.

Which of the following is the most appropriate management for this patient?

(A) Observation
(B) Mammography, ultrasound, and MRI of the breast
(C) CT scan of the neck and panendoscopy of the upper aerodigestive tract
(D) Sputum cytology, CT scan of the chest, and fiberoptic bronchoscopy

## Cancer Question 10

A 50-year-old man is evaluated because of a past history of cancer. He was successfully treated for disseminated non-seminomatous testicular cancer with three courses of cisplatin, etoposide, and bleomycin at age 30 years. He has never had a recurrence, and a review of systems is unremarkable.

Which one of the following routine periodic surveillance tests would you recommend to this patient?

(A) Audiometry
(B) Bone marrow aspiration
(C) CT scans of the chest and abdomen
(D) Urine cytology and gastric endoscopy
(E) Cancer screening appropriate for his age

## Cancer Question 11

A 66-year-old woman is evaluated because of a cough and shortness of breath. She has never smoked cigarettes. On physical examination, her temperature is 37.2 °C (99.0 °F), pulse rate is 82/min, respiration rate is 18/min, and blood pressure is 120/75 mm Hg. She has no palpable cervical, supraclavicular, axillary, or inguinal adenopathy. Her breast examination is normal. She has no hepatosplenomegaly, and her stool is negative for occult blood. A mammogram and Pap smear one month ago were both normal.

Chest radiograph shows a 3-cm mass in the left lower lobe. CT scan of the chest, including the upper abdomen, shows a 3-cm spiculated mass and 2- to 3-cm subcarinal and paratracheal lymph nodes. The liver and the adrenal gland are normal. She undergoes fiberoptic bronchoscopy and mediastinoscopy. Pathologic evaluation shows lung cancer with mediastinal lymph node involvement.

Which of the following is the most likely diagnosis?

(A) Squamous cell carcinoma
(B) Large cell lung cancer
(C) Adenocarcinoma
(D) Small cell lung cancer

## Cancer Question 12

For which one of the following malignancies is a patient taking tamoxifen at higher risk over the next 10 years than age-matched women who have had breast cancer but have never taken tamoxifen?

(A) Endometrial cancer
(B) Lung cancer
(C) Breast cancer
(D) Acute myeloid leukemia
(E) Chest wall sarcoma

## Cancer Question 13

A 64-year-old man is evaluated because of chest and rib pain, anorexia, and headaches. His weight has decreased from 76 to 71 kg (168 to 157 lb) in the past 2 months. A chest radiograph shows a 2-cm right upper lobe mass and a 6-cm mediastinal mass. An abdominal CT scan shows no evidence of liver or adrenal involvement. Histologic examination of a biopsy from the mass shows small cell lung cancer.

In addition to a bone scan and CT scan of the brain, which of the following is the most appropriate next management step for this patient?

(A) Supportive care
(B) Mediastinoscopy
(C) Radiation therapy
(D) Chemotherapy

## Cancer Question 14

A 59-year-old woman is evaluated because of shortness of breath and a fever that has persisted for the past 8 days. She has a cough that is producing thick green sputum. She smoked 1.5 packs of cigarettes per day for 40 years but quit smoking 3 years ago.

On physical examination, her temperature is 38.9 °C (102 °F), pulse rate 118/min, respiration rate 22/min, and blood pressure 120/70 mm Hg. Examination of the chest reveals dullness to percussion in the left upper lobe and decreased breath sounds. A chest radiograph reveals a left upper lobe infiltrate. The patient is treated with a 10-day course of antibiotics with resolution of her fever, but she returns 1 month later with a temperature of 38.7 °C (101.7 °F), cough, and persistent shortness of breath.

What is the most appropriate management for this patient at this time?

(A) Second course of antibiotics
(B) Reevaluate in one month
(C) Pulmonary function tests
(D) Chest radiograph and sputum cytology

## Cancer Question 15

A 68-year-old man is evaluated because of dyspnea on moderate exertion, cough productive of sputum for 1 month, and hemoptysis for 1 week. He smoked one pack of cigarettes per day for 50 years, but quit 3 years ago. He has no fever, chills, sweats, anorexia, or weight loss. The lungs are clear to auscultation and percussion.

A chest radiograph is normal. A PPD skin test is not reactive. Sputum cytology shows no evidence of malignant cells, and acid-fast bacillus stains of the sputum are negative.

Which one of the following is the appropriate management for this patient?

(A) Observation
(B) Antibiotics
(C) Chest CT scan
(D) Chest CT scan and fiberoptic bronchoscopy

## Cancer Question 16

A 54-year-old man develops a cough and shortness of breath. He has smoked two packs of cigarettes per day for 40 years. Physical examination reveals an increased anterior-posterior diameter, and his breath sounds are distant but clear to auscultation and percussion. Examination of the extremities reveals no clubbing, cyanosis, or edema.

Laboratory studies show the following:

| | |
|---|---|
| Serum sodium | 124 meq/L |
| Serum potassium | 4.2 meq/L |
| Serum urea nitrogen | 12 mg/dL |
| Serum creatinine | 0.7 mg/dL |

A chest radiograph and CT scan of the chest reveal a 3-cm right upper lobe mass with enlarged bilateral mediastinal lymph nodes. Following fiberoptic bronchoscopy with biopsy of endobronchial lesions, the patient is diagnosed with lung cancer.

Which of the following is the most likely histologic diagnosis of this patient's lung cancer?

(A) Squamous cell carcinoma
(B) Adenocarcinoma
(C) Adenosquamous carcinoma
(D) Small cell carcinoma
(E) Large cell carcinoma

## Cancer Question 17

A 46-year-old otherwise healthy premenopausal woman is evaluated because of a breast mass, which is excised and found to be a 2-cm infiltrating ductal carcinoma. The tumor is positive for estrogen and progesterone receptors, and the margins are clear of cancer. On axillary lymph node dissection, 3 of 15 nodes are found to contain metastatic disease. The results of a bone scan, CT scan of the chest and liver, and liver function tests are normal.

Which of the following is the best therapy for this patient?

(A) Radical mastectomy
(B) Adjuvant chemotherapy and breast radiation therapy
(C) Tamoxifen
(D) Adjuvant chemotherapy, breast radiation therapy, and tamoxifen

## Cancer Question 18

A 22-year-old man is evaluated because of a growing painless left testicular mass that is solid on ultrasound. The right testicle is normal and serum tumor markers are normal. A left orchiectomy is performed, revealing nonseminomatous germ cell cancer. CT scans of the chest, abdomen, and pelvis are normal, and the patient is asymptomatic. He undergoes a retroperitoneal lymph node dissection. None of the lymph nodes is involved by tumor.

Which one of the following management strategies is most appropriate after the surgery?

(A) Regular follow-up, reserving therapy for disease recurrence
(B) Needle biopsy of the right testicle
(C) Radiation of the right testicle
(D) Adjuvant combination chemotherapy
(E) Adjuvant combination chemotherapy plus radiation to the right testicle

## Cancer Question 19

In which one of the following anatomic areas does melanoma occur most frequently in Asians and African Americans?

(A) Back and upper extremities
(B) Head and neck
(C) Upper and lower extremities
(D) Palms, soles, and mucous membranes
(E) Back and torso

## Cancer Question 20

A 23-year-old woman is evaluated because of the growth (see Figure 14 in the color plates) shown on her arm.

Which of the following is the most likely diagnosis?

(A) Malignant melanoma
(B) Benign melanocytic nevi
(C) Solar lentigo
(D) Seborrheic keratosis

## Cancer Question 21

A 50-year-old man is evaluated because of the growth (see Figure 15 in the color plates) under his eye.

Which of the following is the most likely diagnosis?

(A) Squamous cell carcinoma
(B) Basal cell carcinoma
(C) Interdermal nevus
(D) Sebaceous hyperplasia
(E) Seborrheic keratosis

## Cancer Question 22

A 58-year-old woman has had a cough and increased shortness of breath for 6 weeks. She also reports a 6-lb (2.7-kg) weight loss. Physical examination is unremarkable. Complete blood count and liver function tests are normal. Blood gases show a $Pao_2$ of 88 mm Hg, $Paco_2$ of 38 mm Hg, and pH of 7.4. Chest radiograph shows a 3-cm right mid-lung mass. CT scan of the chest shows a right middle lobe mass 3.3 cm in diameter. Three mediastinal lymph nodes are seen and measure 1 cm, 1.5 cm, and 1.5 cm in diameter, respectively. Bronchoscopy shows a mass in the right middle lobe bronchus. Biopsy specimen shows squamous cell carcinoma.

What is the most appropriate action?

(A) CT scan of the brain and abdomen
(B) Pulmonary function tests
(C) Ventilation and perfusion lung scan
(D) Mediastinoscopy
(E) Preoperative chemotherapy

# Back Pain

## Back Pain Question 1

A 65-year-old previously healthy man is evaluated because of excruciating back pain of 1 week's duration. It radiates predominantly into his right buttock down to his mid-calf, but in the last day he has also noticed intermittent, lancinating pain in his left buttock and leg.

On physical examination, the patient is afebrile. He is in severe pain and moves from supine to sitting position with great difficulty. Straight-leg raising elicits extreme pain in the right knee at 50 degrees of hip flexion. His right ankle jerk is absent, and his left ankle jerk is present but diminished. Dorsiflexion of his right foot cannot be done, and he has mild weakness in his quadriceps on extension of both knees. Sensation is reduced over the buttocks, upper posterior thighs, and perineum as well as on the dorsal surfaces of the feet. Rectal examination reveals decreased anal sphincter tone.

Which of the following is the most appropriate action in this patient's management?

(A) Neuroimaging of the lumbar spine
(B) Bed rest for 3 to 5 days
(C) Spinal manipulation
(D) Bone scan
(E) Spinal traction for 1 week

## Back Pain Question 2

A 60-year-old previously healthy man is evaluated because of nonradiating pain in his lower thoracic spine that began 10 days ago.

He underwent an elective laparoscopic cholecystectomy 6 weeks ago. He required a Foley catheter, and may have had a urinary tract infection. Since surgery, he has had intermittent anorexia and fatigue along with night sweats, and fever. He denies dysuria, urgency or frequency of urination, pain on ejaculation, or hematospermia.

On physical examination, temperature is 37.9 °C (100.2 °F). The abdominal examination reveals a well-healed cholecystectomy scar without drainage or erythema. A loud abdominal bruit is present in the midline. There is mild point tenderness of the lower thoracic spine. Straight-leg raising is negative. Bilateral femoral artery bruits are present. Rectal examination reveals a mildly enlarged, firm, nontender prostate gland.

Which of the following is the most likely diagnosis in this patient?

(A) Metastatic prostate cancer
(B) Aortic aneurysm
(C) Vertebral osteomyelitis
(D) Ankylosing spondylitis
(E) Chronic bacterial prostatitis

## Back Pain Question 3

A 25-year-old woman is evaluated because of a 3-week history of intermittent, moderately severe, localized low back pain. The patient is a nurse, and the pain began after she helped lift a patient but worsened considerably after driving a car for 2 hours. On physical examination, the patient is in moderate pain and changes positions on the examining table with some difficulty. Straight-leg raising is negative, and there are no neurologic deficits.

In addition to heat, analgesics, and activity as tolerated, which one of the following can be recommended to the patient?

(A) Strict bed rest for 10 days
(B) Spinal traction for 1 week
(C) Spinal manipulation
(D) Radiography of the lumbar spine
(E) MRI of the lower spine

## Back Pain Question 4

A 53-year-old woman is evaluated in the emergency department with a 1-week history of increasing back pain. She has a history of "sciatica" about every 3 to 4 months, which lasts a few days and then resolves. The patient had breast cancer 3 years ago, which was treated with surgery and radiation therapy to her right breast. She otherwise is in good health.

On physical examination, she is uncomfortable when she moves but can rest reasonably comfortably when lying flat on her back with her knees bent. Her temperature is 37.5 °C (99.5 °F), pulse rate is 80/min and regular, and blood pressure is 145/80 mm Hg. Palpation of the spine shows tenderness over the lower thoracic region, with some radiation into the left buttocks. On neurologic examination, she has good strength in her arms and legs. She has mild stocking-glove sensory loss below the knee and an absent left patellar reflex.

Which of the following is most appropriate in this patient's management?

(A) Immediate MRI
(B) Hospital admission for observation
(C) Bone scan
(D) Plain radiograph of the spine
(E) Lumbar epidural anesthetic injection

## Back Pain Question 5

A 66-year-old woman is evaluated because of the sudden onset of severe low back pain. On physical examination, there is tenderness in the upper lumbar spine and spasm of the paraspinous muscles. A plain radiograph shows a compression fracture of L1. The serum calcium level and serum protein electrophoresis are normal. She declines treatment with estrogen and is taking no medications.

What is the next best step in this patient's management?

(A) Vitamin D supplementation
(B) Alendronate
(C) Calcium supplementation
(D) Biweekly physical therapy and weight training

## Back Pain Question 6

A 32-year-old white man has a 12-year-history of low back pain. He is otherwise healthy. Anteroposterior and lateral radiographs of his lumbar spine are shown.

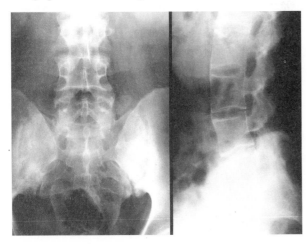

Which of the following is the most likely diagnosis?

(A) Ankylosing spondylitis
(B) Herniated intervertebral disk
(C) Vertebral compression fracture
(D) Vertebral osteomyelitis

## Back Pain Question 7

A 65-year-old man has diffuse metastatic prostate cancer to the thoracic spine, femurs, and ribs has been successfully treated with androgen ablation (goserelin aceteate). Over the last few weeks, however, he has had experienced increased pain in the midthoracic spine and has developed difficulty walking. He denies any sensory changes, incontinence, or changes in bowel habits.

On physical examination, the patient is alert but uncomfortable. He has back pain on palpation at T8, and neurologic examination reveals +3 out of 5 motor strength in the lower extremities. No other neurologic deficit is noted.

Which of the following is the most appropriate management for this patient?

(A) Pain medications and return visit in 2 weeks
(B) High-dose steroids and immediate MRI of the spine
(C) Bone scan
(D) Strontium 89

## Back Pain Question 8

A 78-year-old man is evaluated because of a 3-month history of progressively severe low back pain. The pain is present around the clock but prominent at night, causing him to leave his bed and sleep fitfully in a chair. The pain localizes poorly, with little tendency to radiate. He notes a distinct increase in his long-standing symptom in urinary hesitancy, but no other associated symptoms.

On physical examination, there is saddle anesthesia. The remainder of his examination is normal. All laboratory studies are normal. Radiographs of the lumbosacral spine documents only severe degenerative changes.

Which of the following is the most likely diagnosis?

(A) Centrally herniated nucleus pulposus
(B) Metastatic cancer to the lumbosacral spine
(C) Cauda equina tumor
(D) Bilateral foraminal encroachment by osteophytes
(E) Spinal epidural abscess

## Back Pain Question 9

A 41-year-old woman has had intermittent but disabling low back pain for 10 years. She has normal menstrual cycles and no major medical or surgical problems. Her physical examination was within normal limits, and there was no kyphosis or skeletal deformities. Routine laboratory studies were normal. Radiographs of the spine revealed osteopenia but no compression fractures. A bone mineral density study using dual-energy x-ray absorptiometry (DEXA) yielded lumbar spine and upper femur values 2.9 and 3.0 standard deviations below peak mean bone density for young women (T-score), respectively.

In addition to providing for a calcium intake of 1000 to 1500 mg per day and vitamin D, 800 IU, which of the following should be prescribed for her bones?

(A) Aspirin
(B) Slow-release sodium fluoride
(C) Estrogens
(D) A bisphosphonate
(E) Synthetic salmon calcitonin

## Back Pain Question 10

A 34-year-old woman is evaluated because of back pain that began 2 days ago when she was bending over cleaning her bathtub. She felt something stretch in her back, and she was seized with severe pain, which is now radiating down the back of her right leg. It is made worse by sneezing or coughing. On physical examination, there is loss of lumbar lordosis. Sensation and strength in the legs are intact. The straight leg-raising test is positive on the right.

After prescribing an analgesic for her pain, which one of the following should be done for this patient?

(A) Magnetic resonance imaging of the lumbar spine
(B) Radiographs of the lumbar spine
(C) Bed rest at home
(D) Physical therapy
(E) Continued activity as tolerated

## Back Pain Question 11

A 24-year-old man with a 7-year history of ulcerative colitis is evaluated because of the insidious onset of low back pain over the past 2 months. The pain is deep in the buttocks, dull in character, and difficult to localize. It awakens him from sleep, and he feels better after walking. The pain alternates from side to side, and sometimes radiates down the back of either thigh. There is no family history of back problems. On physical examination, there is no local tenderness, and there is good range of motion in the lumbar region of the spine. Neurologic examination is normal.

Which of the following is the most likely diagnosis?

(A) Rheumatoid arthritis
(B) Ankylosing spondylitis
(C) Herniated nucleus pulposis
(D) Osteomyelitis
(E) Low back strain

## Back Pain Question 12

A 66-year-old man is evaluated because of worsening pain in his low back pain, which he has had for at least 2 years. Recently the pain has begun radiating down the back of his legs when he walks. The pain increases with walking or standing and decreases when he sits, and he has less pain walking uphill than downhill. He has also noticed difficulty starting his urinary stream. Physical examination shows reduced mobility of the spine in the lumbar region. The straight leg-raising test is negative. Pulses in the feet are 2/4, and ankle reflexes are reduced bilaterally (1/4).

Which of the following is the most likely diagnosis?

(A) Herniated nucleus pulposis
(B) Lumbar spinal stenosis
(C) Ankylosing spondylitis
(D) Atherosclerotic narrowing of the iliac and femoral arteries
(E) L5-S1 spondylolisthesis

# Joint Disease

### Joint Disease Question 1
A 29-year-old woman with hemoglobin SC disease is evaluated because of right shoulder pain and stiffness. She has rarely required transfusions and has had no recent injuries. On physical examination, her vital signs are normal. The patient cannot elevate her right arm more than 20 degrees from her side. There is no tenderness or swelling of the arm. Laboratory studies show the following:

| | |
|---|---|
| Hemoglobin | 10.0 g/dL |
| Reticulocyte count | 4% |
| Leukocyte count | 8500/µL; normal differential |
| Erythrocyte sedimentation rate | Normal |

A radiograph of the right shoulder shows diffuse articular sclerosis, patches of decalcification, and narrowing of the joint space.

Which of the following is the most likely cause of the shoulder pain?

(A) Osteomyelitis
(B) Sickle cell crisis
(C) Aseptic necrosis
(D) Bone marrow infarction

### Joint Disease Question 2
An 18-year-old man is evaluated because of a 2-day history of fever, chills, and migratory arthralgias involving the ankles, knees, elbows, and shoulders. On physical examination there are subcutaneous nodules on the volar surface of both forearms, and a grade 2/6 systolic murmur and an $S_3$ heard at the left ventricular apex. There is no objective evidence of joint disease.

Which of the following additional findings establishes a definite diagnosis of acute rheumatic fever in this patient?

(A) Arthritis
(B) Erythema marginatum
(C) Choreoathetosis
(D) An elevated erythrocyte sedimentation rate
(E) A throat culture positive for group A streptococci

### Joint Disease Question 3
A 66-year-old man is evaluted because of a 3-week history of painful fingers, as shown in the image (see Figure 17 in the color plates).

Which of the following is the most likely diagnosis?

(A) Osteoarthritis
(B) Rheumatoid arthritis
(C) Scleroderma
(D) Psoriatic arthritis
(E) Gout

### Joint Disease Question 4
A 56-year-old woman is evaluated because of pain in her fingers, some joints of which become acutely red and tender at times. Her mother had similar problems. Radiographs of her hands and wrists are shown.

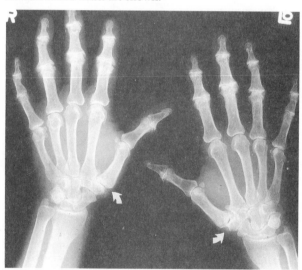

Which of the following is the most likely diagnosis?

(A) Osteoarthritis
(B) Rheumatoid arthritis
(C) Psoriatic arthritis
(D) Gout

## Joint Disease Question 5

A 48-year-old woman is evaluated because of polyarthritis and morning stiffness that lasts for approximately 2 hours. Radiographs of her hands and wrists are shown.

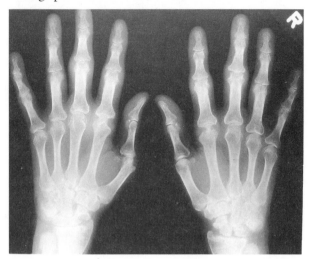

Which of the following is the most likely diagnosis?

(A) Rheumatoid arthritis
(B) Osteoarthritis
(C) Gout
(D) Psoriatic arthritis

## Joint Disease Question 6

A 42-year-old man is evaluated because of pain and swelling in his right knee of 1 week's duration. He relates a 15-year history of intermittent pain and swelling over the middle finger of his left hand as well as recurrent attacks of pain and swelling in his knees. Previous blood tests for the presence of rheumatoid factor have been negative, but antinuclear antibody has been present in low titer (1:160, homogeneous pattern). He has previously been treated for nongonococcal urethritis. On physical examination, there is synovial thickening and mild tenderness over the left third proximal interphalangeal joint. The right knee is tender with effusion, and tenderness is noted at the insertion of the right Achilles tendon. Several scaly plaques are present over the soles of both feet. Aspiration of the knee reveals the presence of an inflammatory effusion (leukocyte count, 20,000/μL—predominantly neutrophils), but Gram's stain and cultures are negative, and no crystals are seen when the fluid is analyzed by polarized microscopy.

Which of the following is the most likely diagnosis?

(A) Gout
(B) Rheumatoid arthritis
(C) Reiter's syndrome
(D) Osteonecrosis
(E) Systemic lupus erythematosus

## Joint Disease Question 7

A 34-year-old white woman from Nantucket, Massachusetts, develops constitutional symptoms and mild swelling in her left inguinal area. Physical examination reveals lymphadenopathy and a few mild skin abrasions over her lower leg. There is no rash, and the patient cannot remember obvious tick exposure. The symptoms resolve spontaneously without therapy.

Approximately 6 weeks later, she develops migratory polyarthralgia, sore throat, left facial palsy, and headache. Physical examination is normal except for a peripheral facial cranial neuropathy. Laboratory analysis is normal, except for mild elevation of serum aminotransferase levels. Rheumatoid factor is positive in a titer of 1:64. Analysis of cerebrospinal fluid reveals mild pleocytosis and a protein level of 80 mg/dL, and a CT scan of the head is normal.

Which of the following tests is most likely to be helpful in establishing the diagnosis?

(A) Rheumatoid factor
(B) Antinuclear antibody
(C) ELISA for antibodies to *Borrelia burgdorferi*
(D) HLA-B27 antigen
(E) Throat culture

## Joint Disease Question 8

A 69-year-old man is evaluated because of arthritis, which he has had for at least 20 years. Physical examination shows markedly decreased range of motion in the small joints of the hands, knees, ankles, elbows, and shoulders. Synovial thickening is present in all palpable joints, and large, subcutaneous nodules are present over the bony prominences of the proximal interphalangeal joints, metacarpophalangeal joints, and elbows. The skin overlying these nodules has broken down in a number of places, and a gritty, chalk-like substance is being extruded.

Which of the following is the most likely diagnosis?

(A) Rheumatoid arthritis
(B) Chronic gouty arthritis
(C) Systemic lupus erythematosus
(D) Inflammatory osteoarthritis
(E) Osteonecrosis

## Joint Disease Question 9

A 24-year-old woman is evaluated because of severe pain and swelling of her right ankle that began last night. She also had fever and chills. Her medical history is positive for a successful cadaveric renal transplantation, which has been maintained with prednisone and cyclosporine therapy.

Physical examination shows an exquisitely tender and swollen right ankle. Arthrocentesis is done, and analysis of the synovial fluid shows 20,000 leukocytes/μL and needle-shaped, negatively birefringent crystals.

What is the most likely factor contributing to the development of intra-articular crystals in this patient?

(A) Hyperoxalemia
(B) Prednisone
(C) Hyperphosphatemia
(D) Cyclosporine
(E) Hypercalcemia

## Joint Disease Question 10

For the past 6 months, a 52-year-old woman has noted recurrent, moderately severe pain and tenderness in the region of the right elbow. The pain occurs mainly with the use of the arm and hand. She has noted no pain or tenderness in other joints. She is otherwise well.

Examination of the right arm shows marked tenderness over the lateral epicondyle. The elbow range of motion is normal, and there is no redness or swelling. Resisted wrist extension exacerbates the elbow pain.

Which one of the following tests is necessary to establish the diagnosis?

(A) Rheumatoid factor
(B) Antinuclear antibodies (ANA)
(C) Erythrocyte sedimentation rate (ESR)
(D) Radiograph of the elbow
(E) No further testing

## Joint Disease Question 11

A 48-year-old white man is evaluated because of 2 years of gradually increasing exercise-related pain in both knees. Within the last 6 months, he has been developing similar complaints in his knuckles. Physical examination reveals bony enlargement of the knees and metacarpophalangeal joints. There is crepitus with motion of both knees and tenderness over the medial joint line of the right knee; there are no effusions. On x-ray, linear radiodensities are noted in the knee menisci bilaterally. Laboratory tests, including serum calcium and uric acid levels, are unremarkable except for a random plasma glucose level of 250 mg/dL, a serum iron level of 250 µg/dL, and a serum iron binding capacity of 400 µg/dL.

Which one of the following additional diseases may be found in this man?

(A) Nephrolithiasis
(B) Liver disease
(C) Uveitis
(D) Interstitial lung disease
(E) Colitis

## Joint Disease Question 12

A 68-year-old woman is evaluated because of pain localized to the medial aspect of the right knee. She has a history of bilateral knee pain on ambulation, which has been well controlled by moderate doses of ibuprofen until the recent episode. Her history is otherwise unremarkable.

Physical examination reveals crepitus and small effusion in both knees. There is a tender area on the medial aspect of the right knee 3 cm below the tibial plateau. Laboratory findings are unremarkable except for a serum uric acid level of 7.9 mg/dL. Radiographic examination of the knees shows a decrease in the joint space of the medial and patellofemoral compartments of both knees, an osteophyte in the medial aspect of the right tibial plateau, and small joint effusions bilaterally.

Which of the following is the most likely diagnosis?

(A) Pseudogout
(B) Anserine bursitis
(C) Gout
(D) Osteochondritis dissecans

## Joint Disease Question 13

A frail, 73-year-old woman is evaluated because of pain in her right shoulder and both knees that has developed over the last 2 years. She states that she cannot use the shoulder well and has severe pain when she moves her right arm and shoulder.

Motion of the right shoulder is decreased to external rotation, and the patient can abduct and elevate her arm to only 80 degrees actively. The shoulder can be further elevated passively 20 more degrees. Small effusions are present in both knees. Radiographs show migration of the humeral head superiorly toward the acromion, calcifications in the soft tissues surrounding the joint capsule of the right shoulder, and destructive erosive changes in the humeral head and both knees. Arthrocentesis of the right shoulder yields a thick, chalky fluid that on polarized microscopy demonstrates abundant, dense, amorphous material, but no birefringent crystals.

Which of the following is the most likely diagnosis?

(A) Frozen shoulder
(B) Basic calcium phosphate disease
(C) Calcium pyrophosphate dihydrate deposition disease
(D) Tophaceous gout
(E) Reflex sympathetic dystrophy

## Joint Disease Question 14

A 55-year-old woman with a 16-year history of rheumatoid arthritis is admitted to the hospital for an elective cholecystectomy. She has numerous joint deformities and recently lost the ability to walk without assistance.

Physical examination shows normal vital signs. Cardiopulmonary examination is normal. The patient has multiple joint deformities with synovitis of the ankles, knees, and wrists. There is limitation of motion of the neck, and marked weakness of her legs.

Which of the following rheumatoid arthritis-associated complications poses the greatest potential surgical risk?

(A) Cervical spine instability
(B) Pulmonary fibrosis
(C) Uveitis
(D) Sjögren's syndrome

## Joint Disease Question 15
A 68-year-old woman is evaluated because of recent swelling near the posterior aspect of the mandible, dryness of both eyes, and pain on motion of the right elbow, both knees, and left ankle. Her history is unremarkable. Physical examination reveals bilateral parotid swelling, diffuse lymphadenopathy, and trace joint effusion in both knees. Schirmer's test shows 8 mm, right eye; 5 mm, left eye (normal, greater than 15 mm/5 min).

Which of the following is the most likely diagnosis?

(A) Systemic lupus erythematosus
(B) Non-Hodgkin's lymphoma
(C) Sarcoidosis
(D) Sjögren's syndrome
(E) Hodgkin's disease

## Joint Disease Question 16
A 31-year-old man is evaluated because of exquisitely painful, recurring episodes of swelling in his left great toe and both ankles. He states that he has one acute episode per month. Between the episodes, he has no symptoms at all. He is asymptomatic now.

The patient's blood pressure is 120/80 mm Hg, pulse rate is 80/min, and temperature is 37 °C (98.6 °F). The physical examination is normal, including the left first metatarsophalangeal joint and ankles. Laboratory evaluation shows a serum uric acid level of 10.5 mg/dL, serum creatinine level of 0.8 mg/dL, and blood urea nitrogen level of 23 mg/dL. Blood counts, hepatic enzymes, and radiographs of the affected joints are normal.

What of the following is the best course of action?

(A) Allopurinol
(B) Colchicine
(C) Intra-articular corticosteroids
(D) A 24-hour urine for uric acid excretion
(E) Observation

## Joint Disease Question 17
A 28-year-old woman is evaluated because of new-onset right knee pain. Three days ago, she noted the onset of pain over the back of the left wrist, which was worse with wrist extension. This resolved spontaneously after 1 day. Yesterday afternoon, she began to feel pain in the right knee. The pain is worse with bending the knee, and it is now difficult

for her to walk. She denies fever or chills. She is sexually active with one partner and is currently having her menstrual period.

On physical examination, she has a temperature of 38.5 °C (101.3 °F), pulse rate of 90/min, respiration rate of 15/min, and blood pressure of 130/70 mm Hg. Range of motion of the right knee is limited because of pain, and there is a small effusion. Examination of the skin reveals two small (2-mm) pustules on the right palm. An attempted arthrocentesis is unsuccessful.

Which of the following is the most appropriate therapy?

(A) Ceftriaxone
(B) High-dose aspirin
(C) Sulfasalazine
(D) Prednisone
(E) Gluten-free diet

## Joint Disease Question 18
A 73-year-old woman is evaluated because of a 6-week history of fever, malaise, hip and shoulder girdle pain, stiffness, and weight loss of 8 kg (17 lb). Additionally, she notes the onset 2 weeks earlier of pain and swelling in her wrists, ankles, and knees. One week before her presentation, she noted the onset of severe, right-sided jaw pain, which occurs predictably whenever she eats.

Physical examination shows a temperature of 38 °C (100.4 °F), pulse rate of 104/min, and blood pressure of 140/80 mm Hg. There is moderate synovitis of her wrists and ankles. The remainder of the examination is unremarkable.

Laboratory studies show the following:

| | |
|---|---|
| Hematocrit | 34% |
| Leukocyte count | 11,400/µL |
| Erythrocyte sedimentation rate | 110 mm/h |

Which of the following is the most likely diagnosis?

(A) Rheumatoid arthritis
(B) Polyarteritis nodosa
(C) Gout
(D) Systemic lupus erythematosus
(E) Giant cell arteritis

## Joint Disease Question 19
A 47-year-old woman with steroid-dependent asthma is evaluated because of a 5-day history of pain in her right knee. Examination shows synovial swelling in the knee with overlying warmth and evidence of an effusion. On arthrocentesis, the synovial fluid leukocyte count is 42,000/µL, with a predominance of neutrophils. Gram stain of synovial fluid shows clumps of gram-positive cocci. Treatment with nafcillin sodium intravenously, is begun. Subsequent synovial fluid culture results are positive for methicillin-sensitive *Staphylococcus aureus*.

Following 5 days of treatment with nafcillin sodium and daily drainage with a 16-gauge needle, the joint remains warm and swollen, and the synovial fluid leukocyte count is 34,000/µL.

What is the most appropriate way to manage this patient?

(A) Discontinue nafcillin, begin vancomycin
(B) Discontinue nafcillin, begin methicillin and gentamicin
(C) Arthroscopic debridement and drainage of the knee joint
(D) Increase nafcillin
(E) Continue current therapy

## Joint Disease Question 20

A 73-year-old man is evaluated because he has not felt well for some time. He does not smoke cigarettes. His major symptom is profound morning stiffness, especially in the shoulders and hips. He denies any headaches, jaw claudication or visual complaints. The joint examination shows mild crepitus of the knees, but no frank synovitis. The remainder of the examination is normal. Laboratory studies show a hematocrit level of 27%, an erythrocyte sedimentation rate of 120 mm/h, and a negative rheumatoid factor.

Which of the following is the next best management option for this patient?

(A) Temporal artery biopsy
(B) Prednisone
(C) Chest radiography
(D) Ibuprofen
(E) Celecoxib

## Joint Disease Question 21

An obese 56-year-old man was evaluated because of severe pain in his left great toe. A diagnosis of gout was made. Since that time he has had four or five more episodes in the last 3 years, and each one has been more painful than the last. The patient is now asymptomatic.

His history is remarkable for mild hypertension, which has been well controlled with atenolol, 50 mg/d, for the about past 2 years. Tests show an elevated uric acid level (9.9 mg/dL) and mild renal dysfunction (serum creatinine level is 1.9 mg/dL; blood urea nitrogen is 25 mg/dL). A 24-hour urine collection contained 1200 mg of uric acid.

Which of the following is the most appropriate treatment for this patient?

(A) Nonsteroidal anti-inflammatory drugs
(B) Allopurinol
(C) Probenecid
(D) Colchicine
(E) Prednisone

## Joint Disease Question 22

A 33-year-old woman is evaluated because of pain in her right ankle. She was working in her garden when she stepped on a rock and twisted her ankle.

The ankle is swollen, especially above the lateral malleolus, but there is no ecchymosis. Because of severe pain, the ankle cannot be moved to assess range of motion. There is tenderness above the lateral malleolus, and the ankle pain is made remarkably worse by trying to invert the foot. Radiograms show no fracture.

Which of the following is the most appropriate management option?

(A) Arthrography
(B) Elevation, ice, and bracing
(C) Inject with glucocorticoids
(D) Casting and crutches

## Joint Disease Question 23

An 18-year-old woman is evaluated because of a 10-day history of joint pain. She has had fever followed by pain and swelling in the knuckles of both hands for 3 days. Her left wrist subsequently became swollen and painful, followed by her left knee. She has a sore throat and two small skin lesions. She is currently menstruating.

Her temperature is 38.6 °C (101.5 °F), pulse rate is 100/min, and blood pressure is 110/70 mm Hg. The posterior oropharynx is slightly red without exudate. There is a red papular skin lesion 0.5 cm in diameter on the left forearm and a small pustule on the left upper chest. There is a large right knee effusion; the knee is red, warm, and tender to palpation and painful on movement. The remainder of the examination, including pelvic, was normal.

Arthrocentesis of the right knee obtained 35 mL of cloudy yellow fluid. No organisms are seen on Gram's stain, synovial fluid leukocyte count is 15,000/µL with 90% polymorphonuclear cells; glucose level is 48 mg/dL (serum glucose is 125 mg/dL); protein is 45 g/dL.

Which of the following is the most likely diagnosis?

(A) HIV infection
(B) Acute rheumatic fever
(C) Hepatitis B virus infection
(D) Disseminated gonococcal infection
(E) Lyme arthritis

## Joint Disease Question 24

A 69-year-old woman with a 5-year history of intermittent left knee pain owing to osteoarthritis is evaluated because of increased knee pain and swelling. She says that she had been walking and climbing stairs more than usual. She developed watery diarrhea around the same time as the knee pain, but there were no chills or fever. She has atrial fibrillation and takes warfarin.

Physical examination shows a temperature of 38 °C (100 °F). There is a large effusion in the left knee, with increased warmth but no redness. There is moderate tenderness and pain on motion. The other joints are unchanged. Left knee radiograph reveals changes of osteoarthritis and an effusion.

Which one of the following should be done next?

(A)  Treat with ciprofloxacin

(B)  Treat with celecoxib

(C)  Perform MRI of left knee

(D)  Perform arthrocentesis

(E)  Treat with intravenous ceftriaxone

## Joint Disease Question 25

A 77-year-old woman is evaluated because of soreness and stiffness in her shoulders, hips, and knees. She has morning stiffness lasting several hours and fatigue lasting all day. Her thumbs and index fingers become numb after holding heavy objects for a few minutes. She also wakes at night with numbness and tingling in these digits. Physical examination shows a pulse rate of 54/min and blood pressure of 140/75 mm Hg. The patient has stiffness and diffuse tenderness of the shoulder girdle, but she has a good range of motion. There is loss of sensation to light touch over both thumbs, but no motor deficit in either hand. There are bilateral small knee effusions with patellofemoral crepitus. Arthrocentesis of the knee produces only 0.5 mL of gelatinous synovial fluid. The leukocyte count is 550/μL (mostly monocytes). The creatine kinase level is 260 U/L.

Which of the following is the most likely cause of her symptoms?

(A)  Polymyalgia rheumatica

(B)  Polymyositis

(C)  Hypothyroidism

(D)  Gout

(E)  Pseudgout

## Joint Disease Question 26

A 70-year-old woman with well-controlled hypertension, a previous episode of diverticulitis, and moderately symptomatic osteoarthritis of the left knee is evaluated for her annual physical examination. Her knee has moderate crepitus and a small effusion but normal alignment, stability, and range of motion. She asks advice about physical activity and exercise.

Which of the following recommendations is best?

(A)  Perform only non weight bearing exercise

(B)  Avoid weight lifting

(C)  Regular walking

(D)  Avoid stair climbing

# Fluid, Electrolyte, and Acid-Base Disorders

**Fluid, Electrolyte, and Acid-Base Disorders Question 1**

A 75-year-old woman is taken to the emergency department after ingesting 50 tablets of enteric-coated aspirin. She has chronic osteoarthritis and type 2 diabetes mellitus. On physical examination, her temperature is 37.8 °C (100 °F), pulse rate is 135/min, respiration rate is 28/min, and blood pressure is 105/65 mm Hg. Blood tests reveal serum sodium 147 meq/L; potassium 2.9 meq/L; chloride 105 meq/L; $CO_2$ 18 meq/L; and glucose 170 mg/dL.

Which of the following best describes her acid-base status?

(A) Metabolic acidosis with respiratory alkalosis
(B) Metabolic acidosis with respiratory acidosis
(C) Metabolic alkalosis with respiratory alkalosis
(D) Metabolic alkalosis with respiratory acidosis

**Fluid, Electrolyte, and Acid-Base Disorders Question 2**

A 28-year-old woman is evaluated because of right flank pain and hematuria. Her blood pressure is 180/98 mm Hg. After being given analgesia and treatment with fluids, she passes a stone, which is shown on subsequent analysis to consist primarily of calcium oxalate.

| | |
|---|---|
| Serum calcium | 11.9 mg/dL |
| Serum phosphorus | 4.1 mg/dL |
| Serum alkaline phosphatase | 92 U/L |
| Serum parathyroid hormone | < 5 pg/mL (normal, 10 to 65 pg/mL) |

Which of the following is the most likely diagnosis?

(A) Idiopathic hypercalciuria
(B) Hyperparathyroidism
(C) Sarcoidosis
(D) Malignancy-associated hypercalcemia

**Fluid, Electrolyte, and Acid-Base Disorders Question 3**

A 55-year-old woman is evaluated because of hypercalcemia. Three years ago, she had a left mastectomy for breast carcinoma, after which she underwent treatment with radiation and adjuvant chemotherapy because 2 of 12 lymph nodes were found to be positive for carcinoma. She has been clinically well since then, but on a routine postoperative check-up 3 months ago, she was found to have a serum calcium level of 10.7 mg/dL. On repeat testing, the serum calcium level is 11.1 mg/dL.

Which of the following is the best first diagnostic step to identify the cause of this patient's hypercalcemia?

(A) Serum parathyroid hormone level
(B) Serum 1,25-dihydroxyvitamin D level
(C) Serum 25-hydroxyvitamin D level
(D) Bone scan

**Fluid, Electrolyte, and Acid-Base Disorders Question 4**

A 76-year-old man is admitted to the hospital with a large pulmonary mass, hilar lymphadenopathy, dehydration, and obtundation. In the emergency department, the following laboratory test results are obtained:

| | |
|---|---|
| Serum calcium | 16.8 mg/dL |
| Serum phosphorus | 3.1 mg/dL |
| Serum creatinine | 2.1 mg/dL |

The most appropriate first-line therapy for this patient is:

(A) Pamidronate, intravenously
(B) Alendronate, orally
(C) Normal saline solution and furosemide
(D) Normal saline solution
(E) Calcitonin, subcutaneously

**Fluid, Electrolyte, and Acid-Base Disorders Question 5**

In a 66-year-old man with a history of low back pain, marked osteopenia is noted on radiographs of the spine. Results of laboratory tests are as follows:

| | |
|---|---|
| Serum calcium | 7.6 mg/dL |
| Serum phosphorus | 1.8 mg/dL |
| Serum albumin | 3.4 g/dL |
| Serum alkaline phosphatase | 240 U/L |

Which of the following is the most likely diagnosis?

(A) Hypogonadism
(B) Osteoporosis
(C) Idiopathic hypoparathyroidism
(D) Vitamin D deficient osteomalacia
(E) Alcoholic liver disease

**Fluid, Electrolyte, and Acid-Base Disorders Question 6**
An 18-year-old man sustains multiple severe injuries in a motorcycle accident and is hospitalized in the surgical intensive care unit. His serum sodium is measured at 152 meq/L. He was in excellent health before the accident and he takes no medications. His urine output is 5 L over 8 h. His medications include intravenous antibiotics and dexamethasone for brain edema; he is being fed by nasogastric tube.

Which one of the following should be measured to evaluate the patient's hypernatremia?

(A) Hemoglobin $A_{1c}$, and plasma glucose
(B) Plasma glucose, serum calcium, and urine and serum osmolality
(C) Hemoglobin $A_{1c}$, serum phosphate, and urine and serum osmolality
(D) Serum cortisol and serum thyroxine

**Fluid, Electrolyte, and Acid-Base Disorders Question 7**
A 44-year-old man has a history of fatigue and poor concentration. As part of a screening chemistry profile, he is found to have a serum calcium level of 10.9 mg/dL and a serum phosphorus level of 2.8 mg/dL. A follow-up parathyroid hormone (PTH) determination is elevated at 75 pg/mL (normal, 10 to 65 pg/mL), and renal function is normal.

Which of the following is the best management option?

(A) Parathyroidectomy
(B) Ultrasonography to screen for kidney stones, and parathyroidectomy if positive
(C) Bone densitometry, and parathyroidectomy if abnormal
(D) Annual measurement of serum calcium, and parathyroidectomy if the calcium level increases
(E) Alendronate

**Fluid, Electrolyte, and Acid-Base Disorders Question 8**
A 53-year-old man with a long history of chronic alcohol abuse comes to the emergency department because of a 3-week history of increasing weakness, anorexia, and a productive cough. On physical examination, the patient is thin and is obviously dyspneic. His pulse rate is 80/min and regular. Blood pressure is 130/70 mm Hg supine, falling to 120/65 mm Hg when he stands. Crackles are heard over the right hemithorax.

Initial laboratory studies revealed normal renal function and serum electrolytes. The patient is hospitalized, and intravenous normal saline is begun. CT of the chest shows a lung mass. CT of the abdomen and pelvis shows an enlarged liver with metastatic lesions, and bilateral adrenal masses. The kidneys appear normal.

Laboratory studies on hospital day 4 show the following:

| | |
|---|---|
| Blood urea nitrogen | 8 mg/dL |
| Serum creatinine | 1.0 mg/dL |
| Serum sodium | 123 meq/L |
| Serum potassium | 3.4 meq/L |
| Serum chloride | 91 meq/L |
| Serum bicarbonate | 20 meq/L |
| Urinary sodium | 110 meq/L |

Which of the following is the most likely cause of the decreasing serum sodium concentration in this patient?

(A) Extracellular fluid volume depletion
(B) Addison's disease
(C) Syndrome of inappropriate antidiuretic hormone (SIADH) secretion
(D) Cirrhosis
(E) Congestive heart failure

**Fluid, Electrolyte, and Acid-Base Disorders Question 9**
A 50-year-old woman with a long history of type 1 diabetes mellitus develops ketoacidosis following an upper respiratory tract infection and fever.

Laboratory studies show the following:

| | |
|---|---|
| Plasma glucose | 1200 mg/dL |
| Serum sodium | 124 meq/L |
| Serum potassium | 4.1 meq/L |
| Serum chloride | 90 meq/L |
| Serum bicarbonate | 10 meq/L |

Along with insulin, isotonic saline is infused to restore extracellular fluid volume, and potassium chloride is given to correct the hypokalemia that later developed. No free water or additional solute was administered.

This patient's serum sodium concentration is most likely to be which of the following after her plasma glucose is restored to 120 mg/dL?

(A) < 120 meq/L
(B) About 124 meq/L
(C) 135 to 145 meq/L
(D) > 149 meq/L

**Fluid, Electrolyte, and Acid-Base Disorders Question 10**
A 35-year-old man with chronic renal failure undergoes hemodialysis three times each week. His compliance has been poor, and he has missed his last dialysis treatment. He now comes to the emergency department because of weakness and nausea.

Laboratory studies show the following:

| | |
|---|---|
| Serum sodium | 128 meq/L |
| Serum potassium | 7.2 meq/L |
| Serum chloride | 95 meq/L |
| Serum bicarbonate | 15 meq/L |

An electrocardiogram shows first-degree heart block, peaked T waves, and wide QRS complexes. While awaiting dialysis, he receives infusions of calcium gluconate, sodium bicarbonate, glucose, and insulin. He also receives oral sodium polystyrene sulfonate (Kayexalate).

Which of these medications is least likely to reduce his serum potassium concentration?

(A) Sodium bicarbonate
(B) Glucose and insulin
(C) Calcium gluconate — *stabilize cardiac membrane*
(D) Sodium polystyrene sulfonate (Kayexalate) — *removes K+ from GI*

**Fluid, Electrolyte, and Acid-Base Disorders Question 11**
A 24-year-old man is taken to the emergency department after being found unresponsive on the floor of his shower. He has a longstanding history of chronic schizophrenia and has required two previous hospitalizations for hyponatremia related to psychogenic water ingestion.

On physical examination, he is still unresponsive. He has bitten his tongue and may be postictal. His pulse rate is 100/min and regular, and blood pressure is 130/80 mm Hg. Physical examination is otherwise unremarkable.

Laboratory studies show the following:

| | |
|---|---|
| Blood urea nitrogen | 12 mg/dL |
| Serum creatinine | 0.8 mg/dL |
| Serum sodium | 108 meq/L |
| Serum potassium | 3.5 meq/L |
| Serum chloride | 80 meq/L |
| Serum bicarbonate | 16 meq/L |

Which of the following is most appropriate for this patient?

(A) Hypertonic (3%) saline
(B) Parenteral furosemide and strict water restriction
(C) Normal saline
(D) Observation and supportive care

**Fluid, Electrolyte, and Acid-Base Disorders Question 12**
A 28-year-old man is taken to the emergency department because of a 4-day history of severe watery diarrhea, vomiting, and poor oral fluid intake. On physical examination, his temperature is 38.0 °C (100.4 °F). His pulse rate is 90/min seated and 124/min standing, and his blood pressure is 120/75 mm Hg seated and 80/50 mm Hg standing. A stool specimen is 1+ positive for occult blood. Examination

is otherwise normal. His blood urea nitrogen is 64 mg/dL and serum creatinine is 1.4. mg/dL.

The elevated blood urea nitrogen:serum creatinine ratio is most likely due to which of the following mechanisms?

(A) Extracellular volume depletion
(B) Increased urea production as a result of gastrointestinal bleeding
(C) Shift of urea from the intracellular space to the extracellular space
(D) Fever

**Fluid, Electrolyte, and Acid-Base Disorders Question 13**
A 48-year-old businessman is diagnosed with an acute myocardial infarction. He has a 5-year history of hypertension and has been treated with hydrochlorothiazide with an excellent response. The patient drinks about two alcoholic beverages daily.

On physical examination, his pulse rate is 80/min and regular, and his blood pressure is 126/80 mm Hg without orthostatic changes. There is no neck vein distention or edema. Cardiac and abdominal examinations are normal.

Laboratory studies show the following:

| | |
|---|---|
| Blood urea nitrogen | 12 mg/dL |
| Serum creatinine | 1.0 mg/dL |
| Serum sodium | 137 meq/L |
| Serum potassium | 3.1 meq/L |
| Serum chloride | 99 meq/L |
| Serum bicarbonate | 28 meq/L |
| Serum calcium | 7.8 mg/dL |
| Serum magnesium | 0.7 mg/dL |

Which of the following is the most appropriate first step in correcting the electrolyte disorder in this patient?

(A) Discontinue hydrochlorothiazide
(B) Administer magnesium sulfate intravenously
(C) Administer calcium gluconate intravenously
(D) Administer volume repletion

**Fluid, Electrolyte, and Acid-Base Disorders Question 14**
A patient is diagnosed with extensive-stage small cell lung cancer with chest, bone, and bone marrow involvement. Serum chemistry examination shows a serum sodium concentration of 122 meq/L. The patient is placed on a fluid restriction of 1000 mL/d for 1 week. The serum sodium concentration increases to 129 meq/L. The patient is then treated with two cycles of etoposide and cisplatin over 6 weeks. A repeat chest radiograph shows the mediastinal adenopathy has largely resolved and the right upper lobe mass has decreased to less than 1 cm in diameter.

Which of the following serum sodium concentrations is most likely in this patient at this time?

(A) 112 meq/L
(B) 118 meq/L
(C) 129 meq/L
(D) 137 meq/L
(E) 148 meq/L

## Fluid, Electrolyte, and Acid-Base Disorders Question 15

A 45-year-old woman with breast cancer metastatic to bone presents with drowsiness, confusion, constipation, polyuria, and increased pain. Two weeks earlier, she had been started on tamoxifen therapy. Physical examination reveals a lethargic middle-aged woman oriented to name only. Blood pressure is 90/60 mm Hg supine and 70/40 mm Hg sitting. Skin and mucous membranes are dry. She had percussion tenderness over the midthoracic spine. Neurologic examination shows no focal findings. Laboratory evaluation reveals a serum calcium of 16.7 mg/dL, blood urea nitrogen of 35 mg/dL, creatinine of 2.2 mg/dL, and phosphate of 4.2 mg/dL.

In addition to intravenous fluids, which one of the following provides optimal management for this patient?

(A) Furosemide and mithramycin
(B) A bisphosphonate
(C) Calcitonin
(D) Oral phosphates
(E) Ibuprofen

## Fluid, Electrolyte, and Acid-Base Disorders Question 16

Acute myocardial infarction is diagnosed in a 62-year-old man with severe chest pain and characteristic electrocardiographic changes. Shortly after admission to the coronary care unit, dyspnea, cyanosis, wheezing, and diffuse rales throughout both lung fields develop. On physical examination, the patient is barely responsive. His pulse is regular at 120/min, and his blood pressure is 90/60 mm Hg. Arterial blood gas values (on room air) are pH, 7.10; $PaCO_2$, 63 mm Hg; and $PaO_2$, 41 mm Hg; the calculated serum bicarbonate level is 20.5 meq/L.

Which of the following best describes his acid-base status?

(A) Respiratory acidosis with no metabolic compensation
(B) Respiratory acidosis with metabolic compensation
(C) Combined respiratory acidosis and metabolic alkalosis
(D) Combined respiratory acidosis and metabolic acidosis
(E) Metabolic acidosis with partial respiratory compensation

## Fluid, Electrolyte, and Acid-Base Disorders Question 17

A 55-year-old man is being evaluated for coronary artery bypass graft surgery. He smoked 2 packs of cigarettes per day for approximately 35 years and stopped 3 months before the evaluation.

The patient is 193 cm (64 in) tall and weighs 128 kg (285 lb), for a body mass index of 43. The cardiac examination shows an $S_4$, but the remainder of the examination is normal. Spirometry gives the following results:

| | |
|---|---|
| Forced vital capacity (FVC) | 2.75 L (83% of predicted) |
| Forced expiratory volume in 1 sec ($FEV_1$) | 1.60 L (59% of predicted) |
| Ratio of $FEV_1$ to FVC | 0.58 (71% of predicted) |
| Forced expiratory flow, midexpiratory | 1.10 L/sec (38% of predicted) phase ($FEF_{25\%-75\%}$) |

$FEV_1$ improves only 4% after administration of a bronchodilator. Arterial blood gas measurements show: $PaO_2$, 66 mm Hg; $PaCO_2$, 52 mm Hg; and pH, 7.46.

Which of the following diagnoses is the most likely primary cause of hypercapnia in this patient?

(A) Chronic obstructive pulmonary disease
(B) Obesity hypoventilation syndrome
(C) Compensation for metabolic alkalosis
(D) Diaphragmatic muscle weakness
(E) Congestive heart failure

A6 =

# Dysuria

## Dysuria Question 1
A 29-year-old woman is evaluated because of dysuria and urinary frequency. She is 35 weeks into an uncomplicated pregnancy. She has had no recent urinary tract infections. She denies flank pain, fever, chills, nausea, or increased contractions. Urine dipstick shows positive leukocyte esterase.

Which one of the following therapies is indicated for this patient?

(A) Ciprofloxacin
(B) Trimethoprim-sulfamethoxazole
(C) Amoxicillin
(D) Doxycycline

## Dysuria Question 2
A 50-year-old man is treated in the emergency department for fever, dysuria, and urinary frequency with trimethoprim-sulfamethoxazole, 160/800 mg twice daily for 10 days. He has relief of his symptoms, but he comes to the office 6 weeks later complaining of intermittent dysuria and painful ejaculation. The prostate gland is mildly enlarged but nontender.

Which of the following oral therapies is the most appropriate treatment at this time?

(A) Trimethoprim-sulfamethoxazole
(B) Doxycycline
(C) Ampicillin
(D) Ciprofloxacin

## Dysuria Question 3
An 80-year-old woman is hospitalized with dysuria, pyuria, mild confusion, fever, and an elevated peripheral blood leukocyte count. Therapy with trimethoprim-sulfamethoxazole is started for a presumed urinary tract infection. The patient's condition is much improved 3 days later, with disappearance of her dysuria and fever and normalization of her leukocyte count. The urine culture and sensitivity results show *Escherichia coli* not sensitive to trimethoprim-sulfamethoxazole, but sensitive to gentamicin and ampicillin.

Which of the following is the most appropriate management for this patient?

(A) Switch to gentamicin
(B) Switch to ampicillin
(C) Make no changes
(D) Switch to ampicillin plus gentamicin
(E) Increase the dosage of trimethoprim-sulfamethoxazole

## Dysuria Question 4
A 72-year-old woman with probable Alzheimer's disease is admitted to the medical service from a long-term care facility for evaluation of a persistent cough. She has a long history of cigarette smoking, and a chest radiograph shows a right hilar mass; bronchoscopy is scheduled for tomorrow morning. She has had an indwelling urinary catheter for 5 years.

On physical examination, her temperature is 37 °C (98.6 °F), pulse rate is 72/min and regular, respiration rate is 14/min, and blood pressure is 140/80 mm Hg. The leukocyte count is 13,800/µL, with 72% polymorphonuclear cells and no band forms. Urinalysis shows 50 leukocytes per high-power field, and Gram's stain of an unspun specimen shows gram-negative rods.

Which one of the following is appropriate management of this patient's bacteruria?

(A) Oral trimethoprim-sulfamethoxazole
(B) Oral ciprofloxacin
(C) No antibiotics; continue clinical observation
(D) An intravenous third-generation cephalosporin
(E) Intravenous trimethoprim-sulfamethoxazole

## Dysuria Question 5
A 16-year-old female adolescent is evaluated because of 2 days of urinary frequency and dysuria. There is no prior history of similar symptoms. She has been well otherwise and is not sexually active. Urinalysis shows 10 to 15 leukocytes and 20 to 30 erythrocytes per high-power field.

Which of the following is the most appropriate management for this patient?

(A) A single dose of a fluoroquinolone
(B) A 3-day course of nitrofurantoin
(C) A 3-day course of trimethoprim-sulfamethoxazole
(D) A 7-day course of trimethoprim-sulfamethoxazole
(E) A 7-day course of nitrofurantoin

## Dysuria Question 6
A 22-year-old male college student is evaluated because of new onset of dysuria. He is sexually active. On physical examination, the patient is afebrile. Examination is normal except for a slight urethral discharge. Urinalysis shows 5 to 10 leukocytes and 0 erythrocytes per high-power field. Gram stain of the urethral discharge reveals polymorphonuclear neutrophils and intracellular, gram-negative diplococci. Results of a serologic test for HIV are pending.

Which of the following is the best management for this patient?

(A) A 3-day course of trimethoprim-sulfamethoxazole

(B) Intramuscular ceftriaxone

(C) Intramuscular ceftriaxone and oral azithromycin

(D) Oral ofloxacin

## Dysuria Question 7

A 29-year-old woman with type 1 diabetes mellitus is evaluated because of a 10-day history of urinary frequency, mild dysuria and fever. She has no history of chills, hematuria, renal stones, or flank pain. Physical examination is normal.

Blood count, serum electrolytes including calcium, and renal function tests are normal. Urinalysis shows: pH 6.5; 2+ heme, trace protein, trace glucose; 5-10 erythrocytes, 40-50 leukocytes/hpf; many bacteria; leukocyte-esterase positive. The urine culture grows > 100,000 colonies of *Proteus mirabilis.*

A plain radiograph of the abdomen and pelvis shows an irregular calcified object measuring $3 \times 5$ cm overlying the right renal shadow. An intravenous pyelogram shows a branched, calcified calculus occupying the upper half of the right renal collecting system with loss of renal parenchymal thickness of the right kidney. The left kidney is normal.

Which of the following stone diseases does this patient most likely have?

(A) Calcium oxalate stone

(B) Calcium phosphate and oxalate stones

(C) Uric acid stone

(D) Triple phosphate (struvite) stone

## Dysuria Question 8

A 24-year-old woman is evaluated because of a 3-day history of dysuria, urgency, and frequency. Yesterday she felt feverish, and this morning she developed nausea, vomiting, chills, and pain in the back.

Physical examination reveals an ill-appearing, clammy white woman with a temperature of 39 °C (102.2 °F), pulse rate of 110/min, and blood pressure of 105/80 mm Hg. She has diffuse left lower quadrant pain and pain on percussion in the left flank. An initial urinalysis shows 50 leukocytes and 30 erythrocytes per high-power field.

A gram stain of the urine will most likely reveal which of the following?

(A) 10 WBC/high power field, 20 epithelial cells/high power field, 20 red blood cells/high power field, gram-positive cocci.

(B) 10 WBC/high power field, 10 red blood cells/high power field, gram-negative bacilli

(C) 10 WBC/high power field, 20 epithelial cells/high power field, 20 red blood cells/high power field, budding yeasts

(D) 10 WBC/high power field, red blood cell casts, gram-negative cocci

(E) 10 WBC/high power field, 20 red blood cells/high power field, gram-positive bacilli

# Acute Renal Failure

## Acute Renal Failure Question 1

A 55-year-old woman was hospitalized because of fever and fatigue. Her medical history revealed the presence of mitral valve prolapse. Blood cultures after admission grew viridans streptococci, and a diagnosis of bacterial endocarditis was made. Intravenous gentamicin and ampicillin were begun. Serum creatinine on admission was 0.6 mg/dL. On day 8, the patient was discharged and placed on home intravenous therapy. Her serum creatinine on discharge was 0.7 mg/dL. On day 16 of therapy, her serum creatinine was 2.2 mg/dL. She is readmitted to the hospital.

On physical examination on admission, temperature is 36.8 °C (98.2 °F). Her pulse rate is 87/min, respiratory rate is 12/min, and blood pressure is 167/98 mm Hg without orthostatic changes. There is a soft systolic murmur at the apex, but no gallop is heard. The rest of her examination is normal.

Laboratory studies show the following:

| | |
|---|---|
| Hematocrit | 35% |
| Leukocyte count | 8500/μL; 65% neutrophils, 30% lymphocytes, 3% monocytes, 2% basophils |
| Blood urea nitrogen | 39 mg/dL |
| Serum creatinine | 2.3 mg/dL |
| Serum sodium | 143 meq/L |
| Serum potassium | 5.5 meq/L |
| Serum chloride | 109 meq/L |
| Serum bicarbonate | 21 meq/L |
| Urinalysis | Specific gravity 1.011; trace protein, no blood or glucose; granular casts but no erythrocyte or leukocyte casts; no bacteria |
| Urinary sodium | 42 meq/L |

Which of the following is the most likely diagnosis?

(A) Prerenal azotemia
(B) Acute interstitial nephritis
(C) Aminoglycoside nephrotoxicity
(D) Rhabdomyolysis
(E) Glomerulonephritis associated with bacterial endocarditis

## Acute Renal Failure Question 2

In the previous case, which of the following is most appropriate at this time?

(A) Intravenous methylprednisolone
(B) Intravenous normal saline with low-dose dopamine
(C) Discontinue gentamicin
(D) Alkalinize the urine with sodium bicarbonate

## Acute Renal Failure Question 3

Which of the following urinalysis findings is most compatible with contrast induced acute tubular necrosis?

(A) Specific gravity 1.012; 20-30 erythrocytes and 15-20 leukocytes/hpf; Hansel's stain positive for eosinophil leukocytes
(B) Specific gravity 1.010; 1-3 leukocytes and 5-10 renal tubular cells/hpf; many pigmented granular casts, occasional renal tubular cell casts; Hansel's stain negative
(C) Specific gravity 1.012; 5-10 erythrocytes and 25-50 leukocytes/hpf; many bacteria; occasional finely granular casts; Hansel's stain negative
(D) Specific gravity 1.020; 10-20 erythrocytes and 2-4 leukocytes/hpf; 1-3 erythrocyte casts/hpf; Hansel's stain negative

## Acute Renal Failure Question 4

In which of the following clinical situations would an increase in the serum creatinine concentration be explained only by a reduction in the glomerular filtration rate?

(A) Use of trimethoprim
(B) Increased muscle mass
(C) Severe extracellular volume contraction
(D) Seizures

## Acute Renal Failure Question 5

A 57-year-old man is evaluated because of oliguria and rapidly increasing serum creatinine and blood urea nitrogen. The microscopic urinalysis (see Figure 20 in the color plates) is shown.

Which of the following is the most likely diagnosis?

(A) Acute tubular necrosis
(B) Acute glomerulonephritis
(C) Acute interstitial nephritis
(D) Nephrotic syndrome

## Acute Renal Failure Question 6

A 25-year-old woman is evaluated because of hypertension, oliguria, and rapidly increasing serum creatinine and blood urea nitrogen. A specimen of her urine (see Figure 21 in the color plates) under light microscopy is shown.

Which of the following is the most likely diagnosis?

(A) Acute tubular necrosis
(B) Acute glomerulonephritis
(C) Acute interstitial nephritis
(D) Nephrotic syndrome

## Acute Renal Failure Question 7

A 19-year-old woman is evaluated because of weakness, easy fatigability, fever, and diarrhea. Her temperature is 37 °C (98.6 °F). Her blood pressure is 148/92 mm Hg. Except for petechiae on both lower extremities, her physical examination is normal.

Laboratory studies show the following:

| | |
|---|---|
| Hemoglobin | 8.4 g/dL |
| Leukocyte count | 15,400/µL |
| Serum creatinine | 2.9 mg/dL |
| Serum alkaline phosphatase | 92 U/L |
| Serum aspartate aminotransferase | 49 U/L |
| Serum alanine aminotransferase | 42 U/L |
| Creatine phosphokinase | 300 U/L |
| Urinalysis: | |
| Protein | 3+ |
| Blood | 3+ |
| Erythrocytes | 20-30 (dysmorphic) per high-power field |
| Lactate dehydrogenase | 600 µL |

Peripheral smear shows schistocytes and decreased platelets.

What is the most likely diagnosis?

(A) Nephrotic syndrome
(B) Systemic vasculiltis
(C) Acute glomerulonephritis
(D) Hemolytic-uremic syndrome
(E) Rhabdomyolysis

## Acute Renal Failure Question 8

A 35-year-old woman is evaluated because of a diagnosis of systemic lupus erythematosus. Over the past 2 years, manifestations of disease have included malar rash, arthralgias and arthritis, and intermittent episodes of pleuritic chest pain. One week ago, the patient developed joint pain for which she was prescribed indomethacin, 50 mg three times daily.

She feels remarkably well. She reports that the chest pain has been markedly reduced by the medication. Physical examination shows only a malar rash.

Laboratory studies reveal a serum creatinine level of 2.3 mg/dL. Two months earlier, the serum creatinine level was 1.0 mg/dL. Urinalysis shows 1+ protein and rare casts containing granulocytes. Other laboratory tests, including complete blood counts and liver enzyme levels, are normal.

Which of the following is the most appropriate intervention for the elevated creatinine?

(A) Prednisone, orally
(B) Methylprednisolone, intravenously daily
(C) Discontinue indomethacin
(D) Prednisone, orally, and cyclophosphamide, intravenously

## Acute Renal Failure Question 9

A 68-year-old man has a 10-year history of hypertension, hypercholesterolemia treated with lovastatin, and intermittent claudication diagnosed 2 years ago. Despite treatment with β-blockers and diuretics, his blood pressure readings are typically 180/100–105 mm Hg. His serum creatinine concentration is 1.6 mg/dL. Enalapril, 10 mg daily, is started, and two weeks later his blood pressure falls to 130/70 mm Hg. His pulse rate is 70/min and there is no orthostatic hypotension. An epigastric bruit is heard on abdominal examination.

Laboratory studies show the following:

| | |
|---|---|
| Blood urea nitrogen | 80 mg/dL |
| Serum creatinine | 3.2 mg/dL |
| Serum potassium | 5.2 meq/L |
| Urinalysis | Normal |

Which of the following is the most appropriate first step in managing this patient's acute renal failure?

(A) Discontinue enalapril
(B) Discontinue the β-blocker
(C) Discontinue lovastatin
(D) Administer intravenous normal saline
(E) Obtain emergent renal arteriography

# Hypertension

**Hypertension Question 1**

An 80-year-old woman is evaluated for hypertension. On physical examination, her blood pressure is 170/92 mm Hg. On each of the next two visits, the blood pressure remains elevated. Her son buys a device to measure her blood pressure at home and gets the same results.

Which of the following will determine the rationale for management of this patient's hypertension?

(A) Her life expectancy is not sufficient for her to benefit from treatment
(B) Antihypertensive therapy will improve her survival
(C) Antihypertensive therapy will decrease her risk of stroke, heart attack, and heart failure
(D) She is more likely to be harmed than benefited by antihypertensive therapy

**Hypertension Question 2**

Which of the following statements is correct regarding an interaction between aspirin and an angiotensin-converting enzyme (ACE) inhibitor?

(A) ACE inhibitors block the breakdown of norepinephrine, and aspirin enhances this effect
(B) ACE inhibitors block the breakdown of bradykinin, and aspirin counteracts this effect
(C) ACE inhibitors have a detrimental effect on the endothelium, and aspirin counteracts this effect
(D) ACE inhibitors enhance platelet aggregation, and aspirin inhibits this effect
(E) ACE inhibitors and aspirin have no known interaction

**Hypertension Question 3**

A 70-year-old man is evaluated because of a 3-month history of angina pectoris with mild exertion despite routine use of prophylactic nitroglycerin. He has had chronic, stable angina pectoris with moderate exertion for many years. Current medications are a β-blocker, isosorbide mononitrate, aspirin, simvastatin, and lisinopril. On physical examination, his resting pulse rate is 50/min, and resting blood pressure is 170/95 mm Hg.

Which one of the following should be increased?

(A) β-Blocker
(B) Lisinopril
(C) Aspirin
(D) Isosorbide mononitrate

**Hypertension Question 4**

A 25-year-old man is evaluated because of several months of episodic sweating, headaches, and palpitations. His medical history includes surgical repair of ankle injuries sustained in a fall while rollerblading 6 months ago; the anesthesiologist noted that the patient's blood pressure fluctuated significantly during the procedure and advised him to be evaluated for possible hypertension.

On physical examination, he is 180 cm (71 in) tall and weighs 72 kg (158 lb); his pulse rate is 80/min, and his blood pressure is 135/80 mm Hg. He has no goiter, lid lag, or tremor. Plasma glucose was normal during an episode of palpitations. His thyroid function tests are normal.

Measurement of which of the following is the best next step in the evaluation of this patient?

(A) Serum insulin and insulin-like growth factor 1
(B) Repeat measurements of blood pressure
(C) Catecholamines in a 24-hour urine sample
(D) Thyroid stimulating hormone (TSH)

**Hypertension Question 5**

A 41-year-old man is evaluated because of easy bruising. His medical history includes recent onset of borderline diabetes mellitus, which is being treated by diet. Review of systems shows a 4.6-kg (10-lb) weight gain, fatigue, muscle weakness, decreased libido, and depression. He uses no drugs, quit smoking 1 year ago, and has been drinking one to two six-packs of beer nightly.

On physical examination, he is 183 cm (72 in) tall and weighs 91 kg (200 lb); his pulse rate is 88/min, and his blood pressure is 150/95 mm Hg. He has a round face and supraclavicular and posterior cervical fullness. He has plethoric facies, tinea versicolor of the chest, no petechiae, and three or four ecchymoses on the extremities. Neurologic examination is normal, except for 3/5 strength in proximal leg muscles.

Which of the following is the most likely diagnosis?

(A) von Willebrand's disease
(B) Platelet dysfunction
(C) Hemochromatosis
(D) Cushing's syndrome
(E) Small vessel vasculitis

## Hypertension Question 6

A healthy 52-year-old woman is evaluated for her routine annual physical examination. On physical examination, she is 162 cm (64 in) tall and weighs 60 kg (130 lb); her pulse rate is 80/min, and her blood pressure is 160/100 mm Hg. On two subsequent days, she has her blood pressure measured and the results are in the same range.

Laboratory studies show the following:

| | |
|---|---|
| Serum sodium | 140 meq/L |
| Serum potassium | 3.3 meq/L |
| Serum creatinine | 0.8 mg/dL |
| Plasma glucose | 78 mg/dL |

Which of the following is the most likely diagnosis?

(A) Primary hyperaldosteronism
(B) Renovascular hypertension
(C) Pheochromocytoma
(D) Bartter's syndrome
(E) Cushing's syndrome

## Hypertension Question 7

A 28-year-old female waitress is evaluated because of an elevated blood pressure (approximately 160/105 mm Hg) for the past 2 to 3 months. The patient feels well. Her mother has hypertension and kidney disease, and a maternal aunt is currently on hemodialysis because of renal failure.

On physical examination, her height is 152 cm (62 in), and weight is 66 kg (145 lb). Her blood pressure is 166/106 mm Hg both seated and standing. The remainder of the examination is normal.

Laboratory studies show the following:

| | |
|---|---|
| Serum creatinine | 0.8 mg/dL |
| Serum sodium | 140 meq/L |
| Serum potassium | 5.0 meq/L |
| Serum chloride | 102 meq/L |
| Serum bicarbonate | 25 meq/L |
| Serum thyroid-stimulating hormone | Normal |
| Urinalysis | Normal |

Which of the following diagnostic studies is most likely to provide information regarding the cause of her hypertension?

(A) Captopril-stimulated renal scan
(B) 24-hour urine determination for vanillylmandelic acid
(C) Renal ultrasonography
(D) Plasma renin activity and aldosterone determinations

## Hypertension Question 8

A 48-year-old woman was found to have primary hypertension 6 months ago. Despite a trial of lifestyle modifications, her blood pressure remained elevated at about 158/96 mm Hg. Therapy with amlodipine, 5 mg daily, was begun.

The patient returns for a follow-up visit 6 weeks after beginning amlodipine. Several blood pressures readings in the office average 152/92 mm Hg. She has also noted progressive ankle edema since therapy was begun.

Which of the following is most appropriate at this time?

(A) No change in therapy
(B) Change to another antihypertensive agent
(C) Increase the amlodipine to 10 mg daily
(D) Recommend a low-salt diet and support hose

## Hypertension Question 9

Which one of the following statements about the measurement of blood pressure is correct?

(A) The risk of hypertensive cardiovascular complications (including left ventricular hypertrophy) correlates more closely with office blood pressure readings than with 24-hour or daytime ambulatory blood pressure readings.
(B) Physicians should routinely measure the office blood pressure of their patients because readings obtained by physicians are lower than those obtained by nurses.
(C) "White coat" hypertension may affect almost 20% of patients with mild office hypertension. Therefore, all patients with this suspected diagnosis should undergo ambulatory blood pressure monitoring with an automated device.
(D) Patients with "white coat" hypertension have a higher systemic vascular resistance and left ventricular mass index than their normotensive counterparts and may have an increased risk of cardiovascular disease.

## Hypertension Question 10

A 22-year-old woman has a 6-week history of headache, malaise, fever, and arthralgias. On physical examination, she has moderate hypertension, bruits over both carotid arteries, and diminished pulses in the upper extremities. The erythrocyte sedimentation rate is 110 mm/h.

Which of the following is the most likely diagnosis?

(A) Thromboangiitis obliterans
(B) Systemic lupus erythematosus
(C) Takayasu's arteritis
(D) Aortic dissection

## Hypertension Question 11

A 56-year-old man is seen for routine follow-up of hypertension. He has no complaints. He denies any recent change in health status or drug use. His has been prescribed a four-drug regimen of diltiazem sustained-release (SR), captopril, atenolol, and hydrochlorothiazide. He is taking all his medications. At his last clinic visit 2 months ago, his pulse rate was 68/min, and his blood pressure was 138/86 mm Hg. He has no other medical problems.

On physical examination, his pulse rate is 86/min and his blood pressure is 194/116 mm Hg. The rest of his physical examination is unremarkable. A stat complete blood count, electrolytes, blood urea nitrogen, creatinine, glucose levels, and urinalysis are all normal.

Which of the following is the most reasonable, immediate office-treatment option?

(A) Captopril and hydrochlorothiazide, orally
(B) Nifedipine, sublingually
(C) Lorazepam, orally
(D) Nitroprusside, intravenously
(E) No change in medications, follow-up in 2 weeks

## Hypertension Question 12
A 43-year-old woman with paroxysmal hypertension is admitted to the hospital. She reports 5 months of intermittent headaches, palpitations, flushing, and dizziness on standing. Outpatient investigations demonstrated markedly elevated urinary catecholamines. A CT scan of the abdomen demonstrates a 5-cm x 5-cm left adrenal mass.

Currently, her pulse rate is 115/min, and her blood pressure is 220/110 mm Hg with a 20 mm Hg systolic orthostatic drop. The remainder of the examination is unremarkable.

Which of the following is the most appropriate initial therapy?

(A) Esmolol, intravenously
(B) Nifedipine, sublingually
(C) Phenoxybenzamine, orally
(D) Intravenous normal saline solution and phenoxybenzamine (orally)
(E) Captopril, orally

## Hypertension Question 13
A 50-year-old man is evaluated because of high blood pressure. On physical examination his blood pressure is 160/90 mm Hg in the right arm and 120/84 mm Hg in the right leg. On auscultation there is an aortic ejection sound, a 2/6 basal midsystolic murmur, and a grade 1/6, high-pitched, early diastolic murmur at the left sternal border.

Which of the following conditions is most likely to be present in this patient?

(A) Essential hypertension with secondary aortic regurgitation
(B) Coarctation of the aorta and a bicuspid aortic valve
(C) Supravalvular aortic stenosis
(D) Isolated aortic regurgitation
(E) Patent ductus arteriosus

## Hypertension Question 14
A 34-year-old woman returns to the office because she has just discovered that she is pregnant. She has chronic essential hypertension, which has been well controlled on enalapril. She has no other medical problems. She does not smoke, use alcohol, or take illicit drugs, and she has no family history of cardiac disease. She has not taken her enalapril since she learned she was pregnant 4 days ago.

On physical examination, her pulse rate is 74/min, and blood pressure is 164/102 mm Hg. Her lungs are clear, and the cardiovascular examination is normal. A urine pregnancy test is positive.

What is the most appropriate management strategy for her hypertension?

(A) Restart enalapril
(B) A low-salt diet
(C) Hydrochlorothiazide
(D) Methyldopa

## Hypertension Question 15
A 47-year-old man who has had type 1 diabetes mellitus for 23 years is found to have hypertension that has been unresponsive to dietary salt restriction. His physical examination shows a blood pressure of 144/94 mm Hg and background retinopathy.

His creatinine, blood urea nitrogen, and potassium are normal. A 24-h urine albumin excretion rate is 152 mg. A second urine sample is also positive for albumin, which measures 85 mg/24 h.

Which one of the following medications should be used to treat this patient's blood pressure?

(A) Thiazide diuretic
(B) Central sympatholytic agent
(C) Angiotensin-converting enzyme (ACE) inhibitor
(D) Calcium-channel blocker

## Hypertension Question 16
A 56-year-old man undergoes a routine physical examination. A funduscopic examination is performed.

What does the funduscopic (see Figure 22 in the color plates) photograph show?

(A) Arteriolar sclerosis and hypertensive retinopathy
(B) Diabetic proliferative retinopathy
(C) Papilledema
(D) Malignant hypertensive retinopathy

## Hypertension Question 17
A 62-year-old hypertensive woman is evaluated because of headaches and confusion. After her vital signs are recorded, a funduscopic examination (see Figure 23 in the color plates) is performed.

Based on the funduscopic examination, which of the following conditions most likely present?

(A) Optic neuritis
(B) Arteriolar sclerosis
(C) Brain tumor
(D) Malignant hypertension

## Hypertension Question 18

A 42-year-old woman is evaluated because of striae, irregular menses, and moderate sustained hypertension of recent onset. A CT scan of the abdomen is obtained.

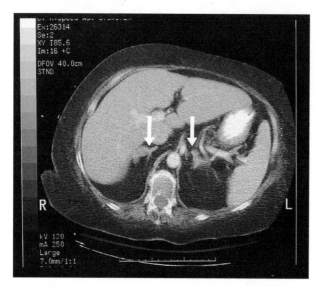

Which of the following is the most likely diagnosis?

(A) Adrenal adenoma
(B) Renal cell carcinoma
(C) Pheochromocytoma
(D) Renal artery fibromuscular dysplasia

## Hypertension Question 19

A 37-year-old man comes to the emergency department complaining of headache and transient visual loss. He has not seen a physician in more than 10 years and takes no medication. He was told many years ago that he had high blood pressure but did not follow up with a health care provider. Initial physical examination shows him to be awake but slightly confused and irritable. He is afebrile. Pulse rate is 72/min, and blood pressure is 268/176 mm Hg. Eyeground examination reveals arteriovenous crossing changes and several hemorrhages, but no papilledema. Cardiac examination shows an $S_4$ gallop; the lungs are clear. There is no peripheral edema.

Laboratory studies reveal normal electrolytes; BUN 32 mg/dL, and serum creatinine is 1.7 mgldL.

Which of the following is the best treatment option?

(A) Nitroprusside, intravenously
(B) Nifedipine, sublingually
(C) Nifedipine and furosemide, orally
(D) Labetalol, orally

## Hypertension Question 20

A 39-year-old woman is referred because of recent onset of hypertension. The patient had two uneventful pregnancies 20 and 17 years ago. Eight months ago, she was placed on a low-dose estrogen contraceptive, 21 days out of 28. At that time, her blood pressure was 136/76 mm Hg.

Six months ago, she was found to have a blood pressure of 140/98 mm Hg. One month ago, her blood pressure was found to be 148/100 mm Hg, and the oral contraceptive was discontinued.

Physical examination revealed a moderately obese woman in no distress. Blood pressure was 144/102 mm Hg. Funduscopic examination was normal. There were no signs of cardiovascular disease on physical examination. Laboratory studies revealed the following: blood urea nitrogen, 12 mg/dL; creatinine, 0.6 mg/dL; normal electrolytes; and glucose. Urinalysis was normal.

Which of the following is the best option for this patient?

(A) Schedule a follow-up appointment in 8 weeks
(B) Order 24-hour ambulatory blood pressure monitoring
(C) Order an echocardiogram
(D) Start therapy with an angiotensin-converting enzyme inhibitor
(E) Start therapy with a calcium-channel blocker

## Hypertension Question 21

A 22-year-old primiparous woman in her thirty-second week of gestation is admitted to the hospital because of epigastric pain, nausea, and vomiting. Physical examination shows a blood pressure of 150/105 mm Hg, puffiness of the eyes, 1+ peripheral edema, and segmental arteriolar narrowing but no hemorrhages or exudates of the fundus; cardiovascular examination is normal.

Laboratory studies show the following:

| | |
|---|---|
| Hematocrit | 40% |
| Leukocyte count | 7000/μL |
| Platelet count | 70,000/μL |
| Blood urea nitrogen | 15 mg/dL |
| Serum uric acid | 8.3 mg/dL |
| Serum creatinine | 1.7 mg/dL |
| Serum bilirubin | 2.7 mg/dL |
| Serum aspartate aminotransferase | 500 U/L |
| Serum lactate dehydrogenase | 500 |
| Serum haptoglobin | 14 mg/dL |
| Urinalysis | 2+ protein, no erythrocytes, no leukocytes |

Peripheral smear shows schistocytes and helmet cells. Reticulocyte count is 5%. Plasma fibrin split products level is 20 mg/mL (normal, <10 mg/mL).

What is the most likely diagnosis?

(A) Thrombotic thrombocytopenic purpura
(B) Malignant hypertension
(C) Acute glomerulonephritis
(D) Acute pancreatitis
(E) Preeclampsia

**Hypertension Question 22**
Which of the following procedures is the most cost-effective for evaluating the cause of high blood pressure in a 55-year-old man with suspected unilateral renovascular hypertension?

(A) Intravenous pyelography
(B) Renal scintigraphy
(C) Post converting enzyme inhibitor scintigraphy
(D) Plasma renin activity
(E) Renal ultrasonography

# Altered Mental Status

## Altered Mental Status Question 1

An 85-year-old woman is evaluated because over the past several years she has had progressive difficulty with her memory. She cites word-finding difficulties, especially for names of celebrities whose faces she recognizes on television. She says she forgets what she went into another room to get. She also reports difficulty keeping track of several things at once.

Physical examination reveals a well-appearing, elderly woman with a pulse rate of 76/min, respiration rate of 16/min, and blood pressure of 115/65 mm Hg without orthostatic changes. Results of the rest of the examination are within normal limits. Her Mini-Mental State Examination score is 28/30; a screening test for depression is negative. Laboratory evaluation reveals a normal serum thyroid-stimulating hormone and vitamin $B_{12}$.

The most appropriate next step in the management of this patient is:

(A) MRI of the brain
(B) Neuropsychologic testing
(C) Antidepressant therapy
(D) Monitor the patient without further work-up

## Altered Mental Status Question 2

An 88-year-old man is hospitalized for pneumonia and poor nutritional intake. He is tachypneic, tachycardic, febrile, and coughing continuously. Physical examination and chest radiograph confirm lobar pneumonia, and antibiotic therapy is begun. The fever resolves promptly and leukocytosis resolves by the third day of treatment. His vital signs return to normal, and the cough nears resolution. He is not treated with any other medications.

On the sixth day in the hospital, the patient becomes inattentive, confused, and drowsy with apparent hallucinations and fluctuating mental status. His vital signs remain normal.

Which one of the following is the most likely cause of this patient's delirium?

(A) Hyponatremia
(B) Meningitis
(C) Alcohol abstinence syndrome
(D) Hypoxemia
(E) Drug reaction

## Altered Mental Status Question 3

An 88-year-old woman is hospitalized because of a urinary tract infection. She has a history of mild dementia, and her husband states that her confusion often worsens at night. She takes no medications at home. Antibiotic therapy is begun in the hospital.

Which one of the following measures is most likely to be effective in avoiding the development of delirium in this patient during her hospital stay?

(A) Place a Foley catheter, restrain the patient physically, and limit fluids after supper.
(B) Provide bright illumination in the room at all times, repeated orientation by the nurses whenever the patient is awake, and benzodiazepine hypnotics at night as needed.
(C) Reduce ambient noise at night, enable the patient to move about during the day, and disimpact earwax if necessary.
(D) Reduce ambient noise, encourage family members to stay with her, and give benzodiazepine hypnotics at night.
(E) Provide visual aids and adaptive equipment for low vision and bedrails and haloperidol at night.

## Altered Mental Status Question 4

An 88-year-old woman is hospitalized after sustaining multiple injuries in a fall. She takes no medications and has no allergies; she does not drink alcohol but does smoke cigarettes. After surgery, she is agitated, angry, and demanding. She is moved to a step-down unit where she roams the halls looking for food and cigarettes. She suffers a near-fall and has two heated discussions 7 days postoperatively.

Which one of the following is the best management option for this patient?

(A) Vest restraint, bedrails, and benzodiazepines titrated to a dosage that causes sedation
(B) Four-point restraints, vest restraint, and 24-hour direct supervision
(C) Benzodiazepines titrated to a dosage that causes sedation
(D) A nonconfrontational approach, low-dose benzodiazepines, and bedrails while in bed
(E) A nonconfrontational approach, limit-setting, avoidance of unnecessary stimulation, and supervision while the patient remains confused

## Altered Mental Status Question 5

A 72-year-old man is evaluated because of progressive urinary incontinence and occasional falls for 1 year. His family has noticed that his concentration, speed of thought, and memory have become gradually impaired over the past 6 months. On physical examination, he has a wide-based stance and takes very short steps. He scores 25/30 on the Mini-Mental State Examination. Funduscopic examination is normal. Neurologic examination discloses no tremor or rigidity in the limbs, but mild generalized bradykinesia is present.

Which of the following is the most likely diagnosis?

(A) Parkinson's disease
(B) Normal-pressure hydrocephalus
(C) Brain tumor
(D) Spinal cord tumor
(E) Multi-infarct dementia

## Altered Mental Status Question 6

A 63-year-old man is brought to the emergency department because of a 4-day history of fever associated with progressive headache, lethargy, and confusion. He recently visited his dentist for routine periodontal care. Physical examination reveals a temperature of 38.2 °C (100.8 °F), papilledema, mild right-sided weakness, and nuchal rigidity.

Which one of the following is the most likely diagnosis?

(A) Bacterial meningitis
(B) Cerebral neoplasm
(C) Aseptic meningitis
(D) Pyogenic brain abscess

## Altered Mental Status Question 7

A 58-year-old man is evaluated because of a 2-year history of forgetfulness that began insidiously and has progressively worsened. He lost his job 1 year ago because of poor work performance. Over the past year, he has become more sedentary and has gained 7 kg (15 lb). He enrolls in various sweepstakes and has accumulated dozens of magazine subscriptions. When friends or relatives visit, he tends to go to another room and watch television. He has no problems with driving. He reports mild insomnia. When asked if he is depressed, he replies, "I don't have anything wrong with me!" He is otherwise healthy. His father had Parkinson's disease. On physical examination, the only notable finding is a score of 25/30 on the Mini-Mental State Examination, but he was able to recall 2 of 3 words after a 5-minute delay.

Which one of the following is the most appropriate management for this patient?

(A) Initiate a trial of a selective serotonin reuptake inhibitor.
(B) Initiate a trial of a cholinesterase inhibitor.
(C) Refer to a psychiatrist for a course of electroconvulsive therapy.
(D) Reassure the patient and his family that nothing is wrong.

## Altered Mental Status Question 8

A 43-year-old man is evaluated because of a 3-month history of increasing apathy, withdrawal, mental slowing, and progressive cognitive decline. He is HIV-seropositive and has had two bouts of *Pneumocystis carinii* pneumonia. Physical examination reveals slowing of rapid movements of the eyes and extremities, diffuse hyperreflexia and hypertonia, and release signs. Cerebrospinal fluid examination is unremarkable except for a protein concentration of 67 mg/dL and an increased IgG level. MRI of the brain demonstrates diffuse cerebral atrophy with ill-defined, nonenhancing, white matter hyperintensities.

Which one of the following is the most likely cause of this patient's symptoms?

(A) Cytomegalovirus encephalitis
(B) Central nervous system toxoplasmosis
(C) HIV-associated cognitive-motor complex
(D) Depression

## Altered Mental Status Question 9

An otherwise healthy 72-year-old woman is evaluated because of forgetfulness for 4 years. Over the past year, she has been struggling to recall names of friends and relatives. She recently drove down a one-way street in the wrong direction and is no longer able to manage her own finances. She denies feelings of depression. Her mother had similar symptoms in her 70s and died in a nursing home at age 79. The patient's physical examination is notable only for a Mini-Mental State Examination score of 23/30. Routine laboratory studies are normal, and an MRI scan of the brain shows moderate diffuse cerebral atrophy.

Which one of the following is the most appropriate management for this patient?

(A) Administer ibuprofen and estrogen
(B) Administer donepezil and vitamin E
(C) Determine cerebrospinal fluid tau and amyloid levels
(D) Determine apolipoprotein E genotype

## Altered Mental Status Question 10

A 58-year-old man is evaluated because of a progressive cognitive decline over the last 6 months. His wife has also noted quick jerking movements of his limbs, particularly when he is startled. There is no family history of a similar disorder, and the medical history is significant only for cigarette smoking. The patient's score on the Mini-Mental State Examination is markedly reduced. Occasional, very brief, lightning-like jerks of the extremities are present.

Which one of the following is the most likely diagnosis?

(A) Multi-infarct dementia
(B) Vitamin B$_{12}$ deficiency
(C) Hypothyroidism
(D) Creutzfeldt-Jakob disease
(E) Normal pressure hydrocephalus

**Altered Mental Status Question 11**

A 33-year-old woman is admitted to the hospital after a seizure. She has a history of chronic renal disease. During the past 3 months, in order to lose weight, she has dieted and increased her exercise time. She had begun to drink ten 12-oz glasses of water each day to keep herself well-hydrated and to reduce her appetite. For 2 days, her roommate noted that she was confused.

On the day of admission her roommate observed her having a tonic-clonic seizure. On physical examination, her temperature was 37 °C (98.6 °F), pulse 90/min, and blood pressure 160/100 mm Hg. She was lethargic and often drifted off to sleep. She could not cooperate for testing of memory and would not read, write, or draw. Her level of alertness and intellectual functions fluctuated considerably during the exam. The only abnormalities on neurologic examination were absent ankle jerks and decreased vibration sense in the toes. A computed tomographic (CT) scan of the head was normal.

Which one of the following is the most likely cause of this patient's encephalopathy?

(A) Hyponatremia
(B) Lupus cerebritis
(C) Hypothyroidism
(D) Vitamin B$_{12}$ deficiency
(E) Viral encephalitis

**Altered Mental Status Question 12**

A 73-year-old woman has had several weeks of forgetfulness, paresthesias in her feet, and unsteady gait. On physical examination, she is fully oriented but has mild impairment of recent memory and is mildly inattentive and irritable. Her gait is unsteady and broad-based, and she is unable to walk tandem. Cranial nerves and strength are normal, but muscle tone is mildly increased in her legs. Sensation to pain, temperature, and touch is mildly decreased bilaterally below the midthoracic area. Sensitivity to vibration is decreased at the ankles and knees, and proprioception is decreased at the toes and ankles. Tendon reflexes are absent at the knees and ankles; plantar responses are extensor.

Her hematocrit is 36%, mean corpuscular volume is 90 fL, leukocyte count is 5400/μL, and platelet count is 200,000/μL. Rare hypersegmented polymorphonuclear leukocytes are seen on the blood smear. Computed tomography of the head and spine shows only mild, diffuse cerebral atrophy.

Which one of the following is the most likely diagnosis?

(A) Spinal cord neoplasm
(B) Tabes dorsalis
(C) Normal-pressure hydrocephalus
(D) Alcohol abuse
(E) Vitamin B$_{12}$ deficiency

# Depression

## Depression Question 1

A 72-year-old woman is seen for a health maintenance evaluation. Her health has been excellent. Six weeks ago, her husband died. She is very concerned that she frequently wakes at night hearing her husband's voice coming from the bedroom in which he died. She goes to the room to check "knowing that he won't be there." Each day she has waves of sadness and thoughts of her husband accompanied by sighing and decreased energy. However, she has been cooking her meals, visiting friends, and going to her bridge club.

Which of following is the most appropriate action to take at this time?

(A) Haloperidol, 1 mg at bedtime
(B) Reassurance that her symptoms are a part of normal grieving
(C) Paroxetine, 10 mg daily
(D) Amitriptyline, 25 mg at bedtime
(E) Referral to a psychologist

## Depression Question 2

A 41-year-old man is being treated for depression. After 4 weeks of treatment with sertraline, 50 mg daily, he is feeling better in terms of sleep problems, appetite, and energy level, and he is finding more pleasure in life. However, he continues to show signs of sensitivity to criticism at work and home and periods of despondency in response to minor problems. Despite his calm exterior, he often feels angry and resentful of demands placed on him at work and home. He has responded well to sertraline at this dosage in the past. This is his third episode of depression in the past 5 years.

Which of the following is the best course of action for this patient at this time?

(A) Increase the sertraline dosage
(B) Add methylphenidate
(C) Switch to bupropion
(D) Switch to a tricyclic antidepressant
(E) Refer for psychotherapy

## Depression Question 3

Which of the following is most appropriate in planning future therapy for the patient in the previous question?

(A) Discontinue antidepressant therapy after 12 weeks
(B) Reduce dose by one half at 12 weeks and discontinue in 6 months
(C) Reduce dose by one half at 12 weeks and continue as maintenance
(D) Maintenance therapy should be continued at full dose of antidepressant
(E) Discontinue antidepressant therapy after 9 months

## Depression Question 4

A 74-year-old woman is evaluated for memory problems. The family is concerned that she has become progressively forgetful over the past 4 years, and they have learned she has not paid her electric bill for 4 months. When she is offered help, she becomes agitated. She describes her only problem as difficulty sleeping over the past 2 months.

The patient completed seventh grade and worked as a home health aid for many years until her retirement 9 years ago. She raised two sons, and her husband died 4 months ago. She now lives alone in her home of 20 years. Both of her parents lived into their 80s, with reported cognitive decline before they died.

On physical examination the patient is friendly and dressed neatly. Her speech is regular but slowed. Neurological examination is normal, and her gait is steady. Her Mini-Mental State Examination score is 20/30. Her responses were as follows: Correct response to year, season, and day; however, she says it is January 31 when it is actually February 1. Correct response to state, town, and county, but does not know medical office building's name, address, or floor. Correct registration of three objects; subtracted serial sevens as 100-93-87-81-73; recalled two of three objects; Repeated "No ifs, ands, or buts" as "No if, and, or but"; completed only two steps of a three-step command; read and obeyed "Close your eyes"; wrote "I feel fine"; correctly copied the intersecting pentagons.

What is the appropriate next step in the management of this patient?

(A) Neuropsychiatric evaluation
(B) Donepezil
(C) Screen for depression
(D) No intervention

## Depression Question 5

A 67-year-old man is evaluated because of slow speech and sadness. He has not shaved in several days, has lost 4.5 kg (10 lb) in the past 3 months, and makes poor eye contact. He has been depressed in the past but is not currently being treated. His wife died 6 months ago, and he has not gotten back to his usual routine and feels socially isolated. When asked how he is doing, he says, "Life isn't what it used to be and I don't see that it ever can be."

Which one of the following is the next most appropriate step?

(A) Increase his social activity
(B) Urgent psychiatric consultation
(C) Prescribe an anxiolytic medication
(D) Reassure the patient

## Depression Question 6

An 82-year-old man is taken for an evaluation by his daughter. She has become concerned about her father's appearance because he has gone from being vibrant and healthy to appearing thin and disheveled. He has also become slightly absent-minded and reclusive. His wife died 6 months ago. He does not have any specific complaints but does admit that his appetite is poor and that food often does not taste good.

On physical examination, he weighs 55 kg (121 lb); he has lost 7 kg (15.5 lb) since his physical examination 1 year ago. His affect is flat. There are no other pertinent findings. Laboratory testing reveals normal complete blood count, serum thyroid-stimulating hormone level, and chemistry profile; stool is negative for occult blood.

Which of the following is the most appropriate course of action in this patient's care?

(A) An antidepressant
(B) A proton-pump inhibitor
(C) Placement in an extended-care facility
(D) Zinc supplement
(E) CT scan of the head

## Depression Question 7

A 16-year-old girl is evaluated because of fatigue. For the past 6 months, she has had little appetite, been bored and irritable, and lost interest in most activities. She is struggling with school and has difficulty concentrating. She drinks alcoholic beverages regularly to relax and to get to sleep, and reports numerous alcoholic binges. She is tired all day, even after 10 hours of sleep. She lives with her parents, and family relationships are strained. She is concerned about her insomnia and difficulty controlling her drinking.

What information would be most important to elicit from the patient in further evaluating her fatigue?

(A) Presence of a rash
(B) Presence of suicidal ideation
(C) Presence of cold intolerance
(D) Presence of vomiting
(E) Relationship of fatigue to her menses

## Depression Question 8

A 45-year-old woman reports feeling "down" more often than not for many years. For brief periods of time, she feels somewhat better, then lapses into her usual mood. She cannot remember feeling really happy for more than 10 years. She says, "It seems like I've been like this for as long as I can remember." Her sleep is intermittently poor, with early morning wakening and difficulty falling asleep. She has recurrent feelings of low self-esteem. Her concentration at work is usually good, and she has enough energy to keep up with her activities at home and work. Her weight is stable. She takes pleasure in her children's accomplishments. She denies suicidal ideation.

Which of the following is the most likely diagnosis in this patient?

(A) Major depression
(B) Atypical major depression
(C) Seasonal affective disorder
(D) Adjustment disorder with depressed mood
(E) Dysthymia

## Depression Question 9

A 39-year-old Vietnamese woman is evaluated because of headache, cough, and difficulty sleeping over the past several months. She has been in the United States for 3.5 years, and her history is obtained through an interpreter. She has seen several physicians and has always had a normal physical examination except for a palpable spleen tip. She has had a variety of diagnostic studies, which yielded no discrete diagnosis. Symptoms have been unrelieved by a variety of herbal remedies, physical traditional remedies (for example, coin rubbing and cupping), and empiric Western therapies (nonsteroidal anti-inflammatory drugs, bronchodilators, and sedative hypnotics).

A CT scan of the brain, blood chemistries, complete blood count, and chest radiography have all been negative or normal. Laboratory study is positive for hepatitis B surface antigen; liver function studies and erythrocyte sedimentation rate are normal. Stools have been repeatedly negative for ova and parasites.

The most likely diagnosis is:

(A) Polymyalgia rheumatica
(B) Depression
(C) Disseminated tuberculosis
(D) Malaria
(E) HIV disease

# Substance Abuse

## Substance Abuse Question 1

A 66-year-old man is seen for a periodic health examination. He acknowledges drinking two glasses of wine with dinner and two mixed drinks each evening at least 5 nights a week. He also notes positive responses to "cut down" and "annoyed" on the CAGE questionnaire. He does not have any history of alcohol withdrawal, the need to use escalating amounts of alcohol to obtain a beneficial response, or interference with his family life or occupation by alcohol.

Which of the following is the most effective plan for this patient?

(A) Ask additional questions on frequency and quantity of alcohol use.
(B) Refer the patient to a 12-step treatment program (i.e. Alcoholics Anonymous).
(C) Provide a brief counseling session and educational materials and arrange a follow-up appointment.
(D) Advise the patient to quit alcohol consumption immediately and prescribe daily naltrexone.

## Substance Abuse Question 2

A 28-year-old man is evaluated in the emergency department with chest pain, tachycardia, diaphoresis, and agitation. He admits to snorting cocaine at a party for the past 2 hours. On physical examination, his temperature is 37.8 °C (100 °F), pulse rate is 166/min, respiration rate is 20/min, and blood pressure is 170/120 mm Hg. His optic fundi are normal; his lungs are clear; and there are no cardiac murmurs. A 12-lead electrocardiogram shows sinus tachycardia.

Which one of the following treatments is indicated in this patient?

(A) Diltiazem
(B) Adenosine
(C) Nifedipine
(D) Propranolol
(E) Diazepam

## Substance Abuse Question 3

A 78-year-old woman is hospitalized following a hip fracture that was sustained while she was decorating her Christmas tree. She is a retired attorney, has no significant medical history, and has been well and active until this injury. She undergoes uneventful operative repair, receiving 2 units of packed red blood cells 12 hours after the fall. Within a few hours, she is moved from the recovery room to the orthopedics ward.

Twelve hours postoperatively, her temperature is 38.2 °C (100.8 °F), pulse rate is 120/min, and respiration rate is 20/min. On physical examination, she is tremulous, distractible, irritable, and disoriented. Results of laboratory studies show a leukocyte count of 12,800/µL. Arterial blood gases, chest radiograph, CT scan of the brain, and urinalysis are normal. There is no sign of wound infection or dislocation of the repaired hip.

Which of the following is the most likely cause of this patient's condition?

(A) Venous thromboembolism
(B) Anesthetic complication
(C) Alcohol withdrawal syndrome
(D) Delayed hemolytic transfusion reaction
(E) Acute hemolytic transfusion reaction

## Substance Abuse Question 4

A 37-year-old man is brought to the emergency room by his landlord for "confusion" and "difficulty walking." He appeared normal 3 days before, but the landlord knows nothing of his personal habits.

On physical examination, he is lethargic, inattentive, apathetic, gives the wrong month and year, and is unable to provide a coherent history. Language function is intact, and he does not appear to be hallucinating. There is bilateral limitation of lateral gaze with horizontally directed nystagmus, but vertical movements and pupillary reflexes are intact. Gait is broad-based and ataxic; he cannot walk tandem or stand with his feet together. Strength and muscle tone are normal, and there is neither tremor nor asterixis. He seems to have decreased appreciation of pinprick and vibration in his feet, and his ankle tendon reflexes are absent. Plantar responses are flexor. His liver is palpable 4 cm below the costal margin.

Which of the following is the most likely diagnosis?

(A) Vitamin $B_{12}$ deficiency
(B) Wilson's disease
(C) Hepatic encephalopathy
(D) Alcohol withdrawal
(E) Wernicke-Korsakoff's disease

## Substance Abuse Question 5

A 25-year-old woman who regularly uses heroin, cocaine, and marijuana is brought unresponsive to the emergency department. Respiratory rate is 5/min and shallow. Pupils are pinpoint; reactivity to light is difficult to discern. Her limbs move symmetrically to noxious stimuli, and the oculocephalic maneuver produces full horizontal eye movements. Following administration of 2 mg of naloxone, she becomes alert but within a few minutes develops lacrimation, yawning, rhinorrhea, and marked irritability, for which she receives methadone, 10 mg orally. She then has a major motor seizure. Computed tomography of the head, cerebrospinal fluid analysis, and blood glucose level are normal.

Which of the following is the most likely cause of this patient's seizure?

(A) Opiate toxicity
(B) Opiate withdrawal
(C) Cocaine toxicity
(D) Cocaine withdrawal

## Substance Abuse Question 6

A 46-year-old woman with a 20-year history of alcohol abuse presents with abdominal discomfort, nausea, and vomiting. She states that she had been drinking heavily (15 to 20 beers/day and a fifth of vodka every 2 days) and stopped yesterday morning when she noticed worsening right upper quadrant pain and nausea. She has noticed some mild abdominal pain for the past week. She has been vomiting frequently. She has not eaten a full meal for 7 days and had very little oral intake of any kind yesterday.

Physical examination reveals a thin, pale woman with a marked tremor. Her temperature is 36.8 °C (98.2 °F), pulse rate is 120/min, and blood pressure is 90/60 mm Hg. Her liver is palpable 6 cm below the right costal margin, with a span of 14 cm in the right midclavicular line, and the edge is tender.

| | |
|---|---|
| Hemoglobin | 10 g/dL |
| Hematocrit | 30% |
| Leukocyte count | 12,000/μL |
| Mean corpuscular volume | 104 fL |
| Serum electrolytes | |
| Sodium | 136 meq/L |
| Potassium | 3.6 meq/L |
| Chloride | 94 meq/L |
| Bicarbonate | 16 meq/L |
| Aspartate transaminase (AST) | 60 U/L |
| Alanine transaminase (ALT) | 22 U/L |
| Glucose | 150 mg/dL |
| Amylase | 80 U/L |
| Alcohol | 10 mg/dL |
| Urine | 0-2 WBC; 0-2 RBC |
| Trace protein | Positive for ketones |

Abdominal ultrasound reveals an enlarged liver, a gallbladder without stones, and no dilated bile ducts. She receives intravenous thiamine, multivitamins, and benzodiazepines in the emergency department.

Which one of the following intravenous therapies is indicated?

(A) Sodium bicarbonate
(B) Glucose and saline
(C) Insulin
(D) β-Blockers
(E) Corticosteroids

## Substance Abuse Question 7

An 89-year-old woman is brought to your office by her relatives, who noticed that recently the patient's house had become very messy, that she seemed distracted and irritable, and that she was having memory problems. The patient has lived alone and been self-sufficient since the death of her husband 10 years ago. There is no history of the patient having fallen or having suffered any other trauma. She has hypertension and osteoarthritis, for which she has been taking chlorthalidone, 25 mg/d; atenolol, 25 mg/d; and ibuprofen, 800 mg/d.

Physical examination shows a thin woman with temporal muscle wasting. She has decreased short-term memory and appears to lack insight; there are no focal neurologic findings. Laboratory studies show elevated serum alanine aminotransferase and mean corpuscular volume and low-normal serum albumin. You discontinue the patient's medications and ask her relatives to bring her to your office in 1 week.

In the follow-up visit 1 week later, her relatives report that there is no change in her mental status.

What is the most likely cause of the patient's mental deterioration?

(A) Subdural hematoma
(B) Alzheimer's disease
(C) Alcohol abuse
(D) Multi-infarct dementia

**Substance Abuse Question 8**

A 31-year-old man with a 12-year history of injection drug use (heroin) is brought to the emergency room comatose and cyanotic by a friend. His friend reports that he was fine when he saw him last night.

On physical examination, he has a temperature of 36.5 °C (97.7 °F), pulse rate of 120/min, respiration rate of 8/min, blood pressure of 80/60 mm Hg. He has constricted pupils, bilateral rales, and marked cyanosis of his fingertips and lips. He is tachycardic without an $S_3$ gallop, and an electrocardiogram shows sinus tachycardia without ST-segment changes. $O_2$ saturation is 50%. Chest radiograph reveals a normal cardiac silhouette and bilateral infiltrates. He is intubated and placed on a ventilator with high concentrations of oxygen.

What is the most appropriate management for this patient?

(A) Intravenous dopamine
(B) Intravenous digitalis
(C) Intravenous flumazenil
(D) Intravenous furosemide
(E) Intravenous naloxone

**Substance Abuse Question 9**

A 45-year-old man is admitted to the hospital for alcohol detoxification. He has a 3-year history of heavy alcohol abuse, drinking an average of 1 to 1 1/2 pints of vodka per day. He has no other known medical problems but has had one previous episode of alcohol withdrawal a year earlier, in which he experienced a single grand mal seizure. He is on no medications, and his last drink was 12 hours prior to his presentation. On physical examination, he is a somewhat pale, thin man who appears anxious, diaphoretic, and tremulous. His temperature is 37.4 °C (99.4 °F), pulse rate is 110/min and regular, respiration rate is 20/min, and blood pressure is 150/92 mm Hg. The remainder of the examination is normal. There are no physical signs of liver dysfunction or cirrhosis. Three hours after being admitted, the nurse informs you that the patient seems anxious and may be hallucinating.

The most appropriate drug to administer in this situation would be:

(A) Captopril
(B) Chlorpromazine
(C) Phenytoin
(D) Lorazepam
(E) Naltrexone

# Smoking

## Smoking Question 1

A 24-year-old healthy woman is evaluated because her last menstrual period was 2 months ago and a home pregnancy test last evening was positive. She is concerned about the effects her smoking may have on this pregnancy and wishes to quit. She has smoked 1 pack of cigarettes per day for the past 8 years and has never tried to quit.

Which of the following is the best recommendation for this patient?

(A) Negotiate a quit date, offer her literature on quitting, and arrange for a follow-up.
(B) Prescribe a nicotine patch
(C) Prescribe bupropion
(D) Explore the reasons she smokes and educate her about the risks smoking poses to her pregnancy.
(E) Referral to a smoking-cessation program

## Smoking Question 2

A 45-year-old male executive is seen for his annual physical examination and asks about quitting smoking. He has smoked 2 packs of cigarettes per day for the past 25 years. The patient tried to stop smoking on his own 5 years ago without success. He dislikes chewing gum but did try an over-the-counter 21-mg nicotine patch 3 months ago with initial success. However, 1 week after his last patch he began smoking again after a stressful business meeting.

Which of the following is the most appropriate recommendation for this patient?

(A) Advise him to taper his smoking now.
(B) Refer him to a smoking-cessation program.
(C) Refer him to a hypnotist.
(D) Begin bupropion and set a quit date.

## Smoking Question 3

A 60-year-old man with previously established asymptomatic peripheral artery disease has now developed painful tightening of his right gastrocnemius muscle when walking 4 blocks. This finding has been stable for 2 to 3 months. There is no leg pain at rest, and the patient states that the symptom does not significantly affect his lifestyle. The patient smokes cigarettes and has been unable to stop smoking.

Which of the following has the highest priority in managing this patient?

(A) Begin pentoxifylline.
(B) Begin warfarin.
(C) Begin cilostazol.
(D) Reassess his willingness to stop smoking.
(E) Refer the patient to a vascular surgeon.

## Smoking Question 4

A 60-year-old man comes for advice on prevention of pancreatic cancer. The patient has no symptoms. He drinks four cups of coffee and one or two glasses of wine daily, smokes one-and-a-half packs of cigarettes daily, and is employed as a traveling salesman. He has no pertinent medical history and takes no medications. His physical examination reveals moderate obesity. Laboratory studies show a normal complete blood count and normal electrolyte levels.

What is the most appropriate recommendation for this patient?

(A) Begin a strict vegetarian diet.
(B) Stop drinking alcohol.
(C) Stop drinking coffee.
(D) Stop smoking.
(E) Start a weight-control regimen.

## Smoking Question 5

Which one of the following medical interventions is the most effective in preventing lung cancer in a cigarette smoker?

(A) Annual chest radiograph
(B) Annual sputum cytology
(C) β-carotene supplementation
(D) 13-cis retinoic acid supplementation
(E) Nicotine patches

## Smoking Question 6

What percentage of regular cigarette smokers in the United States quit smoking without formal smoking cessation intervention and abstain from smoking for 1 year?

(A) 2%
(B) 6%
(C) 12%
(D) 25%
(E) 40%

# The Healthy Patient

## The Healthy Patient Question 1

Which of the following statements regarding health risks and health maintenance for lesbian women is true?

(A) Women who have sex only with women acquire chlamydia infection and syphilis at rates similar to women who have intercourse with men
(B) Female-to-female transmission of HIV infection does not occur through exposure to vaginal secretions
(C) Lesbian women are at less risk for cervical cancer than women who have sex with both men and women
(D) Bacterial vaginosis is not sexually transmissible in lesbian women
(E) Lesbian women are at similar risk for contracting hepatitis B as gay men and should therefore receive a hepatitis B vaccine

## The Healthy Patient Question 2

A 19-year-old male college student is seen for removal of sutures. He sustained a laceration on the palm of his right hand in a fight in a bar 10 days ago. He was intoxicated at the time and admits to drinking two to three alcoholic beverages each day and several times that much on most weekends. He never uses a designated driver and was once convicted for driving under the influence. He occasionally uses marijuana and has tried cocaine but denies intravenous drug use. He smokes one pack of cigarettes a day. He is heterosexual, reports more than 10 lifetime sex partners, and has unprotected sex when intoxicated. He tends to feels isolated and occasionally depressed. He does not own or carry a gun.

On physical examination, he has a well-healed laceration with intact tendon function. The results of complete blood count and liver function tests are normal. Serology reveals he is not immune to hepatitis A or B and is negative for HIV infection.

Modification of which of the following would be most effective in preventing death in this patient in the next 5 years?

(A) Use of marijuana and cocaine
(B) Drinking and driving
(C) Unsafe sex
(D) Cigarette smoking
(E) Violent conflict resolution

## The Healthy Patient Question 3

In the previous case, which of the following would be most effective in preventing premature death in the patient's lifetime?

(A) Immunization for hepatitis A and B
(B) Avoid drinking and driving
(C) Avoid unsafe sex
(D) Discontinue cigarette smoking
(E) Avoid violent conflict resolution

## The Healthy Patient Question 4

A 52-year-old man requests an opinion about an exercise program as well as a preparticipation examination. He has mild hypertension that has been well controlled with lisinopril therapy and is otherwise healthy. He has no family history of cardiovascular disease. He was a competitive athlete as a young man, but since college he has become increasingly sedentary. He recently agreed to participate in a 50-mile bicycle ride 6 months from now. He wonders if he should have an exercise tolerance test before starting his conditioning program.

In addition to a focused history and physical examination, which one of the following should be done for an optimal evaluation of this patient?

(A) No additional tests
(B) Screening laboratory tests
(C) Screening laboratory tests and an electrocardiogram
(D) Screening laboratory tests, an electrocardiogram, and a graded exercise test

## The Healthy Patient Question 5

An 18-year-old woman is seen at the time of her precollege physical examination. Records from her pediatrician show that she has received 5 doses of diphtheria-pertussis-tetanus vaccine at ages 2, 4, 6, and 18 months and at 5 years; 1 dose of tetanus vaccine at age 12 years; 4 doses of oral polio vaccine at age 2, 4, and 18 months and at 5 years; 2 doses of measles-mumps-rubella vaccine at ages 15 months and 12 years; and 1 dose of varicella vaccine at age 12 years. She has no history of childhood exanthems. She plans to travel through Western Europe before going to college, where she will live off-campus. She is not sexually active. She does not smoke or use alcohol or other recreational drugs. Physical examination is unremarkable.

Which one of the following vaccines is indicated for this patient at this time?

(A) Quadrivalent meningococcal vaccine

(B) Tetanus booster

(C) Hepatitis B vaccine

(D) Second dose of varicella vaccine

(E) Hepatitis A vaccine

## The Healthy Patient Question 6

A 20-year-old woman is seen for a periodic health examination. She is single and sexually active. She lives in an apartment at the edge of a large urban area. She does not smoke, consumes one to two alcoholic beverages per week, and exercises for 30 minutes three times a week. She's cautious about travel at night, always wears seat belts, and takes a daily multivitamin with iron. Her family history is negative for cardiovascular disease and hypercholesterolemia.

On physical examination, she is 157.5 cm (62 in) and weighs 50 kg (110 lb). Blood pressure is 108/68 mm Hg. The rest of the physical examination and a pelvic examination are normal.

What additional interview-based screening and counseling is most appropriate for this patient?

(A) Breast self-examination

(B) Contraceptive use and sexually transmitted disease prevention

(C) Gambling

(D) Eating disorders

## The Healthy Patient Question 7

For the patient in the previous question, what additional physical examination or laboratory screening should be done?

(A) Hearing screening

(B) Vision screening

(C) Chlamydia and gonococcal screening

(D) Serum cholesterol measurement

(E) Urinalysis

## The Healthy Patient Question 8

A 58-year-old woman is seen for her annual Pap smear. She is in good health, has been married for 35 years, and does not smoke. Her only past surgery is a hysterectomy performed 10 years ago for uterine fibroids. The patient has had annual Pap smears, and she has never had an abnormal one. Her most recent test was 1 year ago.

Which of the following is the most appropriate course of action for this patient?

(A) Obtain a vaginal smear now and every 3 years until age 65 years

(B) Continue to perform yearly Pap smears until age 65 years

(C) Continue to perform annual Pap screening indefinitely

(D) Discontinue annual Pap screening

(E) Perform an annual pelvic examination the rest of her life

## The Healthy Patient Question 9

A 51-year-old man is evaluated for pretravel immunization. He is in excellent health and is planning to travel to remote areas of Central America. He received a tetanus booster when he went to college but can recall no other immunizations since. He is in a monogamous relationship with his wife of 30 years and has no history of intravenous drug use. He is unsure whether he had chicken pox. His physical examination is normal.

Which one of the following immunization regimens would be appropriate for this patient?

(A) Tetanus diphtheria, varicella

(B) Tetanus diphtheria, hepatitis A and B, varicella if serology indicates lack of immunity

(C) Tetanus diphtheria, pneumococcus

(D) Tetanus diphtheria, varicella, pneumococcus, hepatitis A and B

(E) No immunizations needed

## The Healthy Patient Question 10

A 66-year-old white man is seen for a periodic health examination. He has severe chronic obstructive pulmonary disease from a 60-pack-year smoking history, and his most recently measured $FEV_1$ is approximately 1 L. He has no other medical problems or urinary symptoms. He is willing to undergo a rectal examination and flexible sigmoidoscopy for colorectal cancer screening and asks about the "prostate blood test."

What should this patient be advised about prostate-specific antigen (PSA) screening?

(A) Advise against PSA screening because his ethnicity and lack of family history lower his risk for cancer

(B) Provide education about the risks and benefits of PSA testing, and base the decision on patient preference and your interpretation of the risk/benefit equation

(C) Advise the patient to undergo PSA screening

(D) Advise against screening because this patient's lack of symptoms lowers the likelihood of cancer

## The Healthy Patient Question 11

A 65-year-old woman is seen for a routine gynecologic examination. She is postmenopausal and has no family history of cancer, but she is especially interested in making sure that she does not have ovarian cancer.

Which of the following is the best approach to screening for ovarian cancer in this patient?

(A) Pap smear every year

(B) Pap smear every 3 years

(C) Pap smear today and a repeat in 1 year

(D) No screening

**The Healthy Patient Question 12**
An 80-year-old woman is new to the practice and comes for her first medical examination. While discussing routine screening issues with her, she says that she has not had a Pap smear in 2 years and wonders if she needs an annual Pap smear. She has been widowed for 10 years and has not been sexually active since the death of her husband. She has never had an abnormal Pap smear.

Which of the following is the appropriate screening recommendation for this patient?

(A) Pap smear every year
(B) Pap smear every 3 years
(C) Discontinue pap smears
(D) Pap smear today and a repeat in 1 year

**The Healthy Patient Question 13**
A 23-year-old professional golfer would like to know what he can do to prevent skin cancer.

Which of the following is the most practical and effective advice regarding the prevention of skin cancer?

(A) Avoid the sun
(B) High-SPF sunscreens
(C) Protective clothing and hats
(D) Keep a "protective" tan all year by going to a tanning salon
(E) Limit tournaments to locations in northern latitudes

**The Healthy Patient Question 14**
A 50-year-old woman is evaluated because of malaise. For the past year or so, she has gradually felt increasing fatigue. She is having trouble sleeping, waking frequently and typically feeling very warm. She reports irritability with her family and wonders what is wrong with her. Her menstrual cycles are becoming irregular, occurring every 45 to 90 days.

Which one of the following treatments is indicated for this patient?

(A) Estrogen replacement therapy
(B) Paroxetine
(C) Multivitamin with iron
(D) Lorazepam

**The Healthy Patient Question 15**
A 56-year-old postmenopausal woman wishes to evaluate her fracture risk and discuss possible preventive therapies.

Which of the following is the best method to evaluate her fracture risk?

(A) Measure parathyroid hormone (PTH)
(B) Measure erythrocyte sedimentation rate
(C) Measure thyroid-stimulating hormone (TSH), and 25-hydroxyvitamin D levels
(D) Perform a serum protein electrophoresis
(E) Measure bone density

**The Healthy Patient Question 16**
Which one of the following cancers is most amenable to office-based prevention interventions in patients at average risk of developing cancer?

(A) Pancreatic
(B) Colorectal
(C) Gastric
(D) Bladder
(E) Liver

**The Healthy Patient Question 17**
Which one of the following potential confounding effects is not addressed by randomization in a definitive cancer-screening trial of volunteer study subjects with cancer mortality end points?

(A) Lead time bias
(B) Length bias
(C) Overdiagnosis
(D) Selection bias
(E) Generalizability

**The Healthy Patient Question 18**
Which one of the following is the most reliable end point in assessing the screening efficacy in a randomized cancer trial?

(A) Cause-specific cancer mortality
(B) Overall mortality
(C) Case fatality ratio
(D) Survival of patients diagnosed with cancer
(E) Incidence of late-stage cancer

**The Healthy Patient Question 19**
Which one of the following screening tests is best supported by the medical literature and would be most likely to improve cancer-specific mortality if instituted on a regular basis in the office setting?

(A) Testicular cancer palpation
(B) Instruction on breast self-examination
(C) Fecal occult blood testing
(D) Oral cavity examination
(E) Annual chest radiograph

# Diabetes Mellitus

**Diabetes Mellitus Question 1**

Which one of the following provides a definitive diagnosis of type 2 diabetes mellitus?

(A) Symptoms of diabetes plus a random plasma glucose concentration of 160 mg/dL

(B) Hemoglobin $A_{1C}$ level of 7.0% or greater

(C) Fasting plasma glucose concentration of 126 mg/dL or greater

(D) A 2-hour plasma glucose concentration greater than 150 mg/dL during an oral glucose tolerance test

(E) The combination of age greater than 45 years, positive family history of diabetes, and a fasting plasma glucose concentration of 115 mg/dL or greater

**Diabetes Mellitus Question 2**

A 56-year-old woman who has had type 2 diabetes mellitus for 12 years is evaluated because of poorly controlled diabetes. She is obese (body mass index, 32 kg/m²). She takes glyburide, and over the past 6 months, her hemoglobin $A_{1C}$ level has increased from 6.8% to 8.5%, while measurements of her fasting plasma glucose have been greater than 200 mg/dL and postprandial measurements range from 250 to 350 mg/dL. She refuses to take insulin.

Which of following is the best therapy for this patient?

(A) Discontinue glyburide and initiate metformin

(B) Discontinue glyburide and initiate a thiazolidinedione

(C) Continue glyburide and add metformin

(D) Continue glyburide and repeat measurement of hemoglobin $A_{1C}$

(E) Continue glyburide and add acarbose

**Diabetes Mellitus Question 3**

A 42-year-old woman is evaluated because of "chronic fatigue." Among the results of laboratory tests is a random plasma glucose of 226 mg/dL.

Which of the following is the recommended best test to confirm the diagnosis of diabetes mellitus in this patient?

(A) Fasting plasma glucose

(B) Glucose tolerance test

(C) Repeat random plasma glucose

(D) Hemoglobin $A_{1C}$

(E) Fasting plasma insulin and fasting plasma glucose

**Diabetes Mellitus Question 4**

A 29-year-old woman who has had type 1 diabetes mellitus since age 18 years is evaluated because of several episodes of nocturnal hypoglycemia. Her insulin schedule is 24 U NPH/10R before breakfast and 14NPH/10R before supper. Her hemoglobin $A_{1C}$ is 7.2%.

How should the patient's insulin schedule be altered?

(A) Reduce the presupper dose of NPH

(B) Reduce the presupper dose of regular insulin

(C) Reduce the prebreakfast dose of NPH

(D) Reduce the presupper dose of regular insulin and change NPH to bedtime

(E) Reduce the prebreakfast regular insulin and give some regular insulin before lunch

**Diabetes Mellitus Question 5**

In a patient with diabetes mellitus, which one of the following eye disorders is likely to improve with tighter glycemic control?

(A) Glaucoma

(B) Retinal edema

(C) Cataracts

(D) Proliferative retinopathy

**Diabetes Mellitus Question 6**

A 20-year-old woman who has had repeated admissions for diabetic ketoacidosis and was admitted to the hospital 15 hours ago and now has a plasma glucose concentration of 400 mg/dL, and serum ketones are again "strongly positive." She had been doing well on an insulin infusion (5 U/h), fluids, and potassium replacement. When her glucose levels had fallen to 196 mg/dL (see the diabetic laboratory flow sheet below) at midnight, the insulin infusion was stopped and a "sliding scale" initiated.

Diabetes Laboratory Flow Sheet

| Time | Glucose (mg/dL) | Serum Ketones | Potassium (meq/L) | $HCO_2$ (meq/L) |
|---|---|---|---|---|
| 12 noon | 686 | Strongly positive | 6.0 | 6 |
| 3 PM | 424 | Strongly positive | 5.1 | 9 |
| 6 PM | 336 | Moderate | 4.4 | 12 |
| 9 PM | 241 | Slight | 4.6 | 14 |
| 12 midnight | 196 | Absent | 4.8 | 16 |
| 3 AM | 400 | Strongly positive | 5.2 | 14 |

What is the most likely cause of the increase in the patient's plasma glucose concentration at 3 AM?

(A) Subcutaneous insulin was not administered when the infusion was stopped

(B) Inadequate replacement of potassium affected the action of insulin

(C) The patient has an undetected occult infection

(D) The patient has undetected occult hyperthyroidism

(E) The patient is pregnant and resistant to insulin

### Diabetes Mellitus Question 7

A 56-year-old overweight woman has had urinary frequency, nocturia, and dysuria for 5 days. She also reports increasing thirst.

On physical examination, her temperature is normal, she appears dehydrated, and has no costovertebral angle tenderness. Her plasma glucose concentration is 620 mg/dL. Urinalysis reveals 4+ glucose, no ketones, strongly positive protein, and 8 to 10 leukocytes per high-power field. Antibiotic therapy is begun for the urinary tract infection.

Which one of the following therapies is the most appropriate at this time?

(A) Sulfonylurea

(B) Diet and exercise program

(C) Insulin

(D) Metformin

(E) α-Glucosidase inhibitor

### Diabetes Mellitus Question 8

A 64-year-old woman who has had type 2 diabetes mellitus for 8 years is evaluated because of fatigue and irritability. She has been taking combination therapy with glyburide and metformin, and her two most recent hemoglobin $A_{1C}$ measurements were 6.8% and 7.2%. She cannot sleep at night because of severe pain in both feet and ankles; the pain is aggravated when the bed sheets touch her feet, and on occasion the foot pain is accompanied by lancinating pains in both legs. Exercise or movement sometimes eases the pain. On physical examination, both ankle reflexes are absent, and decreased vibratory sensation is noted in both feet.

Which of the following is the most likely diagnosis?

(A) Cauda equina syndrome

(B) Diabetic peripheral neuropathy

(C) L3-L4 herniated disk

(D) Spinal cord infarction

### Diabetes Mellitus Question 9

A 48-year-old man who has had type 1 diabetes mellitus for 28 years had coronary artery bypass grafting 2 days ago. His most recent hemoglobin $A_{1C}$ was 7.2%. In the hospital, he has been on a standard sliding scale where plasma glucose is measured every 4 hours and graduated doses of regular insulin are administered depending on plasma glucose, for example, 5 U for 200/ mg dL; 7 U for 250 mg/dL. Since he has begun eating again, his plasma glucose concentration has fluctuated widely from severe hyperglycemia to hypoglycemia levels. Serum potassium and carbon dioxide values are within the normal range.

In addition to stopping the sliding scale, which one of the following should be done to better control his plasma glucose?

(A) Reinstitute his prehospital insulin schedule

(B) Initiate intermediate-acting insulin with regular insulin supplements

(C) Initiate an insulin infusion

(D) Initiate metformin

### Diabetes Mellitus Question 10

A 64-year-old woman with type 2 diabetes mellitus is evaluated because of nocturia (she urinates three times nightly), a vaginal infection, and progressive fatigue for the past month. She has been obese since early adulthood, and developed diabetes mellitus just after her menopause 17 years ago. Initially she responded well to sulfonylurea therapy, but 3 years ago her hemoglobin $A_{1C}$ values rose progressively to 8.7% and metformin was added to her regimen. Fasting plasma glucose is constantly above 200 mg/dL, and most postprandial values exceed 250 mg/dL.

What is the most appropriate therapy for this patient?

(A) Start morning NPH insulin; maintain sulfonylurea and discontinue metformin

(B) Start morning NPH insulin; maintain metformin and discontinue sulfonylurea

(C) Start bedtime NPH insulin; maintain sulfonylurea and discontinue metformin

(D) Start bedtime NPH insulin; maintain metformin and discontinue sulfonylurea

### Diabetes Mellitus Question 11

A 52-year-old woman was diagnosed with type 2 diabetes mellitus 3 months ago, with a fasting blood glucose of 192 mg/dL and hemoglobin $A_{1C}$ of 8.8%. After completing an educational nutrition and exercise program, she still weighs 104.5 kg (230 lb), and her fasting plasma glucose values are in the 180 to 220 mg/dL range. All presupper values exceed 200 mg/dL, and her hemoglobin $A_{1C}$ is 8.7%.

Which of the following is the best therapy for this patient?

(A) Metformin

(B) Bedtime insulin therapy

(C) An α-glucosidase inhibitor

(D) A thiazolidinedione

**Diabetes Mellitus Question 12**

A 69-year-old man has had well-controlled type 2 diabetes mellitus for 12 years. His therapy consists of metformin with meals; his renal function has been normal. The patient develops severe fatigue and shortness of breath, and an acute anterior myocardial infarction is diagnosed. He is scheduled for a coronary angiography.

Which one of the following should be done with the metformin at the time of the procedure?

(A) Continue metformin
(B) Continue metformin and add regular insulin
(C) Permanently discontinue metformin
(D) Discontinue metformin on the day of the procedure

**Diabetes Mellitus Question 13**

A 31-year-old woman who has had type 1 diabetes mellitus for 12 years is evaluated because of "hypoglycemic reactions" 30 to 45 minutes after eating. She has also recently developed abdominal fullness and belching. Her glycemic control has been good, with hemoglobin $A_{1C}$ values that range from 6.0% to 6.8%. For control of postprandial hyperglycemia, she injects 4 to 6 units of lispro insulin before each meal.

Which of the following is the best explanation for the hypoglycemia?

(A) Diabetic peripheral neuropathy
(B) Diabetic nephropathy
(C) Diabetic gastropathy
(D) Diabetic retinopathy

**Diabetes Mellitus Question 14**

Which one of the following describes the effect of the thiazolidinediones?

(A) Inducing weight loss effect
(B) Decreasing low-density lipoprotein cholesterol
(C) Increasing production of insulin from pancreatic beta cells
(D) Increasing glucose transporter expression

**Diabetes Mellitus Question 15**

A 24-year-old woman who has had type 1 diabetes mellitus for 15 years is evaluated for several episodes of severe hypoglycemia. Her most recent hemoglobin $A_{1C}$ value was 5.4%. This morning she was involved in a motor vehicle accident, and her plasma glucose was measured at 23 mg/dL, although she denied any symptoms of a "reaction."

Hypoglycemia unawareness in this patient most likely is due to which of the following?

(A) Inappropriate timing of insulin injections
(B) Progressive loss of glucagon response to hypoglycemia
(C) Diminished autonomic responses
(D) Defective production of epinephrine in the adrenal medulla
(E) Increased sensitivity of cerebral tissue for glucose

**Diabetes Mellitus Question 16**

A 50-year-old man who has had type 2 diabetes mellitus for 12 years is concerned about becoming dependent on dialysis. His disease has been inadequately controlled (hemoglobin $A_{1c}$ range, 8.7% to 11.8%). His urinalysis is strongly positive for protein, and his serum creatinine concentration has increased from 1.2 to 1.9 mg/dL in the past 8 months. His blood pressure has been 150/90 mm Hg and on occasion as high as 210/120 mm Hg.

Which of the following is the most important factor delaying the onset of dialysis?

(A) Hgb $A_{1c}$ less than 7%
(B) Blood pressure controlled to less than 130/80 mm Hg
(C) LDL cholesterol < 100 mg/dL
(D) Protein-restricted diet
(E) Low-dose aspirin use

**Diabetes Mellitus Question 17**

A 52-year-old woman is found to have a fasting plasma glucose concentration of 168 mg/dL during her annual physical examination. Her lifestyle is sedentary. Obesity has been a problem since early adulthood, and her weight in recent years has ranged from 90 to 103 kg (196 to 226 lb). Her blood pressure has been elevated for the past 18 years, and while taking captopril, it is in the 160/90 to 180/100 range. The hemoglobin $A_{1C}$ level is 8.4%.

After meeting with a dietitian and nurse educator, she starts a calorie-restricted diet and an exercise program; 6 weeks later, she weighs 91.8 kg (202 lb) and her hemoglobin $A_{1C}$ is 8.6%. Other laboratory tests include a total cholesterol of 238 mgldL and a fasting triglyceride level of 278 mgldL.

What is the best hypoglycemic agent for this patient?

(A) Insulin
(B) A sulfonylurea
(C) Metformin
(D) Acarbose
(E) Rosiglitazone

**Diabetes Mellitus Question 18**

Which one of the following statements about diabetic microalbuminuria is correct?

(A) It is indicative of early diabetic nephropathy
(B) Almost all patients with microalbuminuria develop overt nephropathy within 10 years
(C) It does not influence the risk of cardiovascular disease
(D) Optimal therapy includes controlling the blood pressure with nifedipine

**Diabetes Mellitus Question 19**

A 56-year-old man with type 2 diabetes mellitus is evaluated because of polyuria and fatigue. He has a positive family history of diabetes and early coronary artery disease. He gave up cigarettes about 5 years ago but has one or two drinks daily at supper. On physical examination, weight and height are 86 kg (190 lb) and 172 cm (68 in). His blood pressure is 142/88 mm Hg. His fasting plasma glucose level is 190 mg/dL, hemoglobin $A_{1c}$ level is 11.1%, and total fasting cholesterol is 308 mg/dL. A resting electrocardiogram and exercise stress electrocardiogram are normal.

After participating in a cardiovascular fitness program and seeing a dietitian about his diet, he returns 2 months later, having lost 8 kg (17.6 lb). At this point, his fasting plasma glucose level has decreased to 130 mg/dL, hemoglobin $A_{1c}$ has decreased to 9.2%, and fasting cholesterol level is 294 mg/dL.

Which one of the following is the next management step?

(A) Begin an oral sulfonylurea agent
(B) Measure his fasting C-peptide levels
(C) Measure his fasting lipoprotein profile
(D) Restrict his alcohol intake

## Diabetes Mellitus Question 20

A 15-year-old male high-school student is evaluated because of thirst, frequent urination, and a weight loss of 3 kg (7 lb) over a 3-week period. Physical examination shows mild dehydration. His random plasma glucose level measures 468 mg/dL. Urinalysis shows glucosuria and a trace of ketones.

Which one of the following measurements would you ascertain before initiating insulin treatment?

(A) Islet cell and insulin autoantibody titers
(B) Glutamic acid decarboxylase (GAD) antibody titer
(C) Plasma insulin and C-peptide levels, fasting and after glucagon stimulation
(D) None of the above

## Diabetes Mellitus Question 21

A 32-year-old man with type 1 diabetes mellitus develops progressive hypertension and edema. A specimen of his urine under polarized light microscopy is shown.

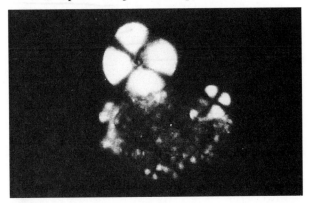

What is the most likely diagnosis?

(A) Pyelonephritis
(B) Nephrotic syndrome
(C) Interstitial nephritis
(D) Hypertensive nephropathy
(E) Bladder cancer

## Diabetes Mellitus Question 22

A 41-year-old man with type 1 diabetes mellitus has a funduscopic examination during a routine office visit. The findings are seen on the funduscopic photograph (see Figure 26 in the color plates).

What does the funduscopic photograph on the left show?

(A) Diabetic background retinopathy
(B) Diabetic proliferative retinopathy
(C) Diabetic macular degeneration
(D) Papilledema

## Diabetes Mellitus Question 23

A 70-year-old woman has developed weakness and numbness of her legs and arms during the past 8 months. The symptoms began with tingling in her feet. Later, severe weakness gradually developed. For 2 years, she has been taking oral hypoglycemic agents to treat diabetes.

On physical examination, the patient has a pulse rate of 70/min and a blood pressure of 120/85 mm Hg. She cannot rise from her chair without pushing off with her arms. She has moderately severe weakness (3/5) of the thigh and lower leg muscles. There is little movement remaining in her feet and toes (1/5). Her hands are also very weak (2/5). She has no deep tendon reflexes in her lower extremities. Vibration sensation and position sense are slightly reduced at the toes and malleoli. Pinprick and touch sensations are normal. Her toes do not move in response to plantar stimulation. Fasting plasma glucose level is 95 mg/dL; the 2-hour postprandial plasma glucose level is 125 mg/dL. $HgbA_{1C}$ is 5.6%.

Which of the following is the most likely diagnosis?

(A) Spinal cord tumor
(B) Polymyositis
(C) Hemispheric stroke
(D) Chronic inflammatory demyelinating polyneuropathy

# HIV Disease

### HIV Disease Question 1
A 30-year-old homosexual man is evaluated because of numerous asymptomatic skin lesions on his face and neck. Physical examination reveals a scaly rash involving the nasolabial folds, eyebrows, and scalp. Results of laboratory tests include a positive HIV antibody and a CD4 count of $50/\mu L$. Several months following the initiation of highly active antiretroviral therapy (HAART), the CD4 count increases to $500/\mu L$, and the viral load is reduced to undetectable levels.

The patient's skin lesions are most likely to:

(A) Remain stable
(B) Slowly progress
(C) Resolve
(D) Become secondarily infected
(E) Transform into a malignancy

### HIV Disease Question 2
A 42-year-old man with HIV infection and a CD4 cell count of $380/\mu L$ is evaluated because of fever, night sweats, and weight loss of 2.2 kg (5 lb). Two months ago, he started an antiretroviral regimen of ritonavir, saquinavir, stavudine, and lamivudine. He has lived in New York City his entire life. He has never used injection drugs and does not currently smoke. The CD4 cell count prior to starting antiretroviral therapy was $240/\mu L$, and a plasma HIV viral load that was 500,000 copies/mL fell below the limit of detection. He takes no other medications. His physical examination is normal except for an enlarged right cervical lymph node. Chest radiograph is normal.

Based on the clinical presentation, which of the following is the most likely diagnosis?

(A) Lymphoma
(B) Histoplasmosis
(C) *Mycobacterium avium* complex infection
(D) *Mycobacterium tuberculosis* infection
(E) Toxoplasmosis

### HIV Disease Question 3
A 43-year-old man comes to the emergency department with a 3-day history of fever and malaise. On physical examination, he has a maculopapular rash and shotty cervical lymphadenopathy. The patient reports that 3 weeks ago he had several high-risk sexual encounters. Three days ago, an enzyme-linked immunosorbent assay (ELISA) for HIV was negative.

Which of the following findings would most likely indicate that this patient has acute HIV infection?

(A) Positive plasma p24 antigen test
(B) Plasma HIV viral load of 600 copies/mL
(C) Western blot showing a single band against p24
(D) Positive repeat ELISA
(E) CD4 cell count of $90/\mu L$

### HIV Disease Question 4
A 39-year-old woman is referred for evaluation because she had a positive enzyme-linked immunosorbent assay (ELISA) and an indeterminate Western blot for HIV when she attempted to donate blood 6 weeks ago. She has been healthy all her life. She lives with her husband and five children. Her husband had gonorrhea 1 year ago and travels extensively in South America. You repeat the ELISA and Western blot. She again has a positive ELISA. The Western blot shows only a single band against gp41 (same as 6 weeks before).

Which of the following is most appropriate at this time?

(A) Reassure the patient that she does not have HIV
(B) Measure her plasma HIV viral load
(C) Perform a specific test for HIV-2
(D) Perform a p24 antigen test
(E) Begin antiretroviral therapy

### HIV Disease Question 5
A 26-year-old surgical resident is placing a central venous line in a patient with advanced HIV infection. During the procedure, the resident sustains a deep percutaneous injury to her gloved hand from the 18-gauge needle that was used to thread the catheter into the vein. She immediately washes the injury. The source patient has a CD4 cell count of $10/\mu L$ and a recent plasma HIV viral load of 300,000 copies/mL. The source patient's prior antiretroviral therapy included stavudine, didanosine, and nevirapine.

Which of the following would be appropriate to offer to the health-care worker?

(A) Zidovudine monotherapy
(B) Zidovudine, lamivudine, and nelfinavir
(C) No therapy
(D) HIV serologic testing

## HIV Disease Question 6

A 32-year-old nurse working in a neonatal intensive care unit sustains a percutaneous injury with HIV-contaminated blood.

Which of the following tests should be done to document occupational exposure to HIV infection?

(A) HIV p24 antigen assay
(B) HIV RNA polymerase chain reaction (PCR)
(C) HIV DNA PCR
(D) HIV enzyme-linked immunosorbent assay (ELISA)

## HIV Disease Question 7

A 36-year-old woman tests positive for HIV antibodies. The patient has a CD4 cell count of 756/µL and a plasma HIV viral load of 2,000 copies/mL. She is asymptomatic, works full time as an investment banker, and travels extensively. Physical examination and results of routine laboratory studies are normal.

Which of the following management options is consistent with current guidelines?

(A) Zidovudine, lamivudine, and abacavir
(B) Zidovudine and lamivudine
(C) Aidovudine, lamivudine, and nevirapine
(D) Observation only

## HIV Disease Question 8

A 27-year-old man is evaluated because of a 1-week history of fever, malaise, pharyngitis, and a diffuse rash. He reports unprotected sex with a new partner 3 weeks earlier. On physical examination, he has tender cervical lymphadenopathy and a tonsillar ulcer.

The results of an HIV enzyme-linked immunosorbent assay (ELISA) are negative; however, the HIV RNA polymerase chain reaction (PCR) is positive at 900,000 copies/mL. The CD4 cell count is 627/µL with a ratio of CD4+/CD8+ cells of 0.63. The patient is reluctant to start treatment.

When should antiretroviral therapy be initiated in this patient?

(A) When the HIV RNA PCR reaches 15,000 copies/mL
(B) When the patient develops oral thrush
(C) When the patient is ready and willing to begin therapy
(D) When the CD4 cell count decreases below 500/µL

## HIV Disease Question 9

A 26-year-old woman with HIV infection is evaluated because of fever, cough, and shortness of breath for the past week. She has not been taking any medications for her HIV infection and has not been receiving regular follow-up care. Her CD4 cell count was 80/µL 1 year ago.

On physical examination, her temperature is 38.5 °C (101.3 °F), pulse rate is 120/min, respiration rate is 18/min, and blood pressure is 120/70 mm Hg. She is breathing comfortably without oxygen but has frequent paroxysms of a dry cough. She has a white exudate on her buccal mucosa, slightly enlarged cervical lymph nodes, and bibasilar dry crackles. The examination is otherwise normal. An induced sputum specimen is sent to the laboratory for staining for *Pneumocystis carinii*. Gram-stained sputum sample shows rare epithelial cells, a few polymorphonuclear cells, and no organisms.

Which of the following tests will be the most helpful in determining which therapy to institute in the next few hours?

(A) Complete blood count with differential
(B) Serum lactate dehydrogenase determination
(C) Measurement of T-cell subsets
(D) Arterial blood gas study

## HIV Disease Question 10

A 47-year-old man with HIV infection is admitted to the hospital in January complaining of shortness of breath and a persistent cough for 2 weeks. He has had a CD4 cell count of 340/µL and a plasma HIV viral load of less than 50 copies/mL. Chest radiograph on admission shows bibasilar infiltrates with a mixed interstitial-alveolar pattern and a right-sided pleural effusion. Oxygen saturation on room air is 92% by pulse oximetry. Fiberoptic bronchoscopy shows a red-purple lesion on the mucosa of the right mainstem bronchus. This lesion is 1 cm in diameter, raised, and nonulcerated. Biopsy specimens from the lesion were not obtained. Results of the bronchoalveolar lavage analysis are pending.

Which of the following is the most likely diagnosis?

(A) Disseminated herpes simplex
(B) Kaposi's sarcoma
(C) Leukocytoclastic vasculitis
(D) Immune thrombocytopenic purpura

## HIV Disease Question 11

A 42-year-old woman with HIV infection is admitted to the hospital with fever, shortness of breath, and hypoxemia. An induced sputum sample is positive for *Pneumocystis carinii*. Therapy with trimethoprim-sulfamethoxazole and prednisone is started. On the sixth day of treatment, she has a temperature to 39 °C (102.2 °F) after being afebrile for the past 3 days. Physical examination shows an erythematous rash on her trunk and extremities that progresses to involve the buccal mucosa and conjunctivae over the next 24 hours. In addition, she has developed diarrhea and moderate nausea.

In addition to stopping the trimethoprim-sulfamethoxazole, which of the following is the most appropriate treatment option for the pneumonia?

(A) Prednisone
(B) Intravenous pentamidine
(C) Aerosolized pentamidine
(D) Oral atovaquone

**HIV Disease Question 12**
A 32-year-old man is evaluated because of painful lesions in the mouth and a history of dysphagia. He was diagnosed with HIV infection 1 year ago but has had no systemic complications of this disease. On physical examination, he has diffusely distributed white plaques and erythema on the tongue. He also has palpable cervical adenopathy.

Which of the following tests should be done first to establish the diagnosis?

(A) Tzanck smear
(B) Potassium hydroxide preparation
(C) Biopsy
(D) Bacterial culture
(E) Polymerase chain reaction for herpesvirus DNA

**HIV Disease Question 13**
A 27-year-old, HIV-positive man presents with multiple, purple pedunculated nodules on his skin. He says that these lesions have spread rapidly and have a tendency to bleed. In the previous 2 weeks, he has had intermittent fevers and general malaise.

The most likely diagnosis is:

(A) Kaposi's sarcoma
(B) Pyogenic granulomas
(C) Bacillary angiomatosis
(D) Secondary syphilis
(E) Cutaneous cryptococcosis

**HIV Disease Question 14**
A 30-year-old man with recently diagnosed HIV infection is evaluated because of the lesion (see Figure 30 in the color plates) shown on the inside of his mouth.

Which of the following is the most likely diagnosis?

(A) Oral hairy leukoplakia
(B) Lichen planus
(C) Leukoplakia
(D) Oral candidiasis

**HIV Disease Question 15**
A 30-year-old man with recently diagnosed HIV infection is evaluated because of the lesion (see Figure 27 in the color plates) shown on the inside of his mouth.

Which of the following is the most likely diagnosis?

(A) Oral hairy leukoplakia
(B) Lichen planus
(C) Leukoplakia
(D) Oral candidiasis

**HIV Disease Question 16**
A 30-year-old, HIV-positive man develops fever, headache, and altered behavior. An MRI scan of his brain is obtained.

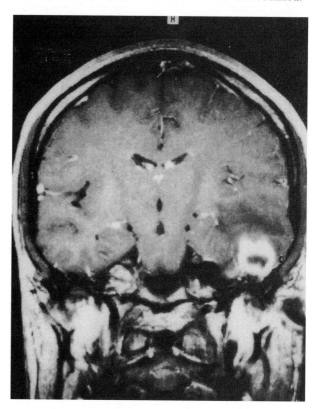

Which of the following is the most likely diagnosis?

(A) HIV dementia
(B) Cerebral toxoplasmosis
(C) Cerebral edema
(D) Thromboembolic stroke
(E) Central nervous system lymphoma

## HIV Disease Question 17

A 45-year-old man who is HIV positive has had fever, headaches, and lethargy for the past 2 weeks. Physical examination reveals an ill-appearing man who is arousable only to loud voices. Diffuse spasticity, hyperreflexia, and bilateral, upward-going plantar reflexes are present. A contrast-enhanced CT scan of the brain is obtained.

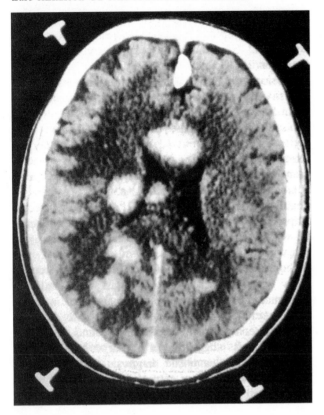

Which of the following is the most likely diagnosis?

(A) HIV dementia
(B) Cerebral toxoplasmosis
(C) Cerebral edema
(D) Thromboembolic stroke
(E) CNS lymphoma

## HIV Disease Question 18

A 27-year-old man is evaluated because of a witnessed grand mal seizure. The patient is alert and oriented but does not remember the seizure. He was found to be HIV-infected 8 years ago and had a CD4 cell count of 175/µL 1 month ago when he was seen for renewal of his prescriptions. He is taking didanosine , fluconazole, and trimethoprim-sulfamethoxazole. Review of the medical records reveals that an IgG serology for *Toxoplasma* species was negative 2 months previously.

His physical examination reveals hairy leukoplakia and a mild weakness in his right leg. Computed tomography (CT) of the head reveals two large lesions in the left parietal area. The lesions are 3 cm and 2 cm in size, respectively, and enhance slightly with contrast medium. There is edema surrounding each lesion.

Which of the following is the best management option?

(A) A trial of trimethoprim-sulfamethoxazole
(B) A trial of trimethoprim-sulfamethoxazole with dexamethasone
(C) A CT-guided needle brain biopsy
(D) An open brain biopsy
(E) *Toxoplasma* antibody

## HIV Disease Question 19

A 40-year-old man with HIV infection is admitted to the hospital because he has had fever, cough, dyspnea, and weight loss for the past 3 weeks. He takes no medications. Physical examination shows a temperature of 38.7 °C (101.7 °F), oral thrush, crackles at both lung bases, and a violaceous skin lesion consistent with Kaposi's sarcoma.

Laboratory studies show the following:

| | |
|---|---|
| Hematocrit | 33% |
| Leukocyte count | 3200/µL |
| CD4 cell count | 144/µL |

Arterial blood studies on room air:

| | |
|---|---|
| $PaO_2$ | 69 mm Hg |
| $PaCO_2$ | 30 mm Hg |
| pH | 7.52 |

Chest radiograph shows diffuse, bilateral interstitial infiltrates. A sample of induced sputum is negative on stains for *Pneumocystis carinii*, acid-fast bacilli, and bacterial organisms.

What is the most appropriate next step in the evaluation of the patient?

(A) Bronchoscopy with bronchoalveolar lavage
(B) Gallium lung scanning
(C) Empiric trial of trimethoprim-sulfamethoxazole
(D) Ventilation-perfusion lung scanning
(E) CT scan of the chest

## HIV Disease Question 20

A 50-year-old man is evaluated because of a 3-month history of fevers, weight loss, night sweats, and a productive cough. The patient denies injection drug use or high-risk homosexual activity but admits to a history of multiple heterosexual encounters involving prostitutes.

On physical examination, the patient has a temperature of 39 °C (102.2 °F) and bilateral supraclavicular and axillary adenopathy. Laboratory findings include an absolute CD4 cell count of 350/µL and a positive HIV serology. A chest radiograph shows bilateral interstitial infiltrates. An acid-fast organism is isolated from sputum and bronchoalveolar lavage fluid.

Which of the following acid-fast organisms is the most likely cause of this patient's infection?

(A) *Mycobacterium avium-intracellulare* complex
(B) *Rhodococcus equi*
(C) *Mycobacterium tuberculosis*
(D) *Nocardia* species
(E) *Cryptosporidium* species

## HIV Disease Question 21

A 32-year-old homosexual man is evaluated because of a painful anal ulcer. His latest CD4 lymphocyte count was 214/µL and his viral load was 3450 copies/mL on combination therapy with stavudine, didanosine, and nelfinavir. His weight has been stable, and he denies symptoms of fever, night sweats, or diarrhea. On physical examination, he is not in any acute distress. He is afebrile. There is no skin rash. He has some lymphadenopathy in the cervical region but no enlarged lymph nodes elsewhere. Examination of the anal area reveals a clean, tender ulcer measuring 2 cm x 3 cm at the anal verge. The edges of the ulcer are serpiginous but not raised, and there are no papules or vesicles. Rectal examination is painful but otherwise unremarkable, and there is no mucus or pus on the glove. The rest of his physical examination is unremarkable.

Which of the following will be most useful in diagnosing the cause of the anal ulceration?

(A) Viral culture
(B) Biopsy
(C) Polymerase chain reaction (PCR) for human papillomavirus
(D) VDRL
(E) Bacterial culture

## HIV Disease Question 22

A 35-year-old woman was recently diagnosed with HIV infection. Her CD4 count is 150/µL, and her HIV viral load is 160,000 copies/mL. She starts antiretroviral therapy with zidovudine, lamivudine, and indinavir. In addition, she starts prophylaxis for *Pneumocystis carinii* pneumonia with trimethoprim-sulfamethoxazole. She is evaluated 10 days later because of fever to 40 °C (104 °F). On physical examination, she looks extremely unwell. She is febrile and has a diffuse, pruritic, macular, blanching, erythematous eruption that is maximal on the chest and abdomen. She denies any respiratory symptoms, and examination of the heart and lungs is normal.

Laboratory studies include a hemoglobin of 11.2 g/dL and leukocyte count of 4,200/dL with no eosinophils.

Which of the following is the most likely cause of her fever?

(A) *Pneumocystis carinii* pneumonia
(B) Disseminated *Mycobacterium avium* infection
(C) Hypersensitivity reaction to zidovudine
(D) Hypersensitivity reaction to trimethoprim-sulfamethoxazole
(E) Bacterial pneumonia

# Answers, Critiques,
# and Bibliographies

# Cough

## Cough Question 1
### Answer: A

**Educational Objective:** *Manage persistent nonproductive cough.*

Postnasal drip syndrome is the most common cause of persistent cough, followed by asthma and gastroesophageal reflux. In the absence of symptoms or signs suggesting the latter two causes, and with some abnormality of the nasal mucosa detected, a treatment trial of decongestant-antihistamine is the best method both to establish the diagnosis and treat the condition. Treatment trials of proton-pump inhibitors or inhaled bronchodilators might be appropriate if the trial of decongestant-antihistamine is unsuccessful, or if the history and physical examination suggest the presence of asthma or gastroesophageal reflux.

Additional tests, including chest computed tomography, bronchoscopy, sinus radiographs, or methacholine challenge, are commonly ordered, but such tests have a low yield in the absence of specific clinical findings suggesting lung or sinus disease.

### Bibliography
1. **Palombini BC, Villanova CA, Araujo E, Gastal OL, Alt DC, Stolz DP, Palombini CO**. A pathogenic triad in chronic cough: asthma, postnasal drip syndrome, and gastroesophageal reflux disease. Chest. 1999;116:279-84. PMID: 10453852

## Cough Question 2
### Answer: A

**Educational Objective:** *Follow a step-by-step approach to managing a cough in a patient receiving an angiotensin-converting enzyme inhibitor.*

Cough secondary to an angiotensin-converting enzyme (ACE) inhibitor can occur at any time during the course of therapy. However, prior to stopping a drug that has adequately controlled this patient's blood pressure, other sources of cough should be excluded. Cough can be a manifestation of heart failure, and an echocardiogram can determine if there has been disease progression. A CT scan of the chest is not warranted unless a chest radiograph shows unsuspected pathologic findings. A cough due to an ACE inhibitor may not resolve for up to 2 weeks after drug discontinuation. There is no evidence of a pneumonic process that would warrant bronchoscopy or a course of antibiotics at this time. Pulmonary function tests may be indicated if a pulmonary cause is suspected for a persistent cough. However, progression of cardiac disease should be ruled out first.

### Bibliography
1. **Aurup P**. Tackling ACE-inhibitor cough. Lancet. 1997;350:1854-5. PMID: 9428279

## Cough Question 3
### Answer: B

**Educational Objective:** *Evaluate patients with chronic cough.*

The single most common cause of chronic cough in adults is postnasal drip syndrome. In one study, it accounted for 41% of all causes of cough. Postnasal drip can be due to sinusitis, allergic rhinitis, perennial nonallergic rhinitis, postinfectious rhinitis, vasomotor rhinitis, drug-induced rhinitis, or environmental irritant-induced rhinitis. It should be considered a possible diagnosis when patients describe a sensation of having something drip down into the throat, a frequent need to clear the throat, or frequent nasal discharge. It should also be considered when a physical examination of the nasopharynx or oropharynx reveals mucoid or mucopurulent secretions or a cobblestone appearance to the mucosa. If the history or physical examination suggests postnasal drip syndrome, sinus radiographs, computed tomographic (CT) scans of the sinuses, and an allergy evaluation should be considered. However, in this case the patient had no suggestion of postnasal drip syndrome.

Asthma, characteristically associated with measurable airway hyperresponsiveness, is the second most common cause of chronic cough. Asthmatic cough is likely caused by the underlying inflammatory process stimulating sensory nerves serving the cough reflex. Asthma should be considered a possible cause of cough in patients with episodic wheezing and shortness of breath. However, cough may be the sole presenting manifestation of asthma, and in one study 28% of asthmatic patients who presented with cough had no other symptoms or signs of asthma. Since this is a common cause of cough alone and previous pulmonary function testing did not suggest a cause, bronchoprovocation challenge should be obtained as the next best test to arrive at a definitive diagnosis. Bronchoprovocation testing involves assessing bronchial reactivity by measuring the $FEV_1$ before and after challenging the patient with increasing doses of a pharmacologic bronchoconstrictor (methacholine or histamine) or stimulus such as cold air or exercise that can cause bronchoconstriction. After this treatment, a decrease in the $FEV_1$ of 15% to 20% is an indication of bronchial hyperresponsiveness, which is the hallmark of bronchial asthma.

Gastroesophageal reflux is the third most common cause of chronic cough and accounts for about 21% of all cases. Gastroesophageal reflux should be considered the cause of chronic cough when patients complain of heartburn, a sour taste in their mouth, or regurgitation; when upper gastrointestinal contrast radiographs show reflux of barium to the mid-esophagus or higher; when esophagoscopy shows esophagitis; or when esophageal pH monitoring shows cough to be associated with reflux episodes even in the absence of gastrointestinal symptoms. Because the patient had no gastrointestinal symptoms and the definitive test, which is esophageal pH monitoring, is invasive and usually done only in some centers, this should be performed when other more common causes have been excluded.

Other causes of cough are chronic bronchitis, bronchiectasis, use of angiotensin-converting enzyme inhibitors, bronchogenic and metastatic carcinomas, sarcoidosis, left ventricular failure, and aspiration from a Zenker's diverticulum. Only when the most common conditions have been ruled out or seem unlikely should other less common conditions be seriously considered, and then a CT scan of the chest, fiberoptic bronchoscopy, and/or echocardiography should be obtained.

### Bibliography

1. **Irwin RS, Curley FJ, French CL**. Chronic cough. The spectrum and frequency of causes, key components of the diagnostic evaluation, and outcome of specific therapy. Am Rev Respir Dis. 1990;141:640-7. PMID: 2178528
2. **Irwin RS, Curley FJ**. The treatment of cough. A comprehensive review. Chest. 1991;99:1477-84. PMID: 2036833

## Cough Question 4
## Answer: B

**Educational Objective:** *Understand the pathogenesis, epidemiology, and clinical findings of the interstitial disorders.*

Idiopathic pulmonary fibrosis (IPF) is the most common interstitial form of pneumonia and often is associated with nail clubbing. Asbestosis is commonly associated with nail clubbing but is unlikely in this case because of lack of exposure. Although there is some concern about asbestos in school buildings, exposures in schools are rarely at the level necessary to cause asbestosis. Other interstitial forms of pneumonia are less common and do not have associated nail clubbing. Acute interstitial pneumonia is more rapidly progressive than is IPF. Respiratory bronchiolitis associated interstitial pneumonia and desquamative interstitial pneumonia are rare among persons who do not smoke. Nonspecific interstitial pneumonia is less common and occurs among younger patients but is otherwise clinically indistinguishable from IPF. Bronchiolitis obliterans organizing pneumonia and desquamative interstitial pneu-

monia often present an alveolar pattern on chest radiographs. Sarcoidosis usually has less prominent auscultatory findings and a variety of radiographic patterns.

Bacterial pneumonia is unlikely considering the long duration of symptoms and absence of fever. The pulmonary function tests and chest x-ray are not compatible with pulmonary embolism or congestive heart failure.

### Bibliography

1. **Katzenstein AL, Myers JL**. Idiopathic pulmonary fibrosis: clinical relevance of pathologic classification. Am J Respir Crit Care Med. 1998;157:1301-15. PMID: 9563754

## Cough Question 5
## Answer: B

**Educational Objective:** *Review common clinical features of occupational asthma and understand the best management of occupational asthma.*

The patient has adult-onset asthma. He is middle-aged, does not smoke, has no history of allergies or asthma, and has a cough, wheezing, and reversible airflow obstruction. The exposure to chemicals in the workplace suggests occupational asthma. Auto-body repair with spray painting is an occupation commonly associated with asthma induced by workplace exposure. In this environment, urethane paint containing isocyanates is the likely sensitizing agent. Once someone is sensitized, smaller and smaller inhalational exposures can trigger asthmatic reactions. It can be stated with relative certainty that with continued exposure to the offending asthmagen in the workplace, this patient's symptoms will worsen over time. Coughing often is an early manifestation of occupational asthma; chest tightness, wheezing, and shortness of breath are likely to follow if exposure continues.

Withdrawal from the workplace exposure is an important first step both in diagnosing occupational asthma and in controlling it. Symptoms of occupational asthma routinely improve during a week away from work and then recur when the person returns to work. Occupational asthma often resolves entirely after removal from the workplace. However, it does not always do so. Prognostic indicators favoring recovery after cessation of exposure include short duration of symptoms before diagnosis and withdrawal, less severe abnormality of lung function at time of diagnosis, and, in some studies, a milder degree of bronchial hyperresponsiveness.

Standard antiasthma therapies, such as bronchodilators and inhaled glucocorticoids, are effective in controlling occupational asthma and constitute standard care. Radioallergosorbent tests to detect specific IgE antibodies are unreliable in assessing occupational asthma. The test often is not available for the specific, suspected sensitizing agent. Even when the tests are available, a positive result indicates only sensitization and does not give conclusive evidence of disease caused by the agent. In any case, the suspected agent for this patient, who is exposed to spray paint, is isocyanates, not anhydrides. Measuring carbon monoxide diffusing capacity has no role in the management of occupational asthma.

**Bibliography**

1. **Chan-Yeung M, Malo JL.** Occupational asthma. N Engl J Med. 1995;333:107-12. PMID: 7777015

## Cough Question 6
## Answer: D

**Educational Objective:** *Recognize cough-variant asthma and prescribe appropriate therapy.*

The patient has postviral airways hyperresponsiveness syndrome. This is also sometimes called *cough-variant asthma.* Inhalation of glucocorticoids, such as budesonide, is the therapy of choice for mild persistent asthma, even if mild. β-Antagonists and angiotensin-converting enzyme inhibitors are not likely to help; in fact, either of these types of drugs may worsen the patient's condition. Because the chest radiographic findings are normal and because the results of a sputum culture are negative, bacterial infection is unlikely, and antibiotics are not beneficial. Dextromethorphan and glyceryl guaiacolate may provide some symptomatic relief as cough suppressants for nonspecific coughing, but they have not been shown to be of benefit for coughing due to asthma. Nocturnal symptoms often are used to differentiate mild intermittent from mild persistent asthma and are indications for inhaled glucocorticoid therapy.

**Bibliography**

1. **Cheriyan S, Greenberger PA, Patterson R.** Outcome of cough variant asthma treated with inhaled steroids. Ann Allergy. 1994;73:478-80. PMID: 7998659

2. **Folkerts G, Busse WW, Nijkamp FP, Sorkness R, Gern JE.** Virus-induced airway hyperresponsiveness and asthma. Am J Respir Crit Care Med. 1998;157:1708-20. PMID: 9620896

# Dyspnea

## Dyspnea Question 1
### Answer: D

**Educational Objective:** *Recognize that coronary artery disease is a common cause of heart failure in the United States.*

Although it may be tempting to treat this patient symptomatically, it is important to assess the presence of coronary artery disease, particularly because she has new-onset heart failure. In the SOLVD trial, more than 40% of patients with heart failure had coronary artery disease as a causative factor. Coronary disease could be causing this patient's heart failure, even in the absence of chest pain. It is precisely this group of patients with impaired ventricular function who could benefit from revascularization if triple-vessel coronary artery disease is found. Therefore, coronary angiography is appropriate. A myocardial biopsy may be indicated if there is no coronary artery disease and a systemic disorder, such as amyloidosis, is suspected. Even if an inflammatory process is found, there is no evidence that anti-inflammatory agents will ultimately affect outcome. If dyspnea persists after adequate therapy, a pulmonary assessment may be indicated. However, it should not be the initial diagnostic test at this time.

### Bibliography
1. **Gheorghiade M, Bonow RO.** Chronic heart failure in the United States: a manifestation of coronary artery disease. Circulation. 1998;97:282-9. PMID: 9462531

## Dyspnea Question 2
### Answer: C

**Educational Objective:** *Recognize a patient with acute aortic regurgitation due to infective endocarditis.*

This patient has acute aortic regurgitation due to infective endocarditis. A classic finding on physical examination is a diastolic murmur at the left sternal border. The murmur often is lower pitched and shorter in duration than the murmur of chronic regurgitation because of the lower pressure difference between the aorta and the left ventricle in diastole. In patients with acute regurgitation, the left ventricular end-diastolic pressure is markedly elevated as a result of the regurgitate volume entering a small, noncompliant left ventricle. In patients with severe acute regurgitation, the pressures at end-diastole in the aorta and left ventricle are equal. Early mitral valve closure results in a diminished $S_1$.

Only aortic valve insufficiency will produce the clinical findings present in this patient. Pericarditis may be associated with fever and a friction rub but no murmur whereas septic pulmonary emboli and aortitis may present as fever without changes in heart sounds or murmur. Myocarditis is an unlikely diagnosis in an intravenous drug user. The optimal treatment for acute aortic regurgitation is prompt surgical valve replacement.

### Bibliography
1. **Dervan J, Goldberg S**. Acute aortic regurgitation: pathophysiology and management. Cardiovasc Clin. 1986;16:281-8. PMID: 3742525
2. **Vlessis AA, Hovaguimian H, Jaggers J, Ahmad A, Starr A.** Infective endocarditis: ten-year review of medical and surgical therapy. Ann Thorac Surg. 1996;61:1217-22. PMID: 8607686

## Dyspnea Question 3
### Answer: C

**Educational Objective:** *Recognize exertional dyspnea as an anginal equivalent, especially in patients with diabetes mellitus.*

One must be especially suspicious of an anginal equivalent in patients with diabetes mellitus because these patients may be insensitive to anginal discomfort. Thus, exercise electrocardiography should be done. The normal lung and cardiac examination makes chronic obstruction pulmonary disease, pulmonary fibrosis, and aortic stenosis unlikely. Dilated cardiomyopathy is possible but less likely than coronary artery disease, and less treatable. In this patient, a therapeutic trial of nitrates and prophylactic nitroglycerin is indicated. In a patient with diabetes mellitus and hypertension, addition of an angiotensin-converting enzyme (ACE) inhibitor is recommended to treat elevated blood pressure and prevent progressive vascular disease. Even in the absence of hypertension, low-dose ACE inhibitor therapy is effective in reducing the risk of death, myocardial infarction, or heart failure in patients at risk for these events. Renal and ocular complications of diabetes mellitus are also reduced.

### Bibliography
1. **Ilia R, Carmel S, Carlos C, Gueron M**. Relation between shortness of breath, left ventricular end diastolic pressure and severity of coronary artery disease. Int J Cardiol. 1995;52:153-5. PMID: 8749875
2. **Yusuf S, Sleight P, Pogue J, Bosch J, Davies R, Dagenais G**. Effects of an angiotensin-converting-enzyme inhibitor, ramipril, on cardiovascular events in high-risk patients. The Heart Outcomes Prevention Evaluation Study Investigators. N Engl J Med. 2000;342:145-53. PMID: 10639539

## Dyspnea Question 4
## Answer: C

**Educational Objective:** *Recognize salient features of the acute respiratory distress syndrome.*

The acute respiratory distress syndrome (ARDS) is defined by the acute onset of diffuse pulmonary infiltrates in the absence of elevated left atrial pressure (that is, pulmonary capillary wedge pressure $\leq 18$ mm Hg). The onset is usually precipitous and rapidly progressive rather than gradual. There is a spectrum of illness, ranging from acute lung injury with a $PaO_2/FiO_2$ ratio $\leq 300$, to ARDS with a $PaO_2/FiO_2$ ratio $\leq 200$. Acute lung injury and ARDS occur in the United States at a rate of about 70/100,000 and 7/100,000, respectively. Multiple precipitating causes of ARDS have been identified; most common are sepsis and the systemic inflammatory response syndrome, followed by gastric acid aspiration, severe trauma, multiple transfusions, drug ingestions, and near-drowning states.

ARDS results from damage to the alveolar epithelium and capillary endothelium, which results initially in alveolar inflammation, hyaline membrane formation, and edema. Immediately after this acute phase, resolution of the alveolar process begins, with organization of the alveolar exudate and beginning fibrosis. Most patients who survive the acute phase develop resolution of the alveolar exudate and re-epithelialization of the alveolar surfaces with minor, long-term functional impairment. However, a small proportion of these patients develop severe, unrelenting pulmonary fibrosis, respiratory failure, and death due to this process. Based on this latter observation, glucocorticoid therapy has been tried as a means of preventing progressive fibrosis. Results of the first randomized trial of methylprednisolone suggest that outcome could be improved with glucocorticoids.

The mortality rate (40% to 45%) of ARDS remains substantial. Multiple interventions have been tried as potential therapies. Reasonably effective therapeutic measures include the use of positive end-expiratory pressure (PEEP), which may prevent the repetitive opening and closing of small, damaged airway units that can facilitate lung damage. PEEP often significantly improves arterial oxygenation and may allow the inspired oxygen requirement to be reduced. Recently, small tidal volumes (rather than large volumes) have been shown to be associated with better outcomes. Judicious fluid management is also reasonable; however, overhydration can increase extravascular lung water and should be avoided. Additional therapeutic modalities have been investigated, including other anti-inflammatory therapies (cytokine antagonists, ibuprofen, prostaglandin E1), extracorporeal carbon dioxide removal, permissive hypercapnia, and aerosolized surfactant, but most have not been effective. Potentially successful measures currently being evaluated include prone positioning, inhaled nitric oxide, and glucocorticoids.

**Bibliography**
1. **Luce JM**. Acute lung injury and the acute respiratory distress syndrome. Crit Care Med. 1998;26:369-76. PMID: 9468178
2. **Meduri GU, Headley AS, Golden E, Carson SJ, Umberger RA, Kelso T, et al**. Effect of prolonged methylprednisolone therapy in unresolving acute respiratory distress syndrome: a randomized controlled trial. JAMA. 1998;280:159-65. PMID: 9669790

## Dyspnea Question 5
## Answer: C

**Educational Objective:** *Recognize and diagnose cor pulmonale and severe tricuspid regurgitation.*

The clue to the correct answer in this patient lies in the history and physical examination. There are symptoms of increasing hypervolemia in the presence of chronic obstructive pulmonary disease that strongly support the diagnosis of cor pulmonale.

In addition, the murmur and $S_3$ that increase with inspiration are typical in right sided cardiac conditions. Metastatic carcinoma or alcoholic cirrhosis would not produce these cardiac findings. Aortic stenosis is likely to be associated with an early systolic murmur heard at the base of the heart with radiation to the carotid arteries and down the left sternal border. The murmur would not change in intensity with inspiration. The findings of chronic obstructive pulmonary disease and right sided heart failure make coronary artery disease an unlikely diagnosis.

**Bibliography**
1. **Lembo NJ, Dell'Italia LJ, Crawford MH, O'Rourke**. Bedside diagnosis of systolic murmurs. N Engl J Med. 1988;318:1578-8. PMID: 2897627

## Dyspnea Question 6
## Answer: D

**Educational Objective:** *Recognize the appearance of a hydropneumothorax on a chest radiograph and understand its cause.*

Spontaneous pneumothorax is a relatively common event among healthy young persons. The radiographic abnormality is characterized by the loss of normal lung markings in the periphery of the hemithorax and the presence of a well-defined, visceral pleural line at some point between the chest wall and the hilum. Spontaneous pneumothorax occurs when a subpleural bleb ruptures into the pleural space, an event that commonly occurs during exertion. The presence of air within the pleural space allows the lung to collapse toward the hilum. Frequently, a small amount of bleeding accompanies rupture of the bleb and produces a characteristic appearance of a flat-line junction between the air and the fluid that collects at the base of the hemithorax; this is known as a hydropneumothorax. Large pneumothoraces require insertion of a chest tube to drain the pleural space and reexpand the lung. An initial chest radiograph showing shift of the mediastinum away from the side of the pneumothorax indicates the development of a tension pneumothorax and requires immediate chest tube insertion.

**Bibliography**

1. **Sahn SA, Heffner JE**. Spontaneous pneumothorax. N Engl Med. 2000;342:868-74. PMID: 10727592

## Dyspnea Question 7
## Answer: C

**Educational Objective:** *Recognize the syndrome of silo filler's disease.*

Silo filler's disease results from inhalation of oxides of nitrogen, including nitrogen dioxide, which tends to accumulate at the top of tall storage silos. The oxides of nitrogen are generated soon after the silo is filled with fresh silage that is subsequently used for animal feed. Nitrogen dioxide, when dissolved in the aqueous film that lines the respiratory tract, becomes nitric acid and produces a chemical pneumonitis. When the farmer enters the top of the silo to level the silage or prepare it for mechanical unloading, exposures can be quite high. The chemical pneumonitis of silo filler's disease must be differentiated from farmer's lung, which is an immunologic reaction to molds or thermophilic actinomycetes that grow in hay during the storage season. Exposure to this organic material occurs when farmers spread the hay for animal feed during the winter. Hypersensitivity pneumonitis can then occur 6 to 8 hours after exposure.

Viral pneumonia could produce symptoms similar to those described but is not as likely, given the recent exposure to fresh silage.

Pneumothorax often occurs during heavy physical exertion, but the time interval between working in the silo and onset of the symptoms makes this choice unlikely.

Allergic bronchopulmonary aspergillosis is caused by hypersensitivity to ubiquitous *Aspergillus* organisms and is characterized by recurrent, severe asthmatic symptoms. A single episode such as that described here is unlikely to be due to this disease.

**Bibliography**

1. **Kokkarinen JI, Tukiainen HO, Terho EO**. Recovery of pulmonary function in farmer's lung. A five-year follow-up study. Am Rev Respir Dis. 1993;147:793-6. PMID: 8466111
2. **Zhaoming W, Lockey RF**. A review of allergic bronchopulmonary aspergillosis. J Investig Allergol Clin Immunol. 1996;6:144-51. PMID: 8807504
3. **Grover JA, Ellwood PA**. Gases in forage tower silos. Ann Occup Hyg. 1989;33:519-33.

## Dyspnea Question 8
## Answer: D

**Educational Objective:** *Select the appropriate postexacerbation management for asthma.*

Acute exacerbations of asthma that do not respond to the written home management plan developed by the physician and patient are dangerous. The first goal of emergency acute therapy is to bring the attack under control, and criteria such as decreasing symptoms, decreasing respiratory rate, and diminished use of accessory muscles are encouraging. Wheezes are generally still present, even when the patient is improving, coughing, and raising sputum effectively. A rising $PaO_2$, with $PaCO_2$ and pH correcting, also signals an attack under control, and if the $FEV_1$ has improved more than 700 mL and is rising, plans for hospital discharge can be made. If these objective improvements are not present after 4 hours of correct emergency management, hospital admission is appropriate.

If discharge to home is planned, it is necessary to augment the patient's medications to ensure that exacerbation does not occur. Thus, discharge on previous medications is inappropriate. Although increasing inhaled corticosteroids is good, the addition of a short course of tapering oral corticosteroids has been proven to decrease the frequency of exacerbations requiring emergency department or office management and should be done. The patient should be seen in the office soon to develop a new long-term therapy and acute home exacerbation plan.

A single exacerbation is not ample reason to select chronic oral corticosteroid therapy with all its dire effects.

**Bibliography**

1. **Chapman KR, Verbeek PR, White JG, Rebuck AS**. Effect of a short course of prednisone in the prevention of early relapse after the emergency room treatment of acute asthma. N Engl J Med. 1991;324:788-94. PMID: 1997850
2. **Sheffer AL, Taggart US**. National Asthma Education Program. Expert panel report guidelines for the diagnosis and management of asthma. Med Care. 1993;31:MS20-8. PMID: 8450685
3. National Asthma Education and Prevention Program. Expert Panel Report: Guidelines for the Diagnosis and Management of Asthma Update on Selected Topics—2002. J Allergy Clin Immunol. 2002;110(5 Suppl):S141-219. PMID: 12542074

## Dyspnea Question 9
## Answer: A

**Educational Objective:** *Interpret a lung scan and manage a patient appropriately.*

The lung scan is normal, with matched perfusion and ventilation. This lung scan rules out a pulmonary embolism, and another source for the chest pain should be sought. Often asthma does complicate the interpretation of the lung scan, but the problem relates to matched defects in which the airway obstruction decreases the ventilation to an area of the lung.

The consequent hypoxia in that area leads to reduction in blood flow in the same area. These areas are rarely segmental.

### Bibliography

1. Value of the ventilation/perfusion scan in acute pulmonary embolism. Results of the prospective investigation of pulmonary embolism diagnosis (PIOPED). The PIOPED Investigators. JAMA. 1990;263:2753-9. PMID: 2332918

## Dyspnea Question 10
## Answer: C

**Educational Objective:** *Distinguish the etiology of dyspnea.*

The most likely diagnosable cause of this patient's shortness of breath is asthma. Chronic dyspnea in a patient younger than 40 years of age with a normal alveolar-arterial oxygen pressure difference is strongly predictive of bronchial hyperreactivity or hyperventilation syndrome. Studies have shown that in 75% of patients evaluated for chronic dyspnea, the disease has a respiratory cause, and the most common cause is asthma (29%). The best test to prove the diagnosis of asthma in this patient would be the methacholine bronchoprovocation challenge test. Although spirometry may be normal at the time of testing, bronchoprovocation challenge with methacholine or histamine will reveal abnormal airway sensitivity and prove the diagnosis of asthma. Treatment with bronchodilators will relieve the dyspnea, further proving the diagnosis to be correct.

Because the patient had a normal physical examination of the chest and a normal chest radiograph, high-resolution computed tomography would be unlikely to yield further diagnostic information. No stridor was described either by the patient or on physical examination. Therefore, a flow-volume loop would not be useful to diagnose upper airway obstruction as a cause of dyspnea. The flow-volume loop has been found to be less useful than bronchoprovocation challenge in diagnosing asthma. There is little in the history or physical examination to suggest primary heart disease as a cause of dyspnea, although a myocardiopathy can present in this way. Although the single-breath diffusion capacity might intuitively appear to be a good way to diagnose the cause of dyspnea by ruling out an interstitial lung disease, emphysema, or pulmonary vascular disease, comparative studies have not found this test to be very useful in the evaluation of chronic dyspnea, particularly if no crackles are heard on physical examination.

### Bibliography

1. **DePaso WJ, Winterbauer RH, Lusk JA, Dreis DF, Springmeyer SC**. Chronic dyspnea unexplained by history, physical examination, chest roentgenogram and spirometry. Analysis of a seven-year experience. Chest. 1991;100:1293-9. PMID: 1935284
2. **Pratter MR, Curley FJ, Dubois J, Irwin RS**. Cause and evaluation of chronic dyspnea in a pulmonary disease clinic. Arch Intern Med. 1989;149:2277-82. PMID: 2802893

## Dyspnea Question 11
## Answer: A

**Educational Objective:** *Choose the most appropriate initial therapy for the patient with severe sleep apnea syndrome.*

Nasal continuous positive airway pressure (CPAP) has become the standard initial treatment of patients with moderate to severe obstructive sleep apnea syndrome. It is believed to work by splinting open the upper airway. Surgical procedures such as uvulopalatopharyngoplasty and tracheostomy are best considered when more conservative measures such as nasal CPAP are ineffective. Progesterone, which is a respiratory stimulant, is sometimes useful as a means to decrease $Paco_2$ in patients with chronic hypercapnia (especially obese patients, who are frequently said to have "pickwickian syndrome"), but it is not a primary mode of therapy for treating obstructive sleep apnea. The cyclic antidepressant protriptyline may decrease obstructive apneas by suppressing rapid-eye-movement (REM) sleep (when apneas occur most frequently) and by increasing upper airway dilating muscle activity. It can be useful in mild, REM-associated sleep apnea, but anticholinergic side effects are a problem in some patients. Nocturnal, supplemental oxygen may decrease the degree of oxygen desaturation during the apneic episodes but does not decrease the frequency of apneic episodes.

### Bibliography

1. **Shepard JW Jr, Olsen KD**. Uvulopalatopharyngoplasty for treatment of obstructive sleep apnea. Mayo Clin Proc. 1990;65:1260-7. PMID: 2205764
2. **Shepard JW Jr, Olsen KD**. Uvulopalatopharyngoplasty for treatment of obstructive sleep apnea. Mayo Clin Proc. 1990;65:1250-9. PMID: 2205763
3. **Fletcher EC, Munafo DA**. Role of nocturnal oxygen therapy in obstructive sleep apnea. When should it be used? Chest. 1990;98:1497-504. PMID: 2245694
4. **Douglas NJ**. ABC of sleep disorders. The sleep apnoea/hypopnoea syndrome and snoring. BMJ. 1993;306:1057-60. PMID: 8490507

## Dyspnea Question 12
## Answer: E

**Educational Objective:** *Select the appropriate therapy for asthma that is not adequately controlled with a β-agonist used as needed.*

In this patient, the increasing use of a β-agonist inhaler suggests that the patient's asthma is not adequately controlled. Because airway inflammation plays an important role in such patients, anti-inflammatory therapy should be added and used on a regular basis. Options include addition of either an inhaled corticosteroid (beclomethasone, triamcinolone, or flunisolide) or cromolyn, although in adults, corticosteroids are more commonly used.

Inhaled albuterol has not been sufficient to control this patient's asthma for the past 6 weeks, so that continued use of albuterol as a single agent, either as needed or on a regular basis, would not constitute optimal therapy. However, inhaled albuterol should be continued on an as-needed basis to supplement inhaled corticosteroids.

Although inhaled ipratropium bromide, an anticholinergic agent, has been used for management of asthma, its relative effectiveness compared with inhaled β-agonists is greater for chronic obstructive pulmonary disease (chronic bronchitis and/or emphysema) than for asthma. Oral albuterol does not have any advantages over inhaled albuterol but does have an increased frequency of adverse systemic effects, especially tremor.

Monitoring of pulmonary function is an important aspect of asthma management and is more reliable for following the course of the disease than are either symptoms or findings on physical examination. Although spirometry is useful in the office or hospital setting, measurement of peak expiratory flow with a hand-held meter allows direct monitoring by the patient on a regular basis at home.

**Bibliography**

1. **McFadden ER Jr, Gilbert IA**. Asthma. N Engl J Med. 1992;327:1928-37. PMID: 1454088

## Dyspnea Question 13
## Answer: A

**Educational Objective:**   *Manage acute exacerbation of asthma.*

Management of severe exacerbation of asthma or status asthmaticus, which can be defined as an asthma attack placing the patient at risk of respiratory failure, requires rapid assessment and therapy. Beta-agonists administered by metered-dose inhaler (MDI), or by nebulizer for patients unable to cooperate with MDI administration, are a first-line treatment to relieve bronchospasm. Corticosteroids relieve inflammation and prevent relapse over the subsequent 7 to 10 days. Although anticholinergics such as ipratropium bromide are not as potent bronchodilators as beta-agonists, they may have additional benefit in severe asthma exacerbations but should not be depended on to reverse a severe exacerbation.

Mechanical ventilation is indicated for patients failing initial therapy (such as this patient), as determined by findings such as altered mental status, worsening tachypnea, and progressive hypercapnia. Bronchoconstriction impedes exhalation, placing patients at risk for air trapping and barotrauma. Ventilatory settings should include a long expiratory phase, low rate, and low tidal volume to minimize air trapping, even at the expense of an elevated $PaCO_2$ (termed "permissive hypercapnia").

Noninvasive mechanical ventilation (such as bilevel positive airway pressure [BiPAP]) can be useful in patients who refuse intubation but is not reliable in acutely ill patients who are failing medical management. It is used in patients with chronic obstructive pulmonary disease (COPD), not in those with asthma.

Heliox is a helium and oxygen mixture with a low density that reduces airway resistance, facilitating air flow through constricted airways. Because it does not reduce bronchoconstriction or airway inflammation, it may be useful as a temporizing therapy to reduce the work of breathing until more definitive therapies, such as corticosteroids, take effect. Because trials to date evaluating the use of heliox for acute asthma exacerbations have included only small numbers of patients, it is not a routine therapy.

**Bibliography**

1. **Corbridge TC, Hall JB**. The assessment and management of adults with status asthmaticus. Am J Respir Crit Care Med. 1995;151:1296-316. PMID: 7735578
2. **Kass JE, Castriotta RJ**. Heliox therapy in acute severe asthma. Chest. 1995;107:757-60. PMID: 7874949

## Dyspnea Question 14
## Answer: A

**Educational Objective:**   *Recognize an illness resembling asthma following a high-level exposure to an irritant.*

Brooks described the reactive airways dysfunction syndrome (RADS) in 1985. Following a single exposure to a high-level concentration of an irritant vapor, fume, gas, or smoke, patients develop an asthma-like illness. Allergic occupational asthma usually requires a latency period after exposure to a sensitizing agent. Some consider RADS a form of nonallergic occupational asthma. The patient denies a prior history of asthma or bronchitis; therefore, the single, initiating event makes RADS the most likely disease.

**Bibliography**

1. **Alberts WM, Brooks SM**. Advances in occupational asthma. Clin Chest Med. 1992;13:281-302. PMID: 1387352

## Dyspnea Question 15
## Answer: D

**Educational Objective:**   *Evaluate the cause of hypoxemia and pulmonary hypertension.*

The patient has had a problem all his life, and a systolic murmur on examination suggests a congenital cause. Of the choices, the one that best fits the results of the tests is an atrial septal defect. The shunt is left-to-right for the bulk of the patient's life; however, when the increased flow in the pulmonary circuit leads to pulmonary hypertension, the shunt reverses and becomes a right-to-left shunt.

Primary pulmonary hypertension is more common in women than in men. It may show enlarged central pulmonary arteries on chest radiograph, but the peripheral vasculature is "pruned" and not increased. Arteriography should show an abrupt decrease in the vessel size, and the right-to-left shunting should not be present unless an incidental, atrial septal defect is opened by the pulmonary hypertension.

Multiple pulmonary emboli would be diagnosed by the limited arteriogram. Because this is not positive, there is no evidence for multiple pulmonary emboli.

Mitral stenosis would produce a diastolic not systolic murmur, ruling out this diagnosis.

**Bibliography**

1. **Kerut EK, Norfleet WT, Plotnick GD, Giles TD.** Patent foramen ovale: a review of associated conditions and the impact of physiological size. J Am Coll Cardiol. 2001;38:613-23. PMID: 11527606
2. **Palevsky HI, Schloo BL, Pietra GG, Weber KT, Janicki JS, Rubin E.** Primary pulmonary hypertension. Vascular structure, morphometry, and responsiveness to vasodilator agents. Circulation. 1989;80:1207-21. PMID: 2805259

## Dyspnea Question 16
## Answer: C

**Educational Objective:** *Manage increased activity of asthma through environmental modification to reduce indoor antigenic exposures.*

The patient has a history of atopy (asthma, eczema, and seasonal rhinitis and conjunctivitis). Her symptoms of asthma are exacerbated by dust exposure, and skin testing results have confirmed a sensitivity to dust mite antigen. The asthma has worsened in a new living environment, which has the potential for increased exposure to dust mite antigen. A reasonable initial intervention to control the symptoms is institution of measures to reduce dust mite exposure in the dormitory apartment. Taking up the large area rug and using allergy-proof wraps to seal the pillows, mattress, and box springs are effective measures. The patient also should wash her sheets and pillow cases regularly in hot water and avoid dusting or vacuuming without a special micropore vacuum bag. Appropriate filters may help if the dormitory has forced hot air heating.

Allergen immunotherapy for asthma is controversial because of the risks and uncertain benefit. It can be considered in the care of this patient only if environmental control measures and conventional antiasthma medications do not control the asthma. Skin testing for food sensitivities is notoriously inaccurate. The best method of diagnosis is careful dietary record keeping (food diary) and, if necessary, an elimination diet. Oral food challenges in a carefully monitored setting sometimes are performed. The standard for diagnosis of food sensitivities is a double-blind, placebo-controlled oral challenge. Dust mites grow best in warm, moist environments. Maintaining a high indoor relative humidity by running a humidifier in the winter promotes dust mite growth and therefore should be avoided.

**Bibliography**

1. **Cloosterman SG, Scherner TR, Bijl-Hofland ID, Van Der Heide S, Brunekreef B, Van Den Elshout FJ, et al.** Effects of house dust mite avoidance measures on Der p 1 concentrations and clinical condition of mild adult house dust mite-allergic asthmatic patients, using no inhaled steroids. Clin Exp Allergy. 1999;29:1336-46. PMID: 10520054
2. **Sporik R, Hill DJ, Thompson PJ, Carlin JB, Nolan TM, Kemp AS, et al.** The Melbourne House Dust Mite Study: long-term efficiency of house dust mite reduction strategies. J Allergy Clin Immunol. 1998;101(4 Pt 1):451-6. PMID: 9564796

## Dyspnea Question 17
## Answer: C

**Educational Objective:** *Recognize allergic bronchopulmonary aspergillosis for a patient with asthma and pneumonia.*

Several features in the clinical presentation raise the possibility of allergic bronchopulmonary aspergillosis (ABPA) as the cause of unresolved pneumonia. The patient has a subacute febrile illness with a cough productive of "cords" in the sputum (possibly representing bronchial casts). He has underlying asthma, and there are pulmonary infiltrates and profound peripheral blood eosinophilia. Use of marijuana increases the likelihood of inhalational exposure to *Aspergillus* organisms.

A number of diagnostic tests are helpful in establishing a diagnosis of ABPA. The total serum IgE level typically is very high, generally greater than 0.1 mg/dL (1.0 g/L) (normal value, 0.01 mg/dL [0.1 mg/L] or less). Allergy skin testing usually shows a positive immediate response to *Aspergillus* organisms, and sputum culture frequently grows *Aspergillus* organisms. Additional, useful serologic tests include identification of IgG antibody to *Aspergillus* organisms ("*Aspergillus* precipitins") and of IgE antibody specific for *Aspergillus* organisms at radioallergosorbent testing. An assay for *Aspergillus* antigen in the blood is not clinically available, and the results are likely to be negative among patients with ABPA.

Alternative diagnoses can be considered, including mycoplasmapneumonia (serum for cold agglutinins), psittacosis (antibody to *Chlamydia psittaci*), and tuberculosis (sputum for acid-fast bacilli). The first two types of pneumonia were appropriately managed with azithromycin. None of the three types is typically associated with peripheral blood eosinophilia. The peripheral blood eosinophilia is a clue that this patient does not have typical infectious pneumonia.

**Bibliography**

1. **Cockrill BA, Hales CA.** Allergic bronchopulmonary aspergillosis. Annu Rev Med. 1999;50:303-16. PMID: 10073280

## Dyspnea Question 18
## Answer: D

**Educational Objective:** *Diagnose new-onset pulmonary hypertension.*

This young woman has moderate to severe pulmonary hypertension without overt evidence of an underlying cardiac or pulmonary cause. The history, physical findings, and pulse oximetry exclude the possibility of cor pulmonale due to end-stage lung disease.

The diagnosis of pulmonary hypertension is suggested by the presence of a parasternal heave, widely split $S_2$ and an elevated venous pressure. Constrictive pericarditis would not alter the $S_2$ or produce a parasternal heave, but would produce an extra cardiac sound during diastole, the pericardial "knock". Hyperthrophic cardiomyopathy would be associated with a bifid pulse and a systolic murmur that increases with Valsalva, or standing. Coarctation of the aorta would be associated with elevated blood pressure in the arms and lower blood pressure in the legs. It is not associated with a parasternal heave or alteration of the $S_2$.

**Bibliography**

1.  **Rubin LJ**. Primary pulmonary hypertension. N Engl J Med. 1997;336:111-7. PMID: 8988890

## Dyspnea Question 19
## Answer: A

**Educational Objective:** *Identify the major causes of secondary pulmonary hypertension.*

Pulmonary hypertension, generally defined as a mean pulmonary arterial pressure exceeding 25 mm Hg at rest or 30 mm Hg with exertion, can complicate severe cardiac or pulmonary disease. The clinician must first establish the degree and severity of pulmonary hypertension. This often can be accomplished noninvasively by means of transthoracic echocardiography. By exclusion, obesity hypoventilation syndrome with obstructive sleep apnea is the most plausible explanation for the pulmonary hypertension and right heart failure in this case. Further questioning would likely reveal daytime hypersomnolence and a history of severe snoring. Daytime hypoxemia, hypercapnia, and polycythemia would substantiate this suspicion as well. The diagnosis can be established with overnight polysomnography. If the diagnosis is confirmed, treatment with continuous positive airway pressure or bilevel positive airway pressure through a nasal mask can substantially improve the sleep pattern and alleviate hypersomnolence, gas exchange problems, and, to some degree, pulmonary hypertension.

Left ventricular failure is the most common cause of secondary pulmonary hypertension. In this case, it is excluded because of the echocardiographic evidence of normal left ventricular systolic and diastolic function. Chronic obstructive pulmonary disease can be complicated by cor pulmonale, hypoxemia, and hypercapnia, but these complications usually are restricted to patients with a forced expiratory volume in 1 sec less than 50% of predicted. A long-standing atrial septal defect can allow substantial left-to-right intracardiac shunting and increase pulmonary arterial blood flow. The result is pulmonary hypertension. This patient did not have a patent foramen ovale detected by echocardiography.

**Bibliography**

1.  **Kessler R, Chaouat A, Weitzenblum E, Oswald M, Ehrhart M, Apprill M, et al**. Pulmonary hypertension in the obstructive sleep apnoea syndrome: prevalence, causes and therapeutic consequences. Eur Respir J. 1996;9:787-94. PMID: 8726947

# Pneumonia

## Pneumonia Question 1
**Answer: D**

**Educational Objective:** *Recognize the relative value of diagnostic tests used to identify microbial pathogens in patients with community-acquired pneumonia.*

Blood cultures yield positive results in only a small minority of cases; however, owing to their specificity, the positive predictive value is above 90%. This patient is a smoker with chronic obstructive pulmonary disease who has symptoms and signs indicative of community-acquired pneumonia. Although the history of shaking chills may suggest a diagnosis of "typical" pneumonia, the history alone is of limited diagnostic utility in assessing microbial cause. Instead, the history and physical examination should be used to differentiate community-acquired pneumonia from other types of pneumonia, such as those occurring as a result of aspiration, in recently hospitalized patients, or in immunodeficient patients. In addition, the history and physical examination play an important role in the assessment of the severity of pneumonia. The utility of Gram staining and culturing of sputum is controversial. Nevertheless, in the evaluation of uncomplicated community-acquired pneumonia, the positive predictive value of either test remains extremely low.

In this patient, the Gram stain must be interpreted in the context of the moderate number of polymorphonuclear leukocytes and epithelial cells, and two or three presumed bacterial pathogens. These findings would not have a demonstrable effect on initial selection of an antibiotic for this patient. The results of sputum culture are likely a result of contamination from oral flora. The chest x-ray cannot make a bacteriologic diagnosis and therefore is of little help in guiding therapy once a diagnosis of pneumonia is made.

### Bibliography
1. **Chalasani NP, Valdecanas MA, Gopal AK, McGowan JE Jr, Jurado RL**. Clinical utility of blood cultures in adult patients with community-acquired pneumonia without defined underlying risks. Chest. 1995;108:932-6. PMID: 7555163

2. **Niederman MS, Mandell LA, Anzeuto A, Bass JB, Broughton WA, Campbell GD, et al**. Guidelines for the management of adults with community-acquired pneumonia, diagnosis, assessment of severity, antimicrobial therapy, and prevention. American Thoracic Society. Am J Respir Crit Care Med. 2001;163:1730-1754. PMID: 11401897

## Pneumonia Question 2
**Answer: E**

**Educational Objective:** *Select an appropriate empiric antibiotic regimen for a patient with severe community-acquired pneumonia with structural lung disease.*

This patient has severe community-acquired pneumonia (pneumonia severity index class 5) complicated by evidence of bronchiectasis on chest radiograph. Risk factors responsible for this patient's increased risk of mortality include his advanced age, the presence of significant comorbidities, unstable vital signs, significant hypoxia, hyponatremia, and acute renal failure. Although the actual pathogen is not identified in most cases of community-acquired pneumonia, the most common causes are *Streptococcus pneumoniae, Legionella* species, aerobic gram-negative bacilli, *Haemophilus influenzae, Mycoplasma pneumoniae*, and respiratory viruses. *Pseudomonas aeruginosa* is more common among patients with structural lung disease, such as bronchiectasis. Because this patient has life-threatening pneumonia, and especially because he has structural lung disease, coverage of *P. aeruginosa* is recommended. Piperacillin-tazobactam combined with levofloxacin would effectively provide double coverage for *P. aeruginosa* and would cover atypical pathogens. In clinical trials, doxycycline has been shown to be an effective regimen for patients with mild to moderate pneumonia, but concern about resistant pneumococcal species in severe cases and a lack of extended gram-negative spectrum would argue against its use here. Coverage of *Legionella* and *Mycoplasma* species should be a high priority; therefore, ceftriaxone alone is not a viable treatment option. Azithromycin covers *S. Pneumoniae, H. Influenzae*, and most atypicals, but lacks coverage against *P. aeruginosa*. Some strains of *S. pneumoniae* are resistant to ciprofloxacin; levofloxacin has enhanced coverage against *S. pneumoniae* and might be a more appropriate choice.

### Bibliography
1. **Niederman MS, Mandell LA, Anzeuto A, Bass JB, Broughton WA, Campbell GD, et al**. Guidelines for the management of adults with community-acquired pneumonia, diagnosis, assessment of severity, antimicrobial therapy, and prevention. American Thoracic Society. Am J Respir Crit Care Med. 2001;163:1730-1754. PMID: 11401897

2. **Fine MJ, Auble TE, Yeyal DM, Hanusa BH, Weissfeld LA, Singer DE, et al**. A prediction rule to identify low risk patients with community-acquired pneumonia. N Engl J Med. 1997;336:43-250. PMID: 8995086

## Pneumonia Question 3
## Answer: B

**Educational Objective:** *Manage a patient with pneumonia acquired in a nursing home who meets criteria for inpatient management.*

This patient is best managed in the hospital because of risk of a poor outcome as defined by the Pneumonia PORT (Patient Outcomes Research Team) study. He has evidence of dehydration (dry mucous membranes), possibly indicating poor oral intake in addition to insensible fluid losses due to fever. He is therefore a candidate for parenteral treatment with fluid replacement as well as antibiotics. The principal pathogens causing community-acquired pneumonia are *Streptococcus pneumoniae*, *Haemophilus influenzae*, *Moraxella catarrhalis*, and atypical pathogens such as *Legionella* spp. A nursing-home patient also has an increased risk of gram-negative pathogens, such as *Klebsiella pneumoniae*. Ciprofloxacin has less activity than levofloxacin against *S. pneumoniae*, and there have been ciprofloxacin failures in patients with serious pneumococcal infections. Ceftriaxone alone covers *H. influenzae*, *M. catarrhalis*, and most strains of *S. pneumoniae* and *K. pneumoniae* but lacks activity against atypical pathogens. Azithromycin may also be effective coverage, as it is effective against atypical pathogens, some gram negative pathogens, and most strains of *S. pneumoniae*, but increasing resistance of *S. pneumoniae* to macrolides such as azithromycin may be of concern in a severely ill patient. Imipenem has broad-spectrum activity against all of the conventional bacterial pathogens, but lacks activity against atypical pathogens. A combination of ceftriaxone and azithromycin adequately covers all likely pathogens.

### Bibliography

1. **Niederman MS, Mandell LA, Anzeuto A, Bass JB, Broughton WA, Campbell GD, et al**. Guidelines for the management of adults with community-acquired pneumonia, diagnosis, assessment of severity, antimicrobial therapy, and prevention. American Thoracic Society. Am J Respir Crit Care Med. 2001;163:1730-1754. PMID: 11401897

2. **Fine MJ, Auble TE, Yealy DM, Hanusa BH, Weissfeld LA, Singer DE, et al**. A prediction rule to identify low-risk patients with community-acquired pneumonia. N Engl J Med. 1997;336:243-50. PMID: 8995086

3. **Fine MJ, Hough LJ, Medsger AR, Li YH, Ricci EM, Singer DE, et al**. The hosptial admission decision for pateints with community-acquired pneumonia. Results from the pneumonia Patient Outcomes Research Team cohort study. Arch Intern Med. 1997;157:36-44. PMID: 8996039

## Pneumonia Question 4
## Answer: B

**Educational Objective:** *Identify the most appropriate treatment for a patient with bacteremic pneumococcal pneumonia not responding to clarithromycin.*

This patient with bacteremic pneumonia is not improving on therapy with clarithromycin, suggesting a clar-

ithromycin-resistant isolate. Gram-positive cocci in pairs growing from the blood culture suggest pneumococci. Fluoroquinolones with increased activity against pneumococci, such as levofloxacin and sparfloxacin, would be beneficial for this patient.

Clarithromycin and other macrolides, such as erythromycin and azithromycin, bind to the bacterial ribosome and inhibit bacterial protein synthesis. Resistance to macrolides occurs by induction of a methylase enzyme that modifies the ribosome and thereby alters the drug target or by active specific efflux. The first mechanism affects clarithromycin, erythromycin, and azithromycin as well as the nonmacrolide, clindamycin, but the second mechanism affects only the macrolides. Since both resistance mechanisms affect all macrolides in clinical use in the United States, the choice of azithromycin would not be appropriate for a patient failing clarithromycin. Since there is epidemiologic linkage between resistance to macrolides and resistance to penicillin and to trimethoprim-sulfamethoxazole, trimethoprim-sulfamethoxazole would not be appropriate for this patient. Ceftazidime, in contrast to ceftriaxone and cefotaxime, has only limited activity against pneumococci and would therefore be a poor choice.

### Bibliography

1. **Weisblum B**. Macrolide resistance. Drug Resist Updates. 1998;1:29-41.

2. **Doern GV, Pfaller MA, Kugler K, Freeman J, Jones RN**. Prevalence of antimicrobial resistance among respiratory tract isolates of Streptococcus pneumoniae in North America: 1997 results from the SENTRY antimicrobial surveillance program. Clin Infect Dis. 1998;27:764-70. PMID: 9798031

3. **Niederman MS, Mandell LA, Anzeuto A, Bass JB, Broughton WA, Campbell GD, et al**. Guidelines for the management of adults with community-acquired pneumonia, diagnosis, assessment of severity, antimicrobial therapy, and prevention. American Thoracic Society. Am J Respir Crit Care Med. 2001;163:1730-1754. PMID: 11401897

## Pneumonia Question 5
## Answer: D

**Educational Objective:** *Recognize the gram-stained appearance of Haemophilus influenzae.*

This slide depicts *Haemophilus influenzae* in the sputum, which appears as characteristic small, pleomorphic, gram-negative coccobacilli. Other microorganisms mimicking *H. influenzae* include *Neisseria gonorrhoeae*, *Neisseria meningitidis*, and *Moraxella catarrhalis*. These microorganisms are also gram-negative, but characteristically appear as bean-shaped diplococci. Although Gram stains of *N. meningitidis*, *N. gonorrhoeae*, and *M. catarrhalis* are indistinguishable from each other, they are differentiated from *H. influenzae* by their size and shape.

### Bibliography

1. **Yungbluth M**. The laboratory diagnosis of pneumonia. The role of the community hospital pathologist. Clin Lab Med. 1995;15:209-34. PMID: 7671572

## Pneumonia Question 6
## Answer: A

**Educational Objective:** *Recognize gram-positive cocci characteristic of a staphylococcal infection and distinguish these microorganisms from streptococci.*

This image depicts large numbers of leukocytes and gram-positive cocci clustered in groups and tetrads. The clusters are formed because staphylococcal cell division occurs on three planes to form grape-like groups. The microorganisms most likely mimicking staphylococci are streptococci. However, streptococci are more likely to be found as gram-positive bullet-shaped or lancet-shaped pairs. *H. influenzae* and *E. coli* organisms are gram-negative rods and should not be confused with gram-positive cocci.

### Bibliography
1. **Yungbluth M**. The laboratory diagnosis of pneumonia. The role of the community hospital pathologist. Clin Lab Med. 1995;15:209-34. PMID: 7671572

## Pneumonia Question 7
## Answer: B

**Educational Objective:** *Recognize Streptococcus pneumoniae in a gram-stained smear of sputum.*

Although examination of gram-stained sputum can be of diagnostic significance in more than 50% of patients with pneumonia, this study can also be misleading. Reliability is greatest if the sputum is purulent and the gram-stained sample has minimal contamination by upper respiratory tract secretions. This would be reflected by abundant polymorphonuclear leukocytes and many fewer epithelial cells. A predominant microorganism should be seen, except in patients with anaerobic pulmonary infections. On microscopic examination of an optimal specimen (such as the one in this image), gram-positive cocci can be identified as *Streptococcus pneumoniae* (cocci in pairs). *Staphylococcus aureus* would appear as gram-positive cocci in clusters or chains. Plump gram-negative rods suggest *Klebsiella pneumoniae*, whereas coccobacillary forms suggest *Haemophilus pneumoniae*. If the smear meets the above criteria, the sputum sample should be cultured. However, the microscopic examination may actually be more sensitive and specific than the sputum culture.

### Bibliography
1. **Yungbluth M**. The laboratory diagnosis of pneumonia. The role of the community hospital pathologist. Clin Lab Med. 1995;15:209-34. PMID: 7671572

## Pneumonia Question 8
## Answer: B

**Educational Objective:** *Identify the cause of community-acquired pneumonia in a patient with HIV infection and a high CD4 cell count.*

The spectrum of opportunistic infections to which an HIV-infected person is susceptible is a function of host cellular and humoral immunocompetence. In patients with CD4 cell counts greater than $500/\mu L$, conventional pathogens are more common than opportunistic pathogens. Community-acquired pneumonia with typical clinical features is most often caused by encapsulated bacteria, particularly *Streptococcus pneumoniae* and *Haemophilus* species. Risk factors for community-acquired pneumonia in patients with HIV infection include cigarette smoking and using injected drugs.

The typical presentation of bacterial pneumonia caused by encapsulated organisms is the abrupt onset of fever, chills, productive cough, and pleuritic chest pain. Patients with bacterial pneumonia have usually had symptoms for 3 to 5 days, in contrast to patients with *Pneumocystis carinii* pneumonia, whose symptoms have usually been present for several weeks. Focal pulmonary infiltrates and leukocytosis are the laboratory hallmarks of bacterial pneumonia in patients with or without HIV infection. *Pneumocystis carnii* pneumonia generally presents with diffuse interstitial infiltrates.

Mycoplasmal disease is unusual in patients with HIV infection and is unlikely to present with such an abrupt onset of respiratory symptoms or productive cough.

*Legionella pneumophila* is an unusual cause of pneumonia in patients with HIV infection but has been reported in association with nosocomial outbreaks.

*Pseudomonas aerugihosa* infections of the respiratory tract are more commonly seen in patients with more advanced HIV disease who have indwelling venous catheters or in patients who have been hospitalized. *P. aerugihosa* is a very unusual cause of community-acquired pneumonia in patients with CD4 cell counts greater than $500/\mu L$.

### Bibliography
1. **Noskin GA, Glassroth J**. Bacterial pneumonia associated with HIV-1 infection. Clin Chest Med. 1996;17:713-23. PMID: 9016373

## Pneumonia Question 9
## Answer: E

**Educational Objective:** *Understand the relationship between tuberculin skin test and active tuberculosis.*

Tuberculin skin testing is most valuable for assessing symptomatic or asymptomatic infection with *Mycobacterium tuberculosis*. A negative tuberculin skin test does not, however, exclude active tuberculosis. Negative tuberculin skin tests are found in approximately 20% to 25% of all adults with pulmonary tuberculosis. This does not include tests that are improperly performed (for example, with a subcutaneous injection of PPD tuberculin) or inaccurately read. Furthermore, there is a very real possibility of infection and progression to reactivation disease because the prior test was done 6 months earlier. The tuberculin skin test is more likely to be negative if the host is immunosuppressed. Second-strength skin testing (using more antigen in the Mantoux test) is seldom done because it tends to bring out more false-positive results and does not really make the diagnosis of active tuberculosis with any greater certainty.

In patients with cavitary tuberculosis, a reliable diagnosis can be made with expectorated sputum in most cases, thus sparing the patient the need for a bronchoscopy. In this man with classic symptoms and chest radiographic findings, sputum for acid-fast bacilli microscopy should be obtained on an emergent basis. A repeat PPD skin test is unlikely to clarify the issue and gastric acid stains for acid fast bacilli would be considered only if the patient could not produce sputum. Respiratory isolation in such a person is critical to limit nosocomial spread of tuberculosis.

### Bibliography
1. **Huebner RE, Schein MF, Bass JB Jr**. The tuberculin skin test. Clin Infect Dis. 1993;17:968-75. PMID: 8110954

## Pneumonia Question 10
## Answer: C

**Educational Objective:** *Recognize pleural space infection as a complication of pneumonia.*

The sputum smear shows gram-negative coccobacilli consistent with *Haemophilus influenzae*. Although the correlation between sputum Gram stain results and pathogens present within the alveoli is still the subject of some debate, the clinical setting (acute febrile illness in a patient with a history of cigarette and alcohol abuse) and sputum smear both suggest that the initial antibiotic should include coverage for *H. influenzae*. Although this acute presentation would be most common for type b strains of *H. influenzae*, a large proportion of both typeable and nontypeable strains produce β-lactamase and must be treated with agents resistant to that enzyme. However, within 24 hours of initiating therapy, the patient still appears to be toxic and now has findings consistent with development of a right pleural effusion. Extension of pneumonia to involve the pleural space is a relatively common complication of infection with *H. influenzae*, as are bacteremia and intrapulmonary or extrapulmonary abscess formation. Assessment of the pleural space with decubitus views or other imaging procedures is appropriate. If an effusion is confirmed, a diagnostic thoracentesis should be performed to exclude empyema. If an empyema (that is, purulent fluid, positive Gram stain or culture) is present or if the pH is less than 7.1, it should be drained. There is no reason to change antibiotic therapy at this time, nor is there any indication that bronchial hygiene would be facilitated by either intubation or percussion and drainage. CT scan of the chest would yield similar information but is significantly more costly; lateral decubitus films are sufficient to do this. Inhaled β-agonists

may transiently improve respiratory status but will not alter the course of a complicated parapneumonic effusion.

### Bibliography
1. **Takala AK, Eskola J, van Alphen J**. Spectrum of invasive Hemophilus influenzae type b disease in adults. Arch Intern Med. 1990;150:2573-6. PMID: 2244774
2. **Light RW**. Diagnostic principles in pleural disease. Eur Respir J. 1997;10:467-81. PMID: 9042652

## Pneumonia Question 11
## Answer: D

**Educational Objective:** *Select the best empiric therapy for potentially severe community-acquired pneumonia.*

This patient has a community-acquired pneumonia. The tachypnea, magnitude of fever, and leukocyte count suggest a potentially severe pneumonia. The sputum specimen described is inadequate in light of the numerous epithelial cells that were noted. Even with a satisfactory sputum specimen (more than 25 neutrophils and fewer than 5 squamous epithelial cells per low-power field), there is debate about the correlation of organisms identified on Gram stain and organisms actually present at the level of the alveoli. Thus, as in this case, empiric therapy directed at the pathogens most likely to be present in a given clinical situation is required. In a patient of this age with potentially severe community-acquired pneumonia, organisms such as *Streptococcus pneumoniae* and *Haemophilus influenzae* are important potential etiologic agents. It would also be important to cover *Legionella* and *Moraxella* species. Other gram-negative organisms are less likely but also should be considered. Erythromycin will cover *S. pneumoniae* and *Legionella* but would be inadequate for *H. influenzae*, *Moraxella* species, and other gram-negative bacteria. Azithromycin has expanded spectrum against these gram-negative bacteria. Penicillin will not provide any gram-negative coverage or coverage for *Legionella*. First-generation cephalosporins, although they provide good treatment for most gram-positive organisms, have limited use against *H. influenzae* or *Legionella* species. Trimethoprim-sulfamethoxazole probably provides coverage for pneumococci and is effective against *H. influenzae* and *Moraxella* but does not cover *Legionella* species. The combination of azithromycin and a third-generation cephalosporin provides broad coverage for pathogens likely to be encountered in this setting and is a good choice for initial empiric therapy.

### Bibliography
1. **Niederman MS, Mandell LA, Anzeuto A, Bass JB, Broughton WA, Campbell GD, et al**. Guidelines for the management of adults with community-acquired pneumonia, diagnosis, assessment of severity, antimicrobial therapy, and prevention. American Thoracic Society. Am J Respir Crit Care Med. 2001;163:1730-1754. PMID: 11401897

## Pneumonia Question 12
## Answer: B

**Educational Objective:** *Recognize and manage the distinguishing features of bacterial pneumonia and pleural effusion in a patient with HIV infection.*

Patients with HIV infection have a wide variety of respiratory complications. Bacterial pneumonia has now replaced *Pneumocystiscarinii* pneumonia (PCP) as the leading cause of death due to infection among persons with HIV infection. Investigators from the Pulmonary Complications of HIV Infection Study Group have reported that persons with HIV infection contract pneumonia at the rate of 5.5 episodes per 100 person-years. The incidence of pneumonia is only 0.9 per 100 person-years among persons without HIV infection. The more advanced the stage of infection, as documented with CD4 lymphocyte count, the greater is the risk of bacterial pneumonia. The most common pathogens isolated were *Streptococcuspneumoniae, Staphylococcus aureus,* and *Haemophilus influenzae.*

HIV infection confers increased risk of complications of pneumonia, including a higher rate of bacteremia, a twofold higher frequency of parapneumonic effusions, and more frequent need for tube thoracostomy drainage than among persons without HIV infection. The patient in this case has a syndrome of abrupt-onset pneumonia strongly suggestive of bacterial infection with radiographic studies that suggest the presence of lobar consolidation and pleural effusion. Regardless of HIV status, a parapneumonic effusion of this size in the acute presentation of pneumonia warrants thoracentesis. Empiric antibiotic therapy without thoracentesis can allow a complicated effusion to progress. Tube thoracostomy drainage is indicated if thoracentesis shows gross pus or features of a complicated effusion, including pH less than 7.0, glucose level less than 40 mg/dL, or positive result of fluid Gram stain or culture.

Pulmonary tuberculosis is always an important diagnostic consideration in the care of patients with HIV infection and respiratory disease. However, this patient has a clinical syndrome highly suggestive of acute bacterial pneumonia rather than the subacute presentation of pulmonary tuberculosis. If other historical or clinical features were to make the possibility of pulmonary tuberculosis more likely, four-drug chemotherapy for tuberculosis might be instituted early. However, it is not needed before diagnostic sputum and pleural studies are obtained and other diagnostic possibilities are evaluated.

PCP is still a prevalent and potentially lethal complication of HIV infection. This patient has a history of PCP, which puts her at greater-than-average risk of PCP. However, trimethoprim-sulfamethoxazole is extremely effective in the secondary prevention of PCP, and the acute, focal pneumonitis with a pleural effusion is atypical of PCP. Bronchoscopy or induced sputum for this unlikely possibility would not be the best initial management.

### Bibliography

1. **Gil Suay V, Cordero PJ, Martinez E, Soler JJ, Perpina M, Greses JV, et al.** Parapneumonic effusions secondary to community-acquired bacterial pneumonia in human immunodeficiency virus-infected patients. Eur Respir J. 1995;8:1934-9. PMID: 8620965

2. **Hirschtick RE, Glassroth J, Jordan MC, Wicosky TC, Wallace JM, Kvale PA, et al.** Bacterial pneumonia in persons infected with the human immunodeficiency virus. Pulmonary Complications of HIV Infection Study Group. N Engl J Med. 1995;333:845-51. PMID: 7651475

## Pneumonia Question 13
## Answer: C

**Educational Objective:** *Understand the need for objective assessment of the severity of community-acquired pneumonia and the data necessary for informed decision making.*

Community-acquired pneumonia has an average mortality of 14% among hospitalized patients. Physicians who rely on their clinical judgment are not accurate in assessing an individual patient's risk of dying during an episode of pneumonia. Several studies over the past two decades have concluded that the risk of death of community-acquired pneumonia correlates with age, presence of comorbid illness, and existence of cardiovascular compromise. The Pneumonia Severity Index (PSI), developed and tested on a prospective basis, allows clinicians to use readily available clinical information to develop a risk score and stratify a given patient into one of five mortality risk classes.

In this case, the patient's demographic characteristics, medical history, and physical examination data yield a preliminary risk score of 81, which places him in risk class III. With a predicted 30-day mortality rate of 1%, a patient in this category can be considered for outpatient treatment or at most a brief hospital stay. However, the risk scoring is incomplete because no data from laboratory testing has yet been obtained. A sputum specimen can be obtained in less than half of cases of community-acquired pneumonia. Gram stain and culture results may help focus antibiotic therapy once the patient is hospitalized but add little to the data incorporated in the PSI. A blood urea nitrogen level ≤ 30 mg/dL or serum sodium level ≤ 130 mg/L alone would place the patient in risk class IV, and the predicted mortality of approximately 9% would be a stronger argument for admission.

Thoracentesis is not indicated. The effusion does not exceed the 10-mm threshold recommended for thoracentesis in the setting of a parapneumonic effusion. Resting room-air oxygen saturation is incorporated into the PSI. Exercise oximetry has been used in the noninvasive diagnosis of *Pneumocystiscarinii* pneumonia related to HIV infection but has not been studied as a means of assessing the severity of community-acquired pneumonia.

113

### Bibliography

1. **Niederman MS, Mandell LA, Anzeuto A, Bass JB, Broughton WA, Campbell GD, et al.** Guidelines for the management of adults with community-acquired pneumonia, diagnosis, assessment of severity, antimicrobial therapy, and prevention. American Thoracic Society. Am J Respir Crit Care Med. 2001;163:1730-1754. PMID: 11401897

2. **Fine MJ, Auble TE, Yeyal DM, Hanusa BH, Weissfeld LA, Singer DE, et al.** A prediction rule to identify low risk patients with community-acquired pneumonia. N Engl J Med. 1997;336:43-250. PMID: 8995086

## Pneumonia Question 14
## Answer: B

**Educational Objective:** *Understand the diagnostic management of a patient with acute hypersensitivity pneumonitis.*

The patient most likely has acute hypersensitivity pneumonitis (allergic alveolitis) because of the presence of arthralgia, shortness of breath, bilateral crackles, reticular nodular opacities and patchy infiltrates, and exposure to a parakeet for several weeks. Removal of the causative agents is sufficient treatment of patients with mild to moderate symptoms.

Lung tissue may be needed if there is no relief of the symptoms after removal of the causative agent, but it is not necessary with the clinical characteristics of this patient. Psittacosis is extremely unlikely without fever or headache and a sputum for culture and sensitivity is not necessary. Elevated angiotensin-converting enzyme level is associated with sarcoidosis but is not specific. These findings might be consistent with sarcoidosis, but sarcoidosis is less likely in this scenario.

### Bibliography

1. **Schuyler M, Cornier Y.** The diagnosis of hypersensitivity pneumonitis. Chest. 1997;111:534-6. PMID: 9118683

## Pneumonia Question 15
## Answer: C

**Educational Objective:** *Recognize the most likely pathogens responsible for community-acquired pneumonia among patients who are not elderly.*

In most cases of community-acquired pneumonia, the culprit pathogen is never identified. Thus, the recent guidelines promulgated by the American Thoracic Society and the Infectious Disease Society of America have emphasized the need to begin empiric therapy for community-acquired pneumonia as soon as possible and to base it on patient's age, comorbid pulmonary and nonpulmonary illnesses, and severity of illness. This patient has a mild case of community-acquired pneumonia. Because of her age, lack of serious comorbid illness, and cardiovascular and pulmonary stability, application of the Pneumonia Severity Index scoring system would indicate that her risk of dying from this episode is less than 1%. Most patients with this presentation can be treated on an outpatient basis with potent oral antibiotics.

In young adults, *Mycoplasma pneumoniae* and *Chlamydia pneumoniae* are the most likely pathogens. After young adulthood, *Streptococcus pneumoniae* rises to the top of the list of microbes isolated in cases of community-acquired pneumonia. Penicillin-resistant *S. pneumoniae* is a problem in many areas of the United States, and the prevalence varies from locality to locality. Antibiotic resistance in this situation is a relative, not absolute, insensitivity to penicillin that can be overcome in cases of intermediate sensitivity by increasing the dose of penicillin administered. Resistance to other first-line agents for community-acquired pneumonia has been seen in tandem with penicillin resistance, particularly resistance to macrolides, trimethoprim-sulfamethoxazole, and first-generation cephalosporins. *M. pneumoniae*, and *C. pneumoniae* remain potential pathogens in this case, as is *Haemophilus influenzae*, the last particularly important among cigarette smokers, such as this patient. *Legionella pneumophila* may cause pneumonia in a healthy patient, but this is less common than other pathogens in this scenario. It is more likely to result in more severe pneumonia among healthy patients.

*Pseudomonas aeruginosa* organisms often colonize the respiratory tracts of patients with chronic lung disease, such as cystic fibrosis, and patients who have been hospitalized and received multiple courses of antibiotics. *Staphylococcus aureus* is another potentially deadly pathogen but one present mainly in patients with a particular predisposing circumstance, such as age older than 60, head injury, or nosocomial pneumonia, none of which pertain to this patient. The special category of methicillin-resistant *S. aureus* is an important consideration in the care of patients who have been or are currently hospitalized, especially if they are receiving multiple courses of broad-spectrum antibiotics.

Effective therapy would likely be achieved with an advanced generation macrolide, which covers most strains of *S. pneumoniae*, *H. influenzae*, and atypical pathogens such as *M. pneumoniae*, *C. pneumoniae*, and *L. pneumophila* species.

### Bibliography

1. **Bartlett JG, Dowell SF, Mandell LA, File Jr TM, Musher DM, Fine MJ.** Practice guidelines for the management of community-acquired pneumonia in adults. Infectious Diseases Society of America. Clin Infect Dis. 2000;31:422-5. PMID: 10987697

2. **Niederman MS, Mandell LA, Anzeuto A, Bass JB, Broughton WA, Campbell GD, et al.** Guidelines for the management of adults with community-acquired pneumonia. Diagnosis, assessment of severity, antimicrobial therapy, and prevention. American Thoracic Society, Am J Respir Crit Care Med. 2001;163:1730-1754. PMID: 11401897

3. **Fine MJ, Auble TE, Yeyal DM, Hanusa BH, Weissfeld LA, Singer DE, et al.** A prediction rule to identify low risk patients with community-acquired pneumonia. N Engl J Med. 1997;336:43-250. PMID: 8995086

# Chronic Obstructive Pulmonary Disease

**Chronic Obstructive Pulmonary Disease
Question 1
Answer: E**

**Educational Objective:** *Recognize the benefit of long-term oxygen therapy for patients with chronic obstructive pulmonary disease.*

Chronic tissue hypoxia results in diminished exercise capacity, neuropsychiatric problems, cor pulmonale, polycythemia, and weight loss. According to two large randomized, controlled trials, long-term oxygen therapy has been shown to improve survival in chronically hypoxic patients when administered during waking and sleeping hours. Although the specific mechanism of action is not fully known, one important component is the decrease in elevated pulmonary artery pressures that result from hypoxia-induced vasoconstriction. Reimbursement is provided for patients with a resting $PaO_2$ of $\leq 55$ mm Hg (oxygen saturation $\leq 88\%$); in patients showing evidence of cor pulmonale, erythrocytosis or altered mental status with a $PaO_2$ of 55 to 59 mm Hg (saturation 89%); or in patients with exercised-induced oxygen desaturation of 88% or less.

ACE inhibitor therapy is known to improve survival in patients with diminished left ventricular function, but it has not been formally studied in patients with isolated cor pulmonale. Appropriate treatment of cor pulmonale consists of treating the underlying pulmonary process, salt and fluid restriction, and diuretics. Inhaled bronchodilators are used to control symptoms in patients with a bronchospastic component to their disease, but these drugs have not been shown to affect mortality. Inhaled glucocorticoids do not appear to alleviate symptoms or improve the functional status in most patients studied.

### Bibliography

1. **Crockett AJ, Cranston JM, Moss JR, Alpers JH**. A review of long-term oxygen therapy for chronic obstructive pulmonary disease. Respir Med. 2001;95:437-43. PMID: 11421499

2. Continuous or nocturnal oxygen therapy in hypoxemic chronic obstructive lung disease: a clinical trial. Nocturnal Oxygen Therapy Trial Group. Ann Intern Med. 1980;93:391-8. PMID: 6776858

**Chronic Obstructive Pulmonary Disease
Question 2
Answer: B**

**Educational Objective:** *Choose an appropriate tapering regimen for glucocorticoids after the first acute exacerbation of chronic obstructive pulmonary disease.*

Glucocorticoids play an important part of the inpatient management of patients with acute exacerbations of chronic obstructive pulmonary disease. But these drugs have not been shown to be effective in the routine care of patients with stable disease. Based on the results of a large randomized, controlled trial among U.S. veterans, there does not appear to be any advantage in tapering glucocorticoids over 8 weeks compared with over 2 weeks. Although a meta-analysis published in early 1999 suggests a benefit from inhaled glucocorticoids in patients with moderate and severe disease, two recent large randomized clinical trials have failed to confirm these results. A recent Cochrane review, however, concludes that a short course of glucocorticoids following assessment for an acute exacerbation of asthma significantly reduces the number of relapses and decreases β-agonist use without an apparent increase in side effects.

Considering the recent finding about inhaled glucocorticoids, physicians should exercise caution in administering oral glucocorticoids on a continuous basis. Most experts suggest that a response to glucocorticoid therapy during an exacerbation is not an appropriate indication for long-term administration. Instead, these medications should be reserved for patients with recurrent exacerbations whose symptoms cannot be adequately controlled by other means and who have an objectively documented response.

### Bibliography

1. **Niewoehner DE, Erbland ML, Deupree RH, Collins D, Gross NJ, Light RW, et al**. Effect of systemic glucocorticoids on exacerbations of chronic obstructive pulmonary disease. Department of Veterans Affairs Cooperative Study Group. N Engl J Med. 1999;340:1941-7. PMID: 10379017

2. **Vestbo J, Sorensen T, Lange P, Brix A, Torre P, Viskum K**. Long-term effect of inhaled budesonide in mild and moderate chronic obstructive pulmonary disease: a randomized controlled trial. Lancet. 1999;353:1819-23. PMID: 10359405

3. **Postma DS, Kerstjens HA**. Are inhaled glucocorticosteroids effective in chronic obstructive pulmonary disease? Am J Respir Crit Care Med. 1999;160:S66-71. PMID: 10556173

4. **Rowe BH, Spooner CH, Ducharme FM, Bretzlaff JA, Bota GW**. Corticosteroids for preventing relapse following acute exacerbations of asthma. Cochrane Database Syst Rev. 2001;(1):CD000195. PMID: 11279682

## Chronic Obstructive Pulmonary Disease
## Question 3
## Answer: C

**Educational Objective:** *Prevent respiratory virus infections in travelers.*

Extensive recirculation of air on jet planes to save fuel puts air travelers at risk of viral respiratory infections. Viral influenza in the Northern Hemisphere usually peaks in January, the time of this patient's intended travel. The convenience and efficacy of vaccine for influenza, which includes current type A and B strains, warrants immunization of this patient every year before the influenza season begins, and certainly before this trip. Patients who develop influenza despite the vaccine tend to have milder disease. If this patient has not received pneumococcal vaccine, immunization would also be appropriate whether or not she takes this trip. Amantadine and rimantadine can reduce the incidence of viral influenza type A but have undesirable central nervous system side effects in the elderly. Amantadine and rimantadine have comparable effectiveness in the prevention and treatment of influenza A in healthy adults, although rimantadine induces fewer adverse effects than amantadine. These antiviral agents are not effective against viral influenza type B, but this type is less common than type A during peak season. Inhalation of zanamivir, 10 mg daily, appears to be effective prophylaxis against both types A and B influenza but could cause transient-bronchospasm in this patient. Oseltamivir, another neuraminidase inhibitor, is a recently marketed oral drug. Oseltamivir also appears promising in chemoprophylaxis of types A and B viral influenza and is more convenient than zanamivir. Antibacterial prophylaxis for the prevention of acute bronchitis has been disappointing, and there is little evidence that air travel increases the incidence of bacterial pneumonia. Zinc lozenges are ineffective for the treatment of viral coryza and have not been evaluated for use as prophylaxis. Zinc can cause nausea, which would impair the patient's ability to stay well hydrated during her long trip in the desiccated atmosphere of an airplane.

### Bibliography

1. **Jefferson TO, Demicheli V, Deeks JJ, Rivetti D.** Amantadine and rimantadine for preventing and treating influenza A in adults. Cochrane Database Syst Rev. 2002;(3):CD001169. Review. PMID: 12137620

2. **Hayden FG, Atmar RL, Schilling M, Johnson C, Poretz D, Paar D, et al.** Use of the selective oral neuraminidase inhibitor oseltamivir to prevent influenza. N Engl J Med. 1999;341:1336-43. PMID: 10536125

## Chronic Obstructive Pulmonary Disease
## Question 4
## Answer: D

**Educational Objective:** *Select the most efficacious initial approach to evaluation of the patient with chronic obstructive pulmonary disease without a high index of suspicion for sleep apnea.*

This patient presents with a history that is not atypical for patients with chronic obstructive pulmonary disease (COPD) — specifically, poor sleep quality and daytime fatigue. There is probably not an increased prevalence of sleep apnea in patients with COPD, and the patient described does not provide a compelling history for this disorder. This does not exclude the possibility of sleep apnea; however, there are sufficient data to make a clinician concerned about its possibility. For example, morning headaches may be an indicator of nocturnal $CO_2$ retention, and patients with awake hypercapnia are more likely to experience desaturation during sleep. In addition, the patient may be developing right ventricular dysfunction despite sufficient awake oxygen saturation, suggesting the possibility of nocturnal hypoxemia. An adequate $PaO_2$ during wakefulness does not preclude the possibility of significant sleep-related desaturation.

Complete polysomnographic evaluations are time-consuming and expensive and are justified for patients in whom sleep apnea is a significant possibility. Because this patient does not have a typical history for sleep apnea and his symptoms may be unrelated to sleep-related breathing disturbance, complete polysomnography may not be cost-effective. However, the possibility of significant nocturnal oxyhemoglobin desaturation cannot be ignored. Until a validated, less expensive home or ambulatory monitoring tool is developed, it is reasonable to conduct overnight oximetry on the patient. If this reveals significant desaturation, it may warrant complete polysomnography. The use of benzodiazepines to improve sleep quality is not indicated and may be harmful by further imparing nocturnal breathing.

### Bibliography

1. **Phillipson EA, Goldstein RS.** Breathing during sleep in chronic obstructive pulmonary disease. State of the art. Chest. 1984;85:24-30. PMID: 6373177

2. **Klink M, Quan SF.** Prevalence of reported sleep disturbance in a general adult population and their relationship to obstructive airways diseases. Chest. 1987;91:540-6. PMID: 3829746

3. **Bradley TD, Mateika J, Li D, Avenano M, Goldstein RS.** Daytime hypercapnia in the development of nocturnal hypoxemia in COPD. Chest. 1990;97:308-12. PMID: 2298055

4. **Fletcher EC, Donner CF, Midgren B, Zielinski J, Levi-Valensi P, Braghiroli A, et al.** Survival in COPD patients with a daytime Pao2 > 60 mm Hg with and without nocturnal oxyhemoglobin desaturation. Chest. 1992;101:649-55. PMID: 1541127

## Chronic Obstructive Pulmonary Disease
## Question 5
## Answer: D

**Educational Objective:** *Define the bacteriology of an acute exacerbation of chronic bronchitis in a complicated patient at risk for drug-resistant or gram-negative bacterial infection.*

The acute exacerbation of chronic bronchitis (AECB) in this complicated patient should be treated with antibiotic therapy. In earlier trials, the common organisms causing exacerbation were *Haemophilus influenzae, Moraxella catarrhalis,* and pneumococcus, and none of these bacteria were commonly resistant to antibiotics, leading to the conclusion that virtually any broad-spectrum antibiotic would be effective.

In the past decade, antibiotic resistance has become a common problem in patients with AECB. Up to 40% of *H. influenzae* and more than 90% of *M. catarrhalis* organisms produce beta-lactamase enzymes, rendering agents such as ampicillin and amoxicillin ineffective. In addition, pneumococci are increasingly resistant to penicillin. Risk factors for resistant pneumococcus include recent beta-lactam therapy in the past 3 months, age greater than 65 years, immunosuppressive illness, and alcoholism. The patient presented here has multiple risk factors for penicillin-resistant pneumococci, and if infected with the other common organisms, these, too, are likely to be antibiotic-resistant (beta-lactamase-positive). *Mycoplasma pneumoniae* is a common pneumonia pathogen, but its role in AECB has never been established, and it is not a likely pathogen in this patient.

This patient has advanced chronic obstructive pulmonary disease (COPD), and he is likely to have an organism such as *Pseudomonas aeruginosa* in his sputum. Recent studies have shown that this organism is more common than other organisms in patients with an $FEV_1$ < 35% of the predicted value. In addition, a shift to gram-negative and drug-resistant organisms is more likely in patients older than 65 years, those with long-standing COPD, those on corticosteroids, those with comorbidities and those who have had at least four exacerbations in the preceding year. This patient has many of these features, making the more simple organisms less likely to be present, being replaced by *P. aeruginosa* or other gram-negative organisms.

The definition of patient subsets has been shown to correlate with the bacteriology of sputum cultures in AECB, but data are still lacking to prove that if therapy is selected with these bacteriologic data in mind, outcome is improved. Preliminary studies do suggest a therapeutic benefit to stratifying patients, but more definitive outcome studies are needed.

### Bibliography

1. **Saint S, Bent S, Vittinghoff E, Grady D**. Antibiotics in chronic obstructive pulmonary disease exacerbations. A meta-analysis. JAMA. 1995;273:957-60. PMID: 7884956
2. **Eller J, Ede A, Schaberg T, Niederman MS, Mauch H, Lode H**. Infective exacerbations of chronic bronchitis: relation between bacteriologic etiology and lung function. Chest. 1998;113:1542-8. PMID: 9631791

## Chronic Obstructive Pulmonary Disease
## Question 6
## Answer: D

**Educational Objective:** *Diagnose and treat pulmonary hypertension.*

This patient, who is a smoker, has developed obstructive airways disease. He presents to the hospital now with cor pulmonale, which is likely caused by chronic hypoxemia. The arterial blood gas studies document the current level of hypoxemia, and the hematocrit of 57% suggests that hypoxemia has been present for a long time and has led to secondary polycythemia. Chronic hypoxemia is the cause of the pulmonary vasoconstriction, pulmonary hypertension, and cor pulmonale. Thus, oxygen therapy is the treatment of choice and might be expected to alleviate the heart failure, polycythemia, and even the altered mental state. Oxygen therapy should be given at low flow rates by nasal cannula or with a Venturi mask so as to avoid precipitating further carbon dioxide retention.

Pulmonary hypertension is secondary to hypoxemia and will not respond to vasodilators, such as calcium-channel blockers. The lung scan shows nonsegmental matched filling defects that are typically seen in patients with obstructive airways disease and do not suggest pulmonary embolism. Even without a confirming pulmonary arteriogram, the likelihood of pulmonary embolism is quite low thus full-dose unfractionated heparin, therefore, would not be indicated.

Although intravenous methylprednisolone may be useful to treat acute exacerbations of chronic obstructive airways disease, the results take hours to achieve. In addition, this would not be the single best treatment for the pulmonary hypertension secondary to chronic hypoxemia. Phlebotomy would benefit this patient, as oxygen-carrying capacity and rheologic properties of the blood are maximal at hematocrits lower than 57%. Oxygen administration will ultimately reduce the hematocrit and produce the same results by a more physiologic sequence of events.

### Bibliography

1. **Albert RK, Martin TR, Lewis SW**. Controlled clinical trial of methylprednisolone in patients with chronic bronchitis and acute respiratory insufficiency. Ann Intern Med. 1980;92:753-8. PMID: 6770731
2. **Weitzenblum E, Sautegeau A, Ehrhart M, Mammosser M, Pelletier A**. Long-term oxygen therapy can reverse the progression of pulmonary hypertension in patients with chronic obstructive pulmonary disease. Am Rev Respir Dis. 1985;131:493-8. PMID: 3922267

## Chronic Obstructive Pulmonary Disease
## Question 7
## Answer: C

**Educational Objective:** *Assess the need for and benefit from chronic oxygen therapy for advanced chronic obstructive pulmonary disease (COPD).*

This patient has severe chronic obstructive pulmonary disease and he has hypoxemia at both rest and with exertion. He is a patient who qualifies for oxygen therapy for a number of reasons and will likely have multiple benefits from this therapy. Criteria for prescribing long-term oxygen therapy include $PaO_2 < 55$ mm Hg or $SaO_2 < 88\%$, and this patient meets these criteria. In addition, he has exertional desaturation, slight polycythemia, and signs of cor pulmonale with a right-sided $S_3$ and peripheral edema. In the presence of cor pulmonale or a hematocrit $\geq 55\%$ or with congestive heart failure, oxygen should be prescribed, even with a $PaO_2$ of 55 mm Hg to 59 mm Hg or an $SaO_2$ of 89%. When any of these criteria are met, oxygen should be prescribed at rest, with exercise, and during sleep. Data from the oxygen therapy trials have shown that the longer oxygen is administered, the greater the benefits, and that nocturnal oxygen alone is not as helpful as oxygen administered all day long. With a higher oxygen saturation at rest, oxygen should be prescribed only if sleep or exercise desaturation is documented, and then therapy should be given only during these times.

The benefits of long-term oxygen therapy include increase in body weight, reversal of secondary erythrocytosis, improvement in heart failure due to cor pulmonale, enhanced neuropsychologic function, improved exercise capacity, and enhanced survival. In the long-term oxygen therapy trials, longevity increased the longer oxygen was used during a 24-hour period. These trials showed that oxygen therapy improved survival for patients who qualified, compared with no oxygen therapy, and that continuous oxygen therapy was more beneficial than nocturnal therapy alone. When patients have exertional dyspnea, oxygen therapy can prevent transient rises in pulmonary artery pressure, relieve dyspnea, and improve exercise performance. Thus, this patient is likely to have multiple benefits from oxygen therapy, but these benefits will be maximized if oxygen is used continuously, at rest as well as with exercise and during sleep.

### Bibliography

1. Standards for the diagnosis and care of patients with chronic obstructive pulmonary disease. American Thoracic Society. Am J Respir Crit Care Med. 1995;152:S77-S121. PMID: 7582322

## Chronic Obstructive Pulmonary Disease
## Question 8
## Answer: E

**Educational Objective:** *Identify interventions that can modify the anticipated progressive loss of lung function among active cigarette smokers with chronic obstructive pulmonary disease.*

A major determinant of prognosis among patients with chronic obstructive pulmonary disease (COPD) is the severity of airflow obstruction, as measured with forced expiratory volume in 1 sec ($FEV_1$). This patient already has severe airflow obstruction, as indicated by the results of spirometry. Among current cigarette smokers with COPD, lung function generally worsens at an accelerated rate compared with that among persons who do not smoke. Among healthy nonsmoking adults, $FEV_1$ declines with aging at an average rate of approximately 20 to 30 mL per year. Among cigarette smokers with COPD, that rate in general increases twofold to threefold. Recent large-scale studies performed among cigarette smokers with mild to moderate airflow obstruction due to COPD found an average annual decrease in $FEV_1$ of approximately 50 to 60 mL.

With smoking cessation, lung function initially improves over weeks to months, and the improvement is followed by a continued decline in $FEV_1$ comparable with that among nonsmokers. Cigarette smokers with COPD who stop smoking and maintain smoking cessation have better lung function at the end of 5 years of follow-up evaluation than do smokers with COPD who continue to smoke. (It must be remembered that 80% to 85% of cigarette smokers do not experience marked airflow obstruction, and they are not vulnerable to the accelerated decline in lung function that occurs among smokers with COPD.)

It has long been observed that inhaled β-adrenergic agonists, a mainstay in the long-term management of COPD, provide temporary improvement in lung function for many patients with COPD, but they do not alter long-term prognosis. Large-scale, double-blind, placebo-controlled randomized clinical trials have been performed to address whether regular use of inhaled anticholinergic agents or inhaled glucocorticoids might slow lung function decline over time. Over 3 to 5 years investigators observed no long-term benefit of these therapies. An important goal of outpatient pulmonary rehabilitation is improvement in exercise capacity among persons with COPD who suffer general physical deconditioning. Regular exercise does not, however, alter lung function among patients with COPD.

### Bibliography

1. **Anthonisen NR, Connett JE, Kiley JP, Altose MD, Bailey WC, Buist AS, et al**. Effects of smoking intervention and the use of an inhaled anticholinergic bronchodilator on the rate of decline of FEV1: the Lung Health Study. JAMA. 1994;272:1497-505. PMID: 7966841

2. Pauwels RA, Löfdahl CG, Laitinen LA, Schouten JP, Postma DS, Pride NB, et al. Long-term treatment with inhaled budesonide in persons with mild chronic obstructive pulmonary disease who continue smoking. European Respiratory Society Study on Chronic Obstructive Pulmonary Disease. N Engl J Med. 1999;340:1948-53. PMID: 10379018

## Chronic Obstructive Pulmonary Disease
## Question 9
## Answer: C

**Educational Objective:** *Identify risks and benefits of regular use of inhaled glucocorticoids.*

Regular use of inhaled glucocorticoids decreases bronchial hyperresponsiveness by reducing airway inflammation. All of the inhaled glucocorticoids are effective given twice a day, and patient adherence is much improved when the prescribed dosing is twice rather than four times a day. One inhaled glucocorticoid, budesonide, has been shown to be effective with once-daily dosing among persons with mild asthma. The response to any bronchoprovocative stimulus, including exercise, is thereby lessened when bronchial hyperresponsiveness is reduced. However, unlike cromolyn or nedocromil, a glucocorticoid inhaled in a single dose before exercise is not effective in preventing exercise-induced bronchoconstriction.

Systemic absorption of inhaled glucocorticoids appears to be dose dependent. Clinically significant systemic side effects are associated with high doses, especially 1000 or more (g/d. The risk of altered bone mineralization and osteoporosis from long-term exposure to inhaled glucocorticoids remains poorly defined. Longitudinal clinical trials are being conducted.

Use of inhaled glucocorticoids is recommended for management of persistent asthma during pregnancy. Evidence particularly supports the safety of beclomethasone and budesonide in this setting.

### Bibliography

1. Garbe E, LeLorier J, Boivin JF, Suissa S. Inhaled and nasal glucocorticoids and the risks of ocular hypertension or open-angle glaucoma. JAMA. 1997;277:722-7. PMID: 9042844
2. McFadden ER, Casale TB, Edwards TB, Kemp JP, Metzger WJ, Nelson HS, et al. Administration of budesonide once daily by means of turbuhaler to subjects with stable asthma. J Allergy Clin Immunol. 1999;104:46-52. PMID: 10400838
3. Schatz M. Asthma and pregnancy [comment]. Lancet. 1999;353:1202-4. PMID: 10217076

## Chronic Obstructive Pulmonary Disease
## Question 10
## Answer: D

**Educational Objective:** *Confirm diagnostic suspicion of $\alpha_1$-antitrypsin deficiency.*

By far the most common inherited predisposition to the development of emphysema is a deficiency of the antiprotease protein, $\alpha_1$-antitrypsin (also called $\alpha_1$-protease inhibitor). The usual cause of $\alpha_1$-antitrypsin deficiency is production of an abnormal $\alpha_1$-antitrypsin protein that has impaired transport out of the liver with only very small amounts entering the blood. Measurement of the blood level of $\alpha_1$-antitrypsin is the most direct method to identify $\alpha_1$-antitrypsin deficiency. Emphysema develops among persons homozygous for an abnormal gene allele (two different abnormal alleles). Such persons have serum concentrations of $\alpha_1$-antitrypsin protein 10% to 15% of the normal value (normal range for $\alpha_1$-antitrypsin, 76 to 190 mg/dL). In rare instances, patients lack the $\alpha_1$-antitrypsin gene and produce no detectable protein.

$\alpha_1$-Antitrypsin is an acute-phase reactant — the blood level increases in acute inflammatory states. Among patients with $\alpha_1$-antitrypsin deficiency, however, blood levels do not increase into the normal range. Among patients with low levels of $\alpha_1$-antitrypsin, starch gel and immunoelectrophoretic techniques can be used to identify the abnormal gene product. The most common abnormal $\alpha_1$-antitrypsin protein is identified as the protease inhibitor Z or PiZ. Persons homozygous for this abnormal protein have the PiZZ phenotype. $\alpha_1$-Antitrypsin phenotyping is a confirmatory test in the diagnosis of $\alpha_1$-antitrypsin deficiency.

In the absence of advanced disease, chest radiographic findings usually are normal among patients with emphysema. CT of the chest is useful in the diagnosis of emphysema wherein dilated air spaces and bullae undetectable on plain chest radiographs are often depicted. The pattern of distribution of emphysematous changes - a predominance at the lung bases (rather than the usual apical predominance) - may suggest a diagnosis of $\alpha_1$-antitrypsin deficiency. However, blood testing is needed to establish the diagnosis.

Oxygen desaturation with exercise and reduced carbon monoxide diffusing capacity are findings of advanced emphysema. However, they are not specific for emphysema and do not indicate that emphysema, if present, is caused by an inherited protein deficiency. Once a diagnosis of $\alpha_1$-antitrypsin deficiency has been established, it is appropriate to screen close family members for the deficiency. Testing can be conducted with $\alpha_1$-antitrypsin blood level as a screening test and $\alpha_1$-antitrypsin phenotyping by means of electrophoresis for confirmation for those with a reduced blood level.

### Bibliography

1. Wiedemann HP, Stoller JK. Lung disease due to alpha 1-antitrypsin deficiency. Curr Opin Pulm Med. 1996;2:155-60. PMID: 9363132

# Deep Venous Thrombosis

## Deep Venous Thrombosis Question 1
### Answer: D

**Educational Objective:** *Understand the appropriate prophylaxis for deep venous thrombosis in orthopedic procedures.*

Warfarin is recommended for prophylaxis for deep venous thrombosis in patients undergoing total knee replacement. There are several regimens for starting prophylaxis in the perioperative period, including one tablet on the night before surgery, or starting with the first dose on the first day after surgery. The target INR is between 2 to 3.

Although subcutaneous low-molecular-weight heparin in prophylactic doses is a reasonable alternative to warfarin in this setting, full-dose intravenous unfractionated heparin is not recommended. Total knee replacement surgery carries a risk of calf deep venous thrombosis of 40% to 80%, a risk for proximal deep venous thrombosis of 10% to 20%, a risk for clinical pulmonary embolism of 5% to 10%, and a risk for fatal pulmonary embolism of 1% to 5%. Aspirin is not effective for prophylaxis of deep venous thrombosis. The patient should stop taking aspirin 7 days before this procedure to reduce the risk of bleeding complications. Elastic stockings and pneumatic compression are additive for prophylaxis, but are not sufficient for effective prophylaxis in themselves.

### Bibliography

1. **Handoll HHG, Farrar MJ, McBirnie J, Tytherleigh-Strong G, Awal KA, Milne AA, Gillespie WJ**. Heparin, low molecular weight heparin and physical methods for preventing deep vein thrombosis and pulmonary embolism following surgery for hip fractures. Cochrane Database Syst Rev. 2000;(2):CD000305. PMID: 10796339

2. **Clagett GP, Anderson FA Jr, Geerts W, Heit JA, Knudson M, Lieberman JR, et al**. Prevention of venous thromboembolism. Chest. 1998;114(5 Suppl):531S-560S. PMID: 9822062

## Deep Venous Thrombosis Question 2
### Answer: B

**Educational Objective:** *Manage recurrent venous thromboembolism in a patient who is therapeutically anticoagulated.*

This patient had a pulmonary embolism while in the early stages of therapy for recognized venous thrombosis. Heparin therapy is at a dosage in the therapeutic range, and warfarin is not yet therapeutic. The appropriate management strategy would be placement of an inferior vena caval filter, which should prevent recurrent pulmonary embolization. Inferior

vena cava filters are placed fairly easily transcutaneously and have a low incidence of adverse reactions (5%) and very low associated mortality ($\leq 0.1\%$). Potential complications include malpositioning, infection, air embolization during placement, local wound problems (for example, hematoma formation), perforation of the vena caval wall, migration from the site of placement, and rarely induction of venous thrombosis at the site of insertion. Indications for filter placement include contraindication to anticoagulation, anticoagulation failure or complication (such as in this patient), and pulmonary embolism prophylaxis. It has been reported that the risk of venous thrombosis is increased in the 2 years after an inferior vena cava filter is placed. The risk of recurrent venous thrombosis dictates a full course of therapy with anticoagulation unless specifically contraindicated by hemorrhagic diatheses.

Because she is adequately anticoagulated with heparin, there is no need to adjust her heparin dosage. Increasing the dose of warfarin is unlikely to have an immediate effect due to the relatively long time required for warfarin to inhibit its target coagulation factors, and it may lead to supratherapeutic effect with an increased risk of bleeding. Because the patient has a large clot persisting in her leg, simple observation does not further reduce her risk of repeat pulmonary embolism.

### Bibliography

1. **Decousus H, Leizorovicz A, Parent F, Page Y, Tardy B, Girard P, et al**. A clinical trial of vena caval filters in the prevention of pulmonary embolism in patients with proximal deep-vein thrombosis. Prevention du Risque d'Embolie Pulmonaire par Interruption Cave Study Group. N Engl J Med. 1998;338:409-15. PMID: 9459643

2. **Becker DM, Philbrick JT, Selby JB**. Inferior vena cava filters. Indications, safety, effectiveness. Arch Intern Med. 1992;152:1985-94. PMID: 1417371

## Deep Venous Thrombosis Question 3
### Answer: D

**Educational Objective:** *Institute therapy in a patient with suspected venous thromboembolism before additional diagnostic procedures.*

When venous thromboembolism is strongly suspected, the first action taken should be to administer heparin in a therapeutic dose (in the absence of contraindications to anticoagulation) to prevent new clot formation, allow unopposed fibrinolytic activity to facilitate thrombus resolution, and avoid progression into the pulmonary circulation. Therapy should be started before performing confirmatory diagnostic tests such as a ventilation-perfusion scan, pulmonary angiogram or compression ultrasonography of the lower extremities. Subtherapeutic or delayed anticoagulation is associated with unacceptable recurrence rates of venous thromboembolism, and is a common error in the initial phases of treatment. Although relatively less heparin is required to prevent the coagulation cascade from being initiated, more is required after the cascade is under way. Therefore, early administration of an adequate dose is required. For continuous infusions, the activated partial thromboplastin time should be monitored regularly to ensure that the dose is therapeutic. Inadequate initial heparin therapy also has been associated with late recurrences of thromboembolism. Anxiolytic therapy would not be an appropriate as the initial step in this patient's management.

**Bibliography**

1.  **Hull RD, Raskob GE, Brant RF, Pineo GF, Valentine KA.** The importance of initial heparin treatment on long-term clinical outcomes of antithrombotic therapy. The emerging theme of delayed recurrence. Arch Intern Med. 1997;157:2317-21. PMID: 9361572
2.  **Prandoni P, Lensing AW, Cogo A, Cuppini S, Villalta S, Carta M, et al**. The long-term clinical course of acute deep venous thrombosis. Ann Intern Med. 1996;125:1-7. PMID: 8644983

## Deep Venous Thrombosis Question 4
## Answer: A

**Educational Objective:** *Avoid an inappropriate and expensive search for an occult neoplasm in a patient with acute deep venous thrombosis.*

Deep venous thrombosis, particularly in an elderly patient, always raises concern about an underlying neoplasm. Although such patients may have an increased incidence of occult malignancy, several studies have demonstrated that an extensive search for a neoplasm rarely yields positive results. A neoplasm amenable to curative therapy is found even more rarely. Therefore, a nondirected and extensive evaluation of this patient for occult malignancy is very unlikely to identify a treatable neoplasm and is not cost effective. However, any clues obtained from the medical history and a thorough physical examination (including a digital rectal examination) suggestive of a neoplasm should be pursued. In this patient, the extensive smoking history justifies a screening chest radiograph despite the lack of symptoms. Since the patient has no other complaints or findings suggestive of an underlying neoplasm (weight loss, stools positive for occult blood, abdominal pain). Therefore, a more extensive evaluation is not indicated. Measurement of the serum carcinoembryonic antigen level may be useful in following the progression of colon cancer once a diagnosis and baseline carcinoembryonic antigen levels are established but is not sensitive or specific when used as a screening assay.

**Bibliography**

1.  **Cornuz J, Pearson SD, Creager MA, Cook EF, Goldman L**. Importance of findings on the initial evaluation for cancer in patients with symptomatic idiopathic deep venous thrombosis. Ann Intern Med. 1996;125:785-93. PMID: 8928984
2.  **Nordström M, Lindblad B, Anderson H, Bergqvist D, Kjellström T**. Deep venous thrombosis and occult malignancy: an epidemiological study. BMJ. 1994;308:891-4. PMID: 8173368

## Deep Venous Thrombosis Question 5
## Answer: B

**Educational Objective:** *Select the most appropriate therapy to reverse excessive warfarin anticoagulation in a patient with minimal evidence of bleeding.*

This patient has a supratherapeutic INR. The ecchymoses are a minor bleeding complication, but he has a normal hemoglobin level and no evidence of more serious bleeding. The deep venous thrombosis of the left leg is relatively new, and he is at risk of further propagation of the clot if anticoagulation is not maintained. This patient therefore needs to have the warfarin effect lowered without fully reversing the anticoagulation. Vitamin K therapy will correct the INR without the risk associated with transfusing a blood product. Additional vitamin K overrides the warfarin blockade of the γ-carboxylation pathway and results in production of functional clotting factors within hours. The dose of vitamin K determines how much of the warfarin effect will be reversed. A dose of 5 mg of vitamin K will significantly reverse the anticoagulant effect of warfarin within 12 to 24 hours if the patient has good liver function. A 10-mg dose will usually block the warfarin effect completely and interfere with attempts to resume anticoagulation with warfarin. The risk of clotting versus the risk of bleeding determines how much vitamin K to give and how long to withhold the warfarin dose.

For patients such as the one described, the dose of vitamin K should be low enough to allow resumption of anticoagulation with warfarin as soon as the INR has dropped into the therapeutic range. Studies have shown that vitamin K, 1 to 2 mg subcutaneously or 2.5 mg orally, will bring the INR into the therapeutic range without causing overcorrection. Low-dose vitamin K should decrease this patient's INR without placing him at risk for another thrombosis.

Fresh frozen plasma is the most rapid way to replace vitamin K clotting factors and reverse the anticoagulation. However, because of the infectious and allergic risks associated with blood products, fresh frozen plasma is only used to reverse warfarin if a patient has a serious bleeding complication or excessive risk of bleeding. Therefore, giving this patient fresh frozen plasma places him at greater long-term risk than the immediate risk imposed by the excessive anticoagulation.

Intramuscular medications should not be given to patients with a coagulopathy because these patients have a high risk of developing an intramuscular hematoma. Furthermore, bleeding into the muscle will hamper attempts to resume anticoagulation for the underlying thrombosis. This patient's poor oral intake over the last several days will result in low vitamin K stores. Stopping the warfarin with no other therapy (that is, without replacing vitamin K) will result in a slow reversal of the anticoagulant effect and prolong the risk of bleeding.

**Bibliography**
1. **Watson HG, Baglin T, Laidlaw SL, Makris M, Preston FE**. A comparison of the efficacy and rate of response to oral and intravenous Vitamin K in reversal of over-anticoagulation with warfarin. Br J Haematol. 2001;115:145-9. PMID: 11722425
2. **Bussey HI**. Managing excessive warfarin anticoagulation. Ann Intern Med. 2001;135:460-2. PMID: 11560459

## Deep Venous Thrombosis Question 6
## Answer: D

**Educational Objective:** *Review the indications for placement of an inferior vena cava filter in the treatment of pulmonary embolism.*

This patient has multiple pulmonary emboli involving two lobes and two lung segments. The presence of systemic hypotension associated with pulmonary emboli indicates a limited pulmonary vascular reserve due to a large volume of clot, and further emboli could be fatal. Thrombolytic therapy with tissue plasminogen activator (t-PA) or urokinase is warranted but cannot be given 5 days after major abdominal surgery. Either unfractionated or low-molecular-weight heparin is necessary to prevent further clot formation, but the patient remains in jeopardy of additional embolization of any remaining lower-extremity thrombi. This is effectively prevented by inserting a filter into the inferior vena cava (IVC). Indications for IVC filters include intolerance of anticoagulation (recent gastrointestinal or intracranial bleeding, thrombocytopenia), documented failure of anticoagulation, massive pulmonary embolus (as in this patient), or chronic pulmonary hypertension with limited capacity to tolerate additional pulmonary emboli. Oral warfarin is not indicated as initial therapy, primarily because of its slow onset of action and, in addition, there is the risk of development of a transient hypercoagulable state when it is given prior to heparin therapy.

**Bibliography**
1. **Becker DM, Philbrick JT, Selby JB**. Inferior vena caval filters. Indications, safety and effectiveness. Arch Intern Med. 1992;152:1985-94. PMID: 1417371
2. **Decousus H, Leizorovicz A, Parent F, Page Y, Tardy B, Girard P, et al**. A clinical trial of vena caval filters in the prevention of pulmonary embolism in patients with proximal deep-vein thrombosis. Prevention du Risque d'Embolie Pulmonaire par Interruption Cave Study Group. N Engl J Med. 1998;338:409-15. PMID: 9459643
3. **Tapson VF, Witty LA**. Massive pulmonary embolism. Diagnostic and therapeutic strategies. Clin Chest Med. 1995;16:329-40 PMID: 7656544

## Deep Venous Thrombosis Question 7
## Answer: D

**Educational Objective:** *Use the Prospective Investigation of Pulmonary Embolism Diagnosis (PIOPED) algorithm for the diagnosis of pulmonary embolism.*

The ventilation-perfusion scan indicates a high probability for acute pulmonary embolism (PE). Results of the Prospective Investigation of Pulmonary Embolism Diagnosis (PIOPED) indicate that the probability of pulmonary embolism is high enough to warrant therapy for pulmonary embolism with no further diagnostic studies. Treatment with unfractionated heparin or low-molecular-weight heparin is warranted because of the high risk of recurrence and death. The findings at pulmonary angiography would increase the certainty of the diagnosis, but the risk and expense of the procedure are not warranted in this setting. If the level of dimerized plasmin fragment D (D-dimer) is normal, there is a low likelihood of PE if the clinical probability is in the low to intermediate range. The level of D-dimer is not relevant in a high-probability clinical scenario and is likely to be elevated in the postoperative period. Malignant disease of the abdomen is associated with increased risk of PE, but a single occurrence of PE, especially in a high-risk clinical setting, does not justify a search for underlying malignant disease. Although factor V Leiden mutation is associated with recurrent PE, a search for factor V Leiden mutation is not warranted after an isolated occurrence of PE.

**Bibliography**
1. **Ginsberg JS, Wells PS, Kearon C, Anderson D, Crowther M, Weitz JI, et al**. Sensitivity and specificity of a rapid whole-blood assay for D-dimer in the diagnosis of pulmonary embolism. Ann Intern Med. 1998;129:1006-11. PMID: 9867754
2. **Sorensen HT, Mellemkjaer L, Steffensen FH, Olsen JH, Nielsen GL**. The risk of a diagnosis of cancer after primary deep venous thrombosis or pulmonary embolism. N Engl J Med. 1998;338:1169-73. PMID: 9554856
3. Value of the ventilation/perfusion scan in acute pulmonary embolism. Results of the prospective investigation of pulmonary embolism diagnosis (PIOPED). The PIOPED Investigators. JAMA. 1990;263:2753-9. PMID: 2332918

## Deep Venous Thrombosis Question 8
## Answer: B

**Educational Objective:** *Understand the appropriate indications for the use of low-molecular-weight heparin.*

Therapy with low-molecular-weight heparin is expensive but is appropriate in the management of deep venous thrombosis (DVT) and pulmonary embolism (PE) when other forms of therapy are ineffective or contraindicated. Low-molecular-weight heparin also has been used for outpatient management of uncomplicated DVT and PE. Intermittent administration of unfractionated heparin has been used for management of PE but has been rejected in recent years because of higher rates of bleeding and recurrent PE compared with continuous administration of heparin. Warfarin therapy is contraindicated during pregnancy because of its teratogenic and fetopathic properties. Insertion of an intravenous filter is not indicated without great risk of reoccurrence of the PE and the inability to use antithrombotic preventive measures. Compression stockings are not practical for patients with lower extremity fractures.

## Bibliography

1. **Gillis S, Shushan A, Eldor A**. Use of low molecular weight heparin for prophylaxis and treatment of thromboembolism in pregnancy. Int J Gynaecol Obstet.1992;39:297-301. PMID: 1361463

## Deep Venous Thrombosis Question 9
## Answer: D

**Educational Objective:** *Select appropriate testing in patients with primary (genetic) versus secondary (acquired) hypercoagulability.*

This patient requires an evaluation for hypercoagulability state because he has a recurrent thrombosis and because of his young age. The patient's history suggests a genetic cause of hypercoagulability. The most common inherited cause of hypercoagulability in white patients is factor V Leiden mutation, which leads to resistance to activated protein C. Approximately 5% of white patients have this mutation. There are many other inherited causes of hypercoagulability, including genetic deficiencies of protein C, protein S, and antithrombin III. This patient could have had an acquired cause of hypercoagulability, the most common of which is the antiphospholipid antibody syndrome, but this is rarely familial.

## Bibliography

1. **Petri M**. Pathogenesis and treatment of the antiphospholipid antibody syndrome. Med Clin North Am. 1997;81:151-77. PMID: 9012759
2. **Nachman RL, Silverstein R**. Hypercoagulable states. Ann Intern Med. 1993;119:819-27. PMID: 8379603

## Deep Venous Thrombosis Question 10
## Answer: B

**Educational Objective:** *Differentiate between rupture of a popliteal cyst and thrombophlebitis.*

The probable diagnosis in this man is a rupture of a popliteal cyst (Baker's cyst) into the calf, an event that can mimic thrombophlebitis. It is important that the diagnosis be made because anticoagulation in such a patient can lead to excessive bleeding in the calf muscles and adjacent tissues. Ultrasonography is the best and least expensive technique for displaying a popliteal cyst and its rupture or extension into the lower leg; it will also identify deep venous thrombosis. A helpful sign for diagnosis, when it is found, is the appearance of a crescentic ecchymosis beneath one of the malleoli of the ankle. Before recognizing the usefulness of ultrasonography in making the diagnosis, arthrography (radiographic injection into the knee) was used. If ultrasonography results are equivocal, MRI and CT would be additional techniques for imaging a popliteal cyst. Venography is not indicated.

Although joint aspiration and injection of glucocorticoids into the joint would not harm the patient, it would not help in discerning between phlebitis and rupture of a popliteal cyst. Rarely, both thrombophlebitis and a rupture of a popliteal cyst can occur concurrently.

When the diagnosis of a ruptured popliteal cyst is made, intra-articular glucocorticoids can be used to suppress the inflammation and decrease the volume of fluid in the joint. Popliteal cysts develop when excessive intra-articular pressure causes a posterior herniation, often with formation of a one-way valve effect, whereby fluid forced into the cyst cannot return to the joint space. Rarely, synovectomy of the knee is necessary for recurrent cysts. Surgical excision of popliteal cysts is rarely done because the rate of recurrence is high.

## Bibliography

1. **Hench PK, Reid RT, Reames PM**. Dissecting popliteal cyst simulating thrombophlebitis. Ann Intern Med. 1966;64:1259-64. PMID: 5933425
2. **Kraag G, Thevathasan EM, Gordon DA, Walker IH**. The hemorrhagic crescent sign of acute synovial rupture. Ann Intern Med. 1976;85:477-8. PMID: 970778

# Nosocomial Infection

## Nosocomial Infection Question 1
### Answer: B

**Educational Objective:**   *Understand the pathophysiology of catheter-associated urinary tract infections.*

Approximately 20% of hospitalized patients with indwelling urinary catheters develop an infection. Before the development of closed drainage systems, ascension along the internal lumen of the catheter after colonization of the tube of the collecting bag was the most common cause of infection, an outcome that occurred in nearly 100% of patients. With the new systems, extraluminal migration along the outside of the catheter in the periurethral mucous sheath has become the most important route of access into the urinary system. Although this patient's intravenous catheter has been in longer than the recommended 72 hours, it still is an unlikely source for this patient's pyuria. At the age of 23 years, this patient is unlikely to have had colonization of the bladder before her accident.

### Bibliography

1.  **Wong ES, Hooton TM**.Guidelines for prevention of catheter-associated urinary tract infections. Available at http://www.cdc.gov/ncidod/hip/Guide/uritract.htm, 8-25-01. Accessed 10/23/02.
2.  **Warren JW**.Catheter-associated urinary tract infections. Infect Dis Clin North Am. 1997;11:609-22. PMID: 9378926
3.  **Tambyah PA, Halvorson KT, Maki DG**.A prospective study of pathogenesis of catheter-associated urinary tract infections. Mayo Clin Proc. 1999;74:131-6. PMID: 10069349

## Nosocomial Infection Question 2
### Answer: C

**Educational Objective:**   *Understand the appropriate protocol for handwashing.*

Handwashing is the cornerstone of infection control. Indicated after all patient contacts, even with the use of gloves, handwashing requires a minimum of 10 to 15 seconds to be effective. Studies show that physician compliance is approximately 50% lower than that of nursing staff. Antimicrobial-containing products are indicated only in high-risk settings. Unfortunately, most interventions have been shown to have only a short-term impact on physician behavior.

### Bibliography

1.  **Goldmann D, Larson E**. Hand-washing and nosocomial infections. N Engl J Med. 1992;327:120-2. PMID: 1603120
2.  **Boyce JM, Pittet D**. Guideline for Hand Hygiene in Health-Care Settings. Recommendations of the Healthcare Infection Control Practices Advisory Committee and the HICPAC/SHEA/APIC/IDSA Hand Hygiene Task Force. Society for Healthcare Epidemiology of America/Association for Professionals in Infection Control/Infectious Diseases Society of America. MMWR Recomm Rep. 2002;51(RR-16):1-45. PMID: 12418624

## Nosocomial Infection Question 3
### Answer: A

**Educational Objective:**   *Recognize the relative risks of infection of various sites of intravenous lines.*

In view of the incidence of bloodstream infection secondary to intravascular device use, clinicians should to be familiar with the relative risks of different sites and devices. In general, sites that are easily kept dry and clean are preferred. Therefore, access via upper rather than lower extremity, subclavian rather than internal jugular, and forearm or hand rather than wrist approaches should be attempted initially. Internal jugular catheterization is associated with more infections than subclavian, possibly due to closer proximity to oral secretions and greater movement. However, technically, placement of internal jugular catheters is associated with fewer mechanical complications than subclavian catheterization. The precise role of antibiotic-impregnated catheters is yet to be determined. Multiple-lumen catheters have a higher rate of infection than their single-lumen counterparts.

### Bibliography

1.  **Pearson ML**.Guideline for prevention of intravascular device-related infection. Hospital Infection Control Practices Advisory Committee. Infect Control Hosp Epidemiol. 1996;17:438-73. PMID: 8839803
2.  **Farkas JC, Liu N, Bleriot JP, Chevret S, Goldstein FW, Carlet J**.Single- versus triple-lumen central catheter-related sepsis: a prospective randomized study in a critically ill population. Am J Med. 1992:93:277-82. PMID: 1524079

## Nosocomial Infection Question 4
### Answer: D

**Educational Objective:**   *Treat severe hospital-acquired pneumonia.*

This patient has late-onset hospital-acquired pneumonia (> 5 days after admission). It is severe by virtue of the multi-lobar involvement shown on chest radiograph and the need for intubation. *Pseudomonas aeruginosa* is a possible bacterial cause, as are other gram-negative organisms. Other organisms to consider in this scenario include drug-resistant *Streptococcus pneumoniae* (DRSP), *Staphylococcus aureus*, and *Legionella* species. This patient may also be at risk for *M. tuberculosis* and endemic fungi, although these are less likely based on her presentation. To cover *Pseudomonas* appropriately in this critically ill patient, double coverage is indicated. One also should initiate coverage for DRSP and *Legionella*. This can be accomplished with an antipseudomonal beta-lactam and an antipseudomonal fluoroquinolone or imipenem OR an antipseudomonal beta-lactam, an aminoglycoside and a macrolide. A single antipseudomonal penicillin might be inadequate for *P. aeruginosa* and would not reliably cover possible DRSP. An aminoglycoside plus sulfa would also not reliably cover DRSP. Adding clindamycin to an quinolone would provide enhanced coverage against anaerobes, but it lacks antipseudomonal activity.

## Bibliography

1. **Fink MP, Snydman DR, Niederman MS, Leeper KV Jr, Johnson RH, Heard SO, et al**. Treatment of severe pneumonia in hospitalized patients: results of a multicenter, randomized, double-blind trial comparing intravenous ciprofloxacin with imipenem-cilastatin. The Severe Pneumonia Study Group. Antimicrob Agents Chemother. 1994;38:547-57. PMID: 8203853

2. **Niederman MS, Mandell LA, et al**. Guidelines for the Management of Adults with Community-acquired Pneumonia, Diagnosis, Assessment of Severity, Antimicrobial Therapy, and Prevention. Am J Respir Crit Care Med. 2001;163:1730-54. PMID: 11401897

## Nosocomial Infection Question 5
## Answer: E

**Educational Objective:** *Identify the patient who is likely to have intravenous catheter-associated sepsis.*

The available laboratory findings do not suggest a specific focal site of infection, and the presence of a central venous catheter for 6 days in an intensive care unit (ICU) dictates strong consideration of catheter-associated sepsis, for which staphylococci are the most common cause. The absence of inflammatory changes at the site of catheter insertion is not uncommon in the presence of catheter-associated bacteremia. Although some patients with vascular catheter-associated sepsis can be managed without changing the catheter, change or removal of the catheter is preferred whenever possible in an unstable patient to accelerate clearance of bacteremia. The patient has no evidence of meningitis, and the cerebrospinal fluid findings are attributable to the subarachnoid hemorrhage alone. Obtaining a CT scan might be considered to evaluate new intracranial hemorrhage, sinusitis, or postsurgical brain abscess, but these conditions uncommonly produce the sudden onset of fever, hypotension, and striking leukocytosis. Although neurosurgical patients are at risk for pulmonary embolism, oxygen saturation is high and this diagnosis is less

likely. The chest x-ray and urinalysis do not support a diagnosis of pneumonia or cystitis.

## Bibliography

1. **Vallés J, León C, Alvarez-Lerma F**. Nosocomial bacteremia in critically ill patients: a multicenter study evaluating epidemiology and prognosis. Spanish Collaborative Group for Infections in Intensive Care Units of Sociedad Espanola de Medicina Intensiva y Unidades Coronarias (SEMIUC). Clin Infect Dis. 1997;24:387-95. PMID: 9114190

2. **Raad I, Hanna H**. Intravascular catheter related infections: new horizons and recent advances. Arch Intern Med. 2002;162:871-8. PMID: 11966337

## Nosocomial Infection Question 6
## Answer: B

**Educational Objective:** *Identify interventions that can reduce the incidence of nosocomial infection, particularly pneumonia, in mechanically ventilated patients.*

Nosocomial pneumonia is a major cause of morbidity and mortality in mechanically ventilated patients. Various interventions have been suggested to reduce the frequency of this complication. Several studies suggest that in mechanically ventilated patients, the supine position and length of time in that position are risk factors for pulmonary aspiration. Elevation of the patient's head to 45 degrees may reduce aspiration and thereby nosocomial pneumonia. There are no data to support the systemic administration of any antibiotic for prevention of nosocomial infection in the intensive care setting. Antibiotics should be reserved for treatment of an identified process and should be selected to cover the most likely pathogen(s) associated with the process. Selective digestive tract decontamination has been suggested as a means of decreasing bacterial translocation from the gut to other organ systems, but available data are conflicting and do not support widespread use of this approach. Likewise, the role of more limited decontamination (for example, of the oropharynx) is also undefined in the intensive care setting. Available information supports reducing the frequency of ventilator tubing manipulations and changes as a way of decreasing pneumonia. Bacteria colonize the condensate that pools in ventilator tubing, and even careful changing of the tubing potentially causes aspiration of these organisms. Changes less often than every 48 hours or no changes at all appear to be superior to more frequent changes.

## Bibliography

1. **Torres A, Serra-Batlles J, Ros E, Piera C, Puig de la Bellacasa J, Cobos A, et al**. Pulmonary aspiration of gastric contents in patients receiving mechanical ventilation: the effect of body position. Ann Intern Med. 1992;116:540-3. PMID: 1543307

2. **Gastinne H, Wolff M, Delatour F, Faurisson F, Chevret S**. A controlled trial in intensive care units of selective decontamination of the digestive tract with nonabsorbable antibiotics. The French Study Group on Selective Decontamination of the Digestive Tract. N Engl J Med. 1992;326:594-9. PMID: 1734249

3. **Marik PE**. Aspiration pneumonitis and aspiration pneumonia. N Engl J Med. 2001;334:665-71. PMID: 11228282

## Nosocomial Infection Question 7
## Answer: B

**Educational Objective:** *Recognize and appropriately treat aspiration pneumonia.*

The patient has sudden onset dyspnea, hypoxia, fever, and pulmonary infiltrates. Pulmonary embolism should be considered, as the risk of deep venous thrombosis and pulmonary embolism is extremely high among patients with recent stroke. However, the fever and infiltrates are more likely due to pneumonia than pulmonary embolism. Pulmonary edema might also cause an acute decompensation, but again the x-ray is not consistent with this diagnosis.

Aspiration is common in stroke patients whose gag reflex is impaired. It may be difficult to distinguish aspiration pneumonitis from aspiration pneumonia. Pneumonitis is likely caused by exposure of the tracheobronchial tree and pulmonary parenchyma to gastric secretions, resulting in an inflammatory reaction. Pneumonia results when the aspirated material is colonized with bacteria. In a patient in which aspiration is witnessed, suctioning the upper airway is indicated to reduce subsequent aspiration, but deep tracheal suctioning is not indicated and is unlikely to help. Antibiotics may not be indicated in the treatment of aspiration pneumonitis; however, empiric coverage for potential infection is indicated in this case given that the patient is febrile. It is important to cover organisms such as *Streptococcus pneumoniae* and *Haemophilus influenzae*, as these may colonize the upper airway. Given that the patient is a long term resident of a nursing facility, coverage of *Pseudomonas* should be considered. Since the patient is edentulous it is probably unnecessary to cover oral anaerobes. For these reasons, levofloxacin, ceftriaxone, or ceftazidime alone would likely be adequate coverage for this aspiration.

### Bibliography

1. **Marik PE**. Aspiration pneumonitis and aspiration pneumonia. New Engl J Med. 2001;344:665-71. PMID: 11228282

# Myocardial Infarction

## Myocardial Infarction Question 1
## Answer: C

**Educational Objective:** *Recognize a patient for whom an angiotensin-converting enzyme inhibitor should be prescribed after an acute myocardial infarction.*

Left ventricular remodeling refers to changes in the size and shape of the left ventricle that occur following myocardial infarction. As the remaining noninfarcted myocardium enlarges and changes shape, compensatory eccentric hypertrophy occurs, ultimately followed by dilatation and further deterioration of left ventricular function. The treatment of choice for the prevention of remodeling is an angiotensin-converting enzyme (ACE) inhibitor. These drugs improve left ventricular function, reduce both acute and long-term mortality, and reduce the incidence of congestive heart failure and recurrent myocardial infarction in patients treated after an acute myocardial infarction. Treatment should begin as soon as possible following the myocardial infarction (on the first day if feasible).

Antiarrhythmic drugs are no longer used routinely as prophylaxis after acute myocardial infarction as they have been found to cause serious adverse reactions, especially as a result of the proarrhythmic effects of drugs such as quinidine. Angiotensin II antagonists are currently under study for use after an acute myocardial infarction, but no data from large randomized trials with long-term follow-up are currently available. As yet, there is no evidence that they can be substituted for an ACE inhibitor. Calcium-channel blockers generally have not been proved to provide long-term benefit in patients at risk for left ventricular remodeling, recurrent infarction, or sudden death. Short-acting calcium-channel blockers (dihydropyridines) are contraindicated as they have been associated with increase in mortality, and evidence that long-acting calcium-channel blockers are beneficial under these conditions is marginal.

### Bibliography

1. **Pfeffer MA**. ACE inhibition in acute myocardial infarction. N Engl J Med. 1995;332:118-20. PMID: 7990887

2. **Pfeffer MA, Greaves SC, Arnold JM, Glynn RJ, LaMotte FS, Lee RT, et al**. Early versus delayed angiotensin-converting enzyme inhibition therapy in acute myocardial infarction. The healing and early afterload reducing therapy trial. Circulation. 1997;95:2643-51. PMID: 9193433

3. **Sander GE, McKinnie JJ, Greenberg SS, Giles TD**. Angiotensin-converting enzyme inhibitors and angiotensin II receptor antagonists in the treatment of heart failure caused by left ventricular systolic dysfunction. Prog Cardiovasc Dis. 1999;41:265-300. PMID: 10362349

4. **Kizer JR, Kimmel SE**. Epidemiologic review of the calcium channel blocker drugs: An up-to-date perspective on the proposed hazards. Arch Intern Med. 2001;161:1145-58. PMID: 11343438

## Myocardial Infarction Question 2
## Answer: A

**Educational Objective:** *Understand the management of patients with elevated troponin levels and non-Q wave infarction.*

The acute coronary syndromes comprise a spectrum of disorders in which patients have symptoms of unstable angina pectoris. Some patients have elevated cardiac protein levels, such as increased troponin levels indicative of myocardial cell necrosis. Such patients are often classified as having a non-Q-wave myocardial infarction. Recent evidence has shown that elevated troponin levels in patients with an acute coronary syndrome are associated with a poorer 30-day (and even 1-year) prognosis for recurrent myocardial infarction and death. In such a patient, the best approach is to perform coronary angiography to determine if the individual is a candidate for revascularization either by angioplasty (with or without stenting) or by coronary artery bypass surgery. A stress test (either exercise or pharmacologic with an ultrasound or scintigraphic readout) would be expected to be abnormal in such a patient. Conversely, a normal result would raise the suspicion of a false-negative result in a patient with risk factors and an abnormal electrocardiogram associated with chest discomfort at rest. Additionally, exercise testing is contraindicated in the context of recent (< 2 days) myocardial infarction or unstable angina not previously stabilized by medical therapy.

The patient is not a candidate for thrombolytics because he does not have ST elevation in contiguous leads. Patients with ST depressions on ECG, unstable angina or non-Q wave infarctions are not eligible for thrombolytic therapy. Heparin should be initiated to prevent progression of thrombosis at the site of coronary plaque rupture. A platelet GP IIb/IIIa inhibitor such as eptifibatide and tirofiban should also be considered.

### Bibliography

1. **Zaacks SM, Liebson PR, Calvin JE, Parillo JE, Klein LW**. Unstable angina and non-Q wave myocardial infarction: does the clinical diagnosis have therapeutic implications? J Am Coll Cardiol. 1999;33:107-18. PMID: 9935016

2. **Ohman EM, Armstrong PW, Christenson RH, Granger CB, Katus HA, Hamm CW, et al**. Cardiac troponin T levels for risk stratification in acute myocardial ischemia. N Engl J Med. 1996;335:1333-41. PMID: 8857016

3. **Boden WE, O'Rourke RA, Crawford MH, Blaustein AS, Deedwania PC, Zoble RG, et al**. Outcomes in patients with acute non-Q-wave myocardial infarction randomly assigned to an invasive as compared with a conservative management strategy: Veterans Affairs Non-Q-Wave Infarction Strategies in Hospital (VANQWISH) Trial Investigators. N Engl J Med. 1998;338:1785-92. PMID: 9632444

4. Invasive compared with non-invasive treatment in unstable coronary-artery disease: FRISC II prospective randomised multicentre study. FRagmin and Fast Revascularisation during InStability in Coronary artery disease Investigators. Lancet. 1999;354:708-15. PMID: 10475181

## Myocardial Infarction Question 3
## Answer: D

**Educational Objective:** *Understand the low predictive value for syncopal ventricular tachycardia or cardiac arrest of ventricular tachycardia occurring during acute myocardial infarction.*

This patient had an episode of sustained monomorphic ventricular tachycardia during the early stages of an acute inferior (ST elevation in II, III, aVF) and posterior (R wave and ST depression in $V_1$) myocardial infarction. This arrhythmia is likely related to the acute ischemia and usually does not recur. It may also be seen in the context of reperfusion of ischemic myocardium when the thrombolytic agent has effectively dissolved the intracoronary thrombus. Late (> 48 to 72 hours) nonsustained or sustained ventricular tachycardia after a myocardial infarction is more strongly associated with the occurrence of subsequent arrhythmia. This patient can therefore be discharged from the hospital when clinically appropriate; no specific antiarrhythmic therapy is required.

Although amiodarone and sotalol can be prescribed safely in patients with left ventricular dysfunction, prophylactic use in this clinical setting has not been shown to be effective. Similarly, as the risk of recurrent arrhythmia is low, there is no need to implant an automatic implantable cardiac defibrillator, although they have been shown to reduce mortality in patients with ventricular tachycardia/ventricular fibrillation. Diltiazem has rare uses in the management of patients after a myocardial infarction.

### Bibliography

1. **Eldar M, Sievner Z, Goldbourt U, Reicher-Reiss H, Kaplinsky E, Behar S**. Primary ventricular tachycardia in acute myocardial infarction: clinical characteristics and mortality. The SPRINT Study Group. Ann Intern Med. 1992;117:31-6. PMID: 1596045

2. **Tofler GH, Stone PH, Muller JE, Rutherford JD, Willich SN, Gustafson NF, et al**. Prognosis after cardiac arrest due to ventricular tachycardia or ventricular fibrillation associated with acute myocardial infarction (the MILIS Study). Multicenter Investigation of the Limitation of Infarct Size. Am J Cardiol. 1987;60:755-61. PMID: 3661389

## Myocardial Infarction Question 4
## Answer: B

**Educational Objective:** *Recognize the predictive value of the electrocardiogram, selected signs, and diagnostic tests in patients presenting to a hospital with chest pain of possible cardiac origin.*

For patients presenting with chest pain and possible acute myocardial infarction, a normal admission electrocardiogram is highly predictive of an uncomplicated hospital course. Studies have shown a very low incidence (23-times lower risk) of life-threatening cardiac complications for patients with a normal or near-normal electrocardiogram when compared with patients with an abnormal admission electrocardiogram. Admission vital signs and the chest radiograph, although potentially important prognostic predictors, have not been shown to have the same discriminatory capability as the admission electrocardiogram in previous studies. Patients with an acute myocardial infarction may present with a normal admission chest radiograph. Because of the timing of creatine kinase release, a normal serum creatine kinase concentration upon presentation does not preclude an acute myocardial infarction with subsequent cardiac complications. Troponin (T or I) measurement may become the preferred means to screen for myocardial necrosis because of very high specificity and high sensitivity, although its release may be delayed for several hours.

### Bibliography

1. **Lewis WR, Amsterdam EA**. Evaluation of the patient with 'rule out myocardial infarction'. Arch Intern Med. 1996;156:41-5. PMID: 8526695

2. **Brush JE Jr, Brand DA, Acampora D, Chalmer B, Wackers FJ**. Use of the initial electrocardiogram to predict in-hospital complications of acute myocardial infarction. N Engl J Med. 1985;312:1137-41. PMID: 3920520

## Myocardial Infarction Question 5
## Answer: B

**Educational Objective:** *Recognize the best available therapy for acute myocardial infarction in patients with a relative contraindications to thrombolytic therapy.*

In principle, thrombolytic therapy, anticoagulation, aspirin therapy, and percutaneous transluminal coronary angioplasty all would be potentially indicated for this patient. However, possible adverse reactions should modify the therapeutic choices. Because of this patient's recent gastrointestinal bleeding, aspirin and heparin may result in additional risk, but they might be administered if the potential benefit outweighed the risk of bleeding (if the patient continued to have blood in the stool, if the patient is anemic.) However, aspirin and heparin alone will not result in reperfusion of the occluded coronary artery. Only thrombolytic agents and angioplasty can accomplish this. The patient's recent GI bleed constitutes a relative contraindication to lytic therapy. Severe uncontrolled hypertension is another relative contraindication for thrombolytics. Percutaneous transluminal coronary angioplasty is an effective treatment of acute myocardial infarction and may be superior to lytic therapy.

## Bibliography

1. **Weaver WD, Simes RJ, Betriu A, Grines CL, Zijlstra F, Garcia E, et al**. Comparison of primary coronary angioplasty and intravenous thrombolytic therapy for acute myocardial infarction: a quantitative review. JAMA. 1997;278:2093-8. PMID: 9403425

2. A clinical trial comparing primary coronary angioplasty with tissue plasminogen activator for acute myocardial infarction. The Global Use of Strategies to Open Occluded Coronary Arteries in Acute Coronary Syndromes (GUSTO IIb) Angioplasty Substudy Investigators. N Engl J Med. 1997;336:1621-8. PMID: 9173270

3. **Grines CL, Browne KF, Marco J, Rothbaum D, Stone GW, O'Keefe J, et al**. A comparison of immediate angioplasty with thrombolytic therapy for acute myocardial infarction. The Primary Angioplasty in Myocardial Infarction Study Group. N Engl J Med. 1993;328:673-9. PMID: 8433725

## Myocardial Infarction Question 6
## Answer: C

**Educational Objective:** *Know the clinical presenting features of right ventricular myocardial infarction.*

Right ventricular (RV) myocardial infarction should be suspected in this patient because of the moderately elevated jugular venous pressure in a previously normal person in the setting of acute inferior infarction. The right coronary artery (RCA) supplies the inferior wall of the heart as well as the right ventricle; occlusion of the RCA may lead to RV infarction. The right ventricular involvement could be detected by performing electrocardiography with leads on the right chest; ST-segment elevation in $V_4R$ is a highly sensitive and specific sign of right ventricular infarction. Right-sided leads should be checked in all patients with an inferior wall infarction.

Hypotension may develop after administration of a venodilator to patients with right ventricular infarction because of insufficient right-sided filling pressures to maintain right ventricular stroke volume, left ventricular filling pressure, and cardiac output. Expansion of intravascular volume with fluids usually reverses severe hypotension associated with right ventricular infarction and may allow judicious use of nitrates or other vasodilators except in the most severely hemodynamically deranged patients.

Acute mitral regurgitation or ruptured interventricular septum is unlikely because of the absence of a cardiac murmur at the onset of hypotension and the absence of physical findings suggestive of pulmonary edema. Anaphylactic reactions to nitroglycerin have not been reported. Left ventricular failure from myocardial infarction usually occurs with an anterior, not inferior, infarction as was present in the patient described.

## Bibliography

1. **Reeder GS**. Identification and treatment of complications of myocardial infarction. Mayo Clin Proc. 1995;70:880-4. PMID: 7643642

## Myocardial Infarction Question 7
## Answer: A

**Educational Objective:** *Recognize cardiogenic shock in a patient with myocardial infarction.*

This patient has sustained an extensive anterolateral myocardial infarction, demonstrated on the electrocardiogram by ST-segment elevation in leads $V_3$ through $V_6$, I, and aVL. He is in cardiogenic shock with hypotension, pulmonary congestion, and tachycardia.

Cardiogenic shock complicates 5% to 15% of cases of acute myocardial infarction. It occurs in the setting of myocardial infarction-related loss of 40% or more of left ventricular myocardium, acute ischemic valvular insufficiency, acute ventricular septal defect, or myocardial rupture. The optimal approach to cardiogenic shock is prevention by treating the patient with myocardial infarction with prompt coronary reperfusion in an effort to save viable myocardium and prevent the mechanical complications of myocardial infarction.

Thrombolysis in cardiogenic shock results in reperfusion of the infarct-related artery in only 40% to 50% of patients, and thrombolytic therapy has not been demonstrated by any randomized, controlled, prospective study to improve survival of patients with this condition. An analysis from the Global Utilization of Streptokinase and Tissue Plasminogen Activator for Occluded Coronary Arteries (GUSTO-1) trial, an observational study, found that an aggressive strategy of early angiography with coronary revascularization when appropriate was associated with a reduction in mortality in patients with acute myocardial infarction and cardiogenic shock who received thrombolytic therapy. Similarly, there are no randomized, prospective studies of percutaneous transluminal coronary angioplasty (PTCA) alone as initial treatment of cardiogenic shock. It has been suggested, based on uncontrolled studies, that PTCA as primary therapy does reduce both short-term and long-term mortality in this patient population. In the absence of randomized, controlled trials, it has been suggested that PTCA be considered as the initial reperfusion modality for patients who present with cardiogenic shock. For patients who present to hospitals that lack the capability to provide PTCA, rapid administration of thrombolytic therapy followed by transfer to a facility equipped to deliver PTCA would be appropriate.

In addition to coronary reperfusion, the patient with cardiogenic shock should be considered for right heart pressure monitoring with a balloon flotation catheter and intra-arterial pressure monitoring. The patient's degree of hemodynamic instability may indicate the need for intra-aortic balloon counterpulsation or inotropic, vasopressor, or vasodilator therapy.

Ventricular septal rupture has a higher prevalence in first infarction, accounts for 5% of infarct-related deaths, and usually occurs in the first few days following myocardial infarction. It is usually associated with development of a new pansystolic murmur heard along the left sternal border, hypotension, left ventricular failure, and evidence of right ventricular failure. In rare instances, the murmur may be absent.

Papillary muscle rupture occurs more commonly in infarcts involving the posteromedial papillary muscle. This muscle is usually supplied by the right or circumflex coronary artery, not the left anterior descending coronary artery as is involved in this patient.

Early postinfarction pericarditis is common, it usually occurs 2 to 4 days after infarction and is not associated with hemodynamic compromise. It is usually treated with NSAIDs.

### Bibliography

1. **Berger PB, Holmes DR Jr, Stebbins AL, Bates ER, Califf RM, Topol EJ**. Impact of an aggressive invasive catheterization and revascularization strategy on mortality in patients with cardiogenic shock in the Global Utilization of Streptokinase and Tissue Plasminogen Activator for Occluded Coronary Arteries (GUSTO-I) trial. An observational study. Circulation. 1997;96:122-7. PMID: 9236426

2. **Califf RM, Bengtson JR**. Cardiogenic shock. N Engl J Med. 1994;330:1724-30. PMID: 8190135

3. **Goldberg R, Samad N, Yarzebski J, Gurwitz J, Bigelow C, Gore JM**. Temporal trends in cardiogenic shock complicating acute myocardial infarction. N Engl J Med. 1999;340:1162-8. PMID: 10202167

## Myocardial Infarction Question 8
## Answer: C

**Educational Objective:** *Be able to correlate physical examination findings and invasive hemodynamic data in the evaluation and treatment of a patient with hypotension in the setting of acute myocardial infarction.*

This patient has an acute myocardial infarction. Invasive monitoring with pulmonary artery catheterization may be helpful in the management with patients with hypotension and uncertain volume status. The patient's cardiac index is low, meaning that he has mildly decreased left ventricular function. Additionally, the pulmonary capillary wedge pressure, which approximates left ventricular filling pressure, is also low, implying that the patient is relatively hypovolemic. The most important first step is administration of fluids to achieve optimal left ventricular filling pressures of 14 to 18 mm Hg. Administration of cardiac glycosides in this patient is not likely to be helpful and may increase ultimate infarct size by increasing myocardial oxygen demand. Although isoproterenol may raise cardiac output, it may, like cardiac glycosides, increase the eventual infarct size. In addition, because of its vasodilator effects, isoproterenol may worsen hypotension, and it may produce serious ventricular arrhythmias. Because dopamine

in high doses leads to peripheral vasoconstriction, it would not be appropriate.

There is considerable evidence for a beneficial effect of acute intravenous administration of β-adrenergic blocking agents in selected patients with acute myocardial infarction. In this patient, however, the sinus tachycardia is a compensatory response to hypotension and low cardiac output. It would be inappropriate to attempt to lower the heart rate with β-adrenergic blocking agents at this point in his management.

### Bibliography

1. **Ryan TJ, Anderson JL, Antman EM, Braniff BA, Brooks NH, Califf RM, et al**. 1999 update: ACC/AHA guidelines for the management of patients with acute myocardial infarction. A report of the American College of Cardiology/American Heart Association Task Force on Practice Guidelines (Committee on Management of Acute Myocardial Infarction). J Am Coll Cardiol. 1996;28:1328-428. PMID: 10483976

## Myocardial Infarction Question 9
## Answer: A

**Educational Objective:** *Know the pathophysiology of non-Q-wave myocardial infarction and select the most appropriate long-term treatment.*

The patient has sustained an uncomplicated non-Q-wave myocardial infarction. Aspirin therapy at doses of 160 mg daily or greater has been clearly shown to reduce the risk of subsequent myocardial infarction and overall cardiovascular death.

β-Blockers have been shown to be beneficial in the long-term treatment of patients following myocardial infarction if they have evidence of recurrent ischemia or have sustained a Q-wave myocardial infarction. Interestingly, subgroup analysis of the β-blocker trials demonstrated no benefit in patients with small or non-Q-wave myocardial infarctions.

Warfarin may have some beneficial role in prevention of subsequent myocardial infarction; however, there appears to be no benefit over aspirin, which is inexpensive and less complicated to regulate.

Although nitrates may play a role in reducing the level of angina, there are no data to suggest that prophylactic use of nitrates in the setting of an acute myocardial infarction or in the subsequent care of a myocardial infarction patient reduces mortality.

### Bibliography

1. Randomised trial of intravenous streptokinase, oral aspirin, both or neither among 17,187 cases of suspected acute myocardial infarction. ISIS-2. ISIS-2 (Second International Study of Infarct Survival) Collaborative Group. Lancet. 1988;2:349-60. PMID: 2899772

2. **Pfeffer MA, Braunwald E, Moye LA, Basta L, Brown EJ Jr, Cuddy TE**. Effect of captopril on mortality and morbidity in patients with left ventricular dysfunction after myocardial infarction. Results of the survival and ventricular enlargement trial. The SAVE Investigators. N Engl J Med. 1992;327:669-77. PMID: 1386652

3. **Yusuf S, Sleight P, Held P, McMahon S**. Routine medical management of acute myocardial infarction. Lessons from overviews of recent randomized controlled trials. Circulation. 1990;82:II117-34. PMID: 1975522

## Myocardial Infarction Question 10
## Answer: B

**Educational Objective:** *Determine patient eligibility for thrombolytic therapy, which thrombolytic drug should be used in a given situation, and the need for adjunctive heparin.*

Given the fact that the patient has ST elevation in multiple contiguous leads presenting within 12 hours of onset of symptoms, the patient meets eligibility criteria for thrombolytics. Although elderly patients are at high risk of having intracranial bleeding, they also have a higher mortality from their infarctions. It has been clearly demonstrated that elderly patients benefit from thrombolytic therapy; therefore, age alone should not be considered a contraindication.

Three large randomized trials have demonstrated a higher risk of intracranial bleeding with tissue plasminogen activator (tPA) when compared with streptokinase therapy. This has been particularly true in patients who are over the age of 70 or who have hypertension at the time of presentation. Furthermore, accelerated tPA with intravenous heparin may produce lower mortality than streptokinase only in patients who are treated within the first 4 hours after onset of symptoms. Therefore, in this mildly hypertensive 80-year-old patient who is treated more than 4 hours after symptom onset and who is at risk of having an intracranial bleed, streptokinase is the clear choice.

There is no evidence to suggest that intravenous heparin is of any advantage when streptokinase is the thrombolytic drug. In fact, intravenous heparin appears to increase the bleeding complications with streptokinase, without any added reduction in mortality or reinfarction. For these reasons, when using streptokinase, no heparin should be used unless the patient has clear-cut indications, such as left ventricular thrombosis.

### Bibliography

1. **GUSTO Investigators**. An international randomized trial comparing four thrombolytic strategies for acute myocardial infarction. N Engl J Med. 1993;329:673-82. PMID: 8204123

2. In-hospital mortality in clinical course of 20,891 patients with suspected myocardial infarction randomized between alteplase and streptokinase with or without heparin. The International Study Group. Lancet. 1990;336:71-5. PMID: 1975322

3. A randomised comparison of streptokinase vs tissue plasminogen activator vs anistreplase and of aspirin plus heparin vs aspirin alone among 41,299 cases of suspected acute myocardial infarction. ISIS-3. ISIS-3 (Third International Study of Infarct Survival) Collaborative Group. Lancet. 1992;339:753-70. PMID: 1347801

## Myocardial Infarction Question 11
## Answer: E

**Educational Objective:** *Differentiate relative from absolute contraindications to a drug proven to reduce mortality in acute myocardial infarction.*

None of the options is an absolute contraindication to the use of intravenous β-blockers in acute myocardial infarction. The benefits of intravenous β-blocker therapy early in acute infarction is well established, presumably due to both reduction in myocardial oxygen consumption afforded by the negative inotropic and chronotropic actions, and a direct antiarrhythmic effect. Often, this important treatment is withheld in patients with sinus bradycardia (D), diabetes (A), and well-controlled asthma (B); at most, these conditions should be considered relative contraindications, and β-blockers should be administered carefully to most infarcting patients with these concomitant conditions. The increased incidence of bradyarrhythmias in inferior infarcts does not justify withholding β-blockers (C), as these rhythm disturbances tend to be reversible and are easily treated with temporary pacing if symptomatic. Severe systolic heart failure (from massive myocardial damage, right ventricular infarction, or acute valvular regurgitation) and active wheezing from reactive airway disease remain absolute contraindications to β-blockade.

### Bibliography

1. **Ryan TJ, Anderson JL, Antman EM, Braniff BA, Brooks NH, Califf RM, et al**. ACC/AHA guidelines for the management of patients with acute myocardial infarction. A report of the American College of Cardiology/American Heart Association Task Force on Practice Guidelines. (Committee on Management of Acute Myocardial Infarction). J Am Coll Cardiol. 1996;28:1328-428. PMID: 8890834

2. **Olsson G, Held P**. Early intravenous beta blockade and thrombolytics in acute myocardial infarction. Am J Cardiol. 1993;72:156G-60G. PMID: 7904119

3. **Pepine CJ**. Adjunctive pharmacologic therapy for acute myocardial infarction. Clin Cardiol. 1994;17(1 Suppl I):I10-14. PMID: 7908862

# Chest Pain

## Chest Pain Question 1
### Answer: B

**Educational Objective:** *Determine the most cost-effective step in managing patients with chest discomfort of probable esophageal origin.*

Recent cost-effective analysis has confirmed that a trial of acid-suppression therapy with a proton pump inhibitor, commonly employed in practice, is a suitable approach to patients with chest discomfort that is suggestive of gastroesophageal reflux. If the patient's symptoms resolve within 7 days, the trial can be considered successful, and a diagnosis of chest pain of gastrointestinal origin is reasonable. If the symptoms do not completely resolve, or if acid-suppression therapy is necessary for more that 6 to 8 weeks, further diagnostic studies are indicated. Evaluation of pain that is highly suggestive of gastrointestinal origin does not require efforts to "rule out" cardiac disease.

### Bibliography

1. **Ofman JJ, Gralnek IM, Udani J, Fennerty MB, Fass R.** The cost-effectiveness of the omeprazole test in patients with noncardiac chest pain. Am J Med. 1999;107:219-27. PMID: 10492314

2. **Richter JE.** Chest pain and gastroesophageal reflex disease. J Clin Gastroenterol. 2000;30:S39-41. PMID: 10777171

## Chest Pain Question 2
### Answer: A

**Educational Objective:** *Evaluate a woman with chest pain who has a moderate pretest probability of having coronary artery disease.*

According to the American College of Cardiology/American Heart Association's most recent guidelines for exercise testing, a standard treadmill stress electrocardiogram, without an imaging study, remains the best initial diagnostic test in this situation. Although the accuracy of the test is slightly lower in women than in men, its wide availability, well-accepted standardization, and lower cost outweigh the reportedly slightly better specificity of studies utilizing imaging techniques. Also, in comparison to tests using dobutamine or dipyridamole, there is significant prognostic value to subjecting a patient to a standardized exercise protocol and determining exercise tolerance, blood pressure response, and occurrence of symptoms.

Finally, cardiac catheterization as the initial diagnostic step should be reserved for patients with pretest probability high enough to lead to further testing even if a treadmill test, with or without imaging, is negative.

### Bibliography

1. **Gibbons RJ, Balady GJ, Beasley JW, Bricker JT, Duvernoy WF, Froelicher VF, et al.** ACC/AHA guidelines for exercise testing: executive summary. A report of the American College of Cardiology/American Heart Association Task Force on Practice Guidelines (Committee on Exercise Testing).Circulation. 1997;96:345-54. PMID: 9236456

## Chest Pain Question 3
### Answer: B

**Educational Objective:** *Select candidates for evaluation or treatment in a "chest pain center."*

Chest pain centers have become increasingly common as part of hospitals' attempts to manage patients more efficiently and to market themselves. Typically, chest pain protocols that can be carried out in the emergency department, or in a designated "chest pain center," include monitoring of vital signs and cardiac rhythm, serial measurements of cardiac enzymes, and electrocardiograms over a 6- to 12-hour period, and the performance of a diagnostic study such as a treadmill stress test or dobutamine echocardiogram if initial evaluation is negative. Ideal candidates for this approach include low- to moderate-risk patients who are not actively having chest pain. Patients at higher risk, such as those with previous coronary artery procedures and recurrence of typical angina; those with ongoing chest pain suspicious of an acute coronary syndrome, or those with coexisting cardiac conditions such as congestive heart failure, should be admitted to the hospital for further management without the delay of the chest pain protocol. Patients with few or no risk factors and symptoms suggestive of gastrointestinal or musculoskeletal pain can be discharged without the chest pain protocol and managed as outpatients.

### Bibliography

1. **Braunwald ET, Antman EM, Beasley JW, Califf RM, Cheitlin MD, Hochman JS, et al.** ACC/AHA guidelines for the management of patients with unstable angina and non-ST-segment elevation myocardial infarction: executive summary and recommendations: a Report of the American College of Cardiology/American Heart Association Task Force on Practice Guidelines. Circulation. 2000;102:1193-209. PMID: 10973852

## Chest Pain Question 4
### Answer: C

**Educational Objective:** *Recognize the options in treating a patient with an acute myocardial infarction and ST-segment elevation.*

Although some randomized trials of angioplasty (with or without stenting) versus thrombolysis have shown a marginal benefit for the former procedure, most hospitals do not have 24-hour coverage by an experienced team capable of performing this procedure. When the physician's own institution or a nearby hospital has the capability of performing this procedure within 1 hour of notification, the outcome is good and may be superior to thrombolysis in some instances. However, current recommendations indicate that the "door to needle" time should be no more than 30 minutes for the administration of a thrombolytic agent. Time is critical, and, in this patient, optimal results of any revascularization approach are best obtained within the first hour of treatment. The success rate decreases between 1 and 3 hours after symptom onset, and a further decline occurs 3 to 6 hours after the onset of symptoms. In many institutions, thrombolysis is routinely followed within 24 hours by coronary arteriography in anticipation of angioplasty with possible stenting, although current guidelines mandate this approach only for patients with recurrent symptoms or for identification of a reversible defect on stress testing using scintigraphy or echocardiography. Patients with diabetes mellitus are especially prone to a high incidence of restenosis after angioplasty with possible stenting. Until this problem is overcome (possibly with the periprocedural use of platelet glycoprotein IIb/IIIa inhibitors), these patients may be better served by thrombolysis followed by consideration for coronary artery bypass surgery.

### Bibliography

1. Indications for fibrinolytic therapy in suspected acute myocardial infarction: collaborative overview of early mortality and major morbidity results from all randomised trials of more than 1000 patients. Fibrinolytic Therapy Trialists' (FTT) Collaborative Group. Lancet. 1994;343:311-22. PMID: 7905143

2. **Weaver WD, Simes RJ, Betriu A, Grines CL, Zijlstra F, Garcia E, et al**. Comparison of primary coronary angioplasty and intravenous thrombolytic therapy for acute myocardial infarction: a quantitative review. JAMA. 1997;278:2093-8. PMID: 9403425

3. **Berger AK, Schulman KA, Gersh, BJ, Pirzada S, Breall JA, Johnson AE, et al**. Primary coronary angioplasty vs thrombolysis for the management of acute myocardial infarction in elderly patients. JAMA. 1999;282:341-8. PMID: 10432031

4. **Gibson CM**. Primary angioplasty compared with thrombolysis: new issues in the era of glycoprotein IIb/IIIa inhibition and intracoronary stenting. Ann Intern Med. 1999;130:841-7. PMID: 10366375

5. **Grines CL, Cox DA, Stone GW, Garcia E, Mattos LA, Giambartolomei A, et al**. Coronary angioplasty with or without stent implantation for acute myocardial infarction. Stent Primary Angioplasty in Myocardial Infarction Study Group. N Engl J Med. 1999;341:1949-56. PMID: 10607811

## Chest Pain Question 5
## Answer: A

**Educational Objective:** *Recognize the importance of a β-blocker as first-line treatment of chronic ischemic heart disease.*

β-Blockade, which lowers both heart rate and blood pressure, two of the main determinants of myocardial oxygen demand, has been shown to be beneficial in preventing recurrent myocardial infarction, sudden death, and death from progressive heart failure in patients with ischemic heart disease. This patient has an elevated blood pressure and a prior myocardial infarction. She has an area of reversible ischemia documented by scintigraphy. Currently, she is taking insufficient anti-ischemic medication. Diabetes mellitus is not a contraindication to β-blockade in most patients. Symptoms of hypoglycemia are unlikely to be masked in patients who are not on insulin. Hypoglycemia is also unlikely in patients who require insulin and who usually measure their blood glucose values. Indeed, patients with diabetes mellitus, who are at higher risk for the complications of ischemic heart disease, may benefit even more than patients without diabetes from β-blocker therapy.

If the patient cannot tolerate a β-blocker for any reason (for example, central nervous system side effects such as depression, fatigue, or cognitive impairment), a calcium-channel blocker is a reasonable second choice. The long-acting calcium-channel blockers are effective in the treatment of angina pectoris and hypertension but, unlike the β-blockers, have not been consistently shown in controlled studies to prevent the complications of ischemic heart disease. Short-acting calcium-channel blockers should no longer be used in outpatients because of the risks of exacerbating ischemic symptoms and possibly causing increased mortality. A long-acting nitrate preparation is a reasonable addition to this patient's regimen, but by itself is insufficient for the effective treatment either of angina pectoris or hypertension. Long-acting nitrates have not been shown to decrease mortality in patients with ischemic heart disease. Administration of α-blockers has not been shown to improve the prognosis of patients with angina pectoris. Estrogen replacement therapy is contraindicated in most patients with a history of breast cancer. Initiation of estrogen replacement therapy to lower blood lipid levels may increase morbidity and mortality.

### Bibliography

1. **Gibbons RJ, Chatterjee K, Daley J, Douglas JS, Fihn SD, Gardin JM, et al**. ACC/AHA/ACP-ASIM guidelines for the management of patients with chronic stable angina: a report of the American College of Cardiology/American Heart Association Task Force on Practice Guidelines. J Am Coll Cardiol. 1999;33:2092-197. PMID: 10362225

2. **Gottlieb SS, McCarter RJ, Vogel RA**. Effect of beta-blockade on mortality among high-risk and low-risk patients after myocardial infarction. N Engl J Med. 1998;339:489-97. PMID: 9709041

3. Risks and benefits of estrogen plus progestin in healthy postmenopausal women: principal results from the Women's Health Initiative randomized controlled trial. JAMA. 2002;288:321-33. PMID: 12117397

4. **Heidenreich PA, McDonald KM, Hastie T, Fadel B, Hagan V, Lee BK, et al**. Meta-analysis of trials comparing beta-blockers, calcium antagonists, and nitrates for stable angina. JAMA. 1999;281:1927-36. PMID: 10349897

## Chest Pain Question 6
## Answer: C

**Educational Objective:** *Recognize the importance of combined antiplatelet and antithrombotic therapy in patients with acute coronary syndromes.*

Recent trials have indicated that a combination of unfractionated heparin plus a platelet glycoprotein IIb/IIIa inhibitor is superior to heparin alone in reducing morbidity and mortality in patients with acute coronary syndromes. Warfarin has not been shown to be effective in acute coronary syndromes as currently described, although numerous trials have confirmed its utility in long-term therapy after an acute myocardial infarction. However, bleeding complications and the need for frequent venipunctures have made its long-term use unattractive. Clopidogrel is an antiplatelet agent that is used after angioplasty and stenting and serves as an aspirin substitute in patients who are unable to take aspirin. However, it is not indicated for the routine medical therapy for patients with acute coronary syndromes.

**Bibliography**

1. Inhibition of the platelet glycoprotein IIb/IIIa receptor with tirofiban in unstable angina and non-Q-wave myocardial infarction. The Platelet Receptor Inhibition in Ischemic Syndrome Management in Patients Limited by Unstable Signs and Symptoms (PRISM-PLUS) Study Investigators. N Engl J Med. 1998;338:1488-97. PMID: 9599103
2. Inhibition of platelet glycoprotein IIb/IIIa with eptifibatide in patients with acute coronary syndromes. The PURSUIT Trial Investigators. Platelet Glycoprotein IIb/IIIa in Unstable Angina: Receptor Suppression Using Integrilin Therapy. N Engl J Med. 1998;339:436-43. PMID: 9705684

## Chest Pain Question 7
## Answer: D

**Educational Objective:** *Recognize the sequence of risk stratification in patients with new-onset angina pectoris.*

Although this patient could be classified as having unstable angina pectoris, his symptoms are of short duration and are not progressive. Because his symptoms are stable and are precipitated by exertion, a simple exercise treadmill test will provide useful information. The β-blocker should be withheld on the morning of the test. If there is an early positive result (for example, early decline in blood pressure or deep and prolonged ST-segment depression), urgent coronary angiography is indicated. If the patient is able to exercise for longer periods (to stage 4 on the Bruce protocol without electrocardiographic changes), medical therapy is indicated. For in between results, the physician and the patient can weigh the benefits of coronary angiography, which would provide information about anatomy and also about the potential for revascularization following angioplasty (with or without stenting) or coronary artery bypass surgery.

In the absence of acute or progressive symptoms, hospitalization is not warranted. Additional outpatient measures include aggressive treatment of any lipid abnormalities that are found, as data now indicate that such treatment may be as good as or better than revascularization procedures under certain circumstances.

**Bibliography**

1. **Gibbons RJ, Balady GJ, Beasley JW, Bricker JT, Duvernoy WF, Froelicher VF, et al**. ACC/AHA Guidelines for Exercise Testing. A report of the American College of Cardiology/American Heart Association Task Force on Practice Guidelines (Committee on Exercise Testing). J Am Coll Cardiol. 1997;30:260-311. PMID: 9207652
2. **Kuntz KM, Fleischmann KE, Hunink MG, Douglas PS**. Cost-effectiveness of diagnostic strategies for patients with chest pain. Ann Intern Med. 1999;130:709-18. PMID: 10357689
3. **Pitt B, Waters D, Brown WV, van Boven AJ, Schwartz L, Title LM, et al**. Aggressive lipid-lowering therapy compared with angioplasty in stable coronary artery disease. Atorvastatin versus Revascularization Treatment Investigators. N Engl J Med. 1999;341:70-6. PMID: 10395630

## Chest Pain Question 8
## Answer: C

**Educational Objective:** *Understand the use of β-blockers in patients with left ventricular dysfunction or overt heart failure due to chronic ischemic heart disease.*

Calcium-channel blockers have been widely used in the treatment of hypertension and ischemic heart disease. Although there is no longer any role for short-acting calcium-channel blockers, long-acting preparations may still have negative inotropic effects (with the likely exception of newer agents such as amlodipine). Although many patients with heart failure appear to tolerate these agents well, there is no evidence that these agents are beneficial in either heart failure or the prevention of recurrent ischemia. There also appears to be no mortality benefit. Conversely, substantial evidence now exists that β-blockade may be beneficial even in patients with depressed left ventricular function and symptoms of heart failure. The majority of the patients in these studies had ischemic heart disease. Thus, appropriate management for this patient is to discontinue the calcium-channel blocker and begin metoprolol at a low dose (for example, 12.5 mg daily, or less), using a reduction in resting heart rate and blood pressure as targets. Carvedilol, 3.125 mg daily, may also be used as a starting dose. These agents may be increased biweekly to tolerance. The total target dose of metoprolol should not exceed 100 mg daily (or 200 mg of the sustained-release preparation) and that of carvedilol should not exceed 25 mg twice daily in patients weighing less than 85 kg (187 lb) and 50 mg twice daily in patients weighing more than 86 kg (190 lb). This patient would also benefit from the prescription of prophylactic nitroglycerin and the intermittent use of another diuretic such as metolazone.

**Bibliography**

1. **Teerlink JR, Massie BM**. Beta-adrenergic blocker mortality trials in congestive heart failure. Am J Cardiol. 1999;84(9A):94R-102R. PMID: 10568667

2. Packer M, O'Connor CM, Ghali JK, Pressler ML, Carson PE, Belkin RN, et al. Effect of amlodipine on morbidity and mortality in severe chronic heart failure. Prospective Randomized Amlodipine Survival Evaluation Study Group. N Engl J Med. 1996;335:1107-14. PMID: 8813041

3. Cohn JN, Ziesche S, Smith R, Anand I, Dunkman WB, Loeb H, et al. Effect of the calcium antagonist felodipine as supplementary vasodilator therapy in patients with chronic heart failure treated with enalapril: V-HeFT III. Vasodilator-Heart Failure Trial (V-HeFT) Study Group. Circulation. 1997;96:856-63. PMID: 9264493

## Chest Pain Question 9
## Answer: C

**Educational Objective:** *Recognize the clinical presentation of aortic dissection.*

Although chest pain in a 62-year-old man most often is due to an acute coronary syndrome, the nondiagnostic electrocardiogram and the mediastinal widening on the chest radiograph raise the possibility of aortic dissection, especially because the patient has a clinical history of hypertension. Mediastinal widening is not associated with pericarditis, pulmonary thromboembolism, or interventricular rupture. Rapid exclusion (or diagnosis) of aortic dissection is essential. Transesophageal echocardiography has a high sensitivity and specificity for aortic dissection and can be performed rapidly at the patient's bedside. Therapy with a β-blocker to decrease blood pressure and heart rate should be initiated immediately and continued during the transesophageal examination. If an ascending aortic dissection is present, prompt surgical intervention is indicated; therefore, it is inappropriate to wait for cardiac enzyme results. In addition, cardiac enzyme values may be positive with a dissection if the intimal flap involves one of the coronary ostia. Both thrombolytic therapy and heparin are contraindicated to prevent further bleeding or rupture if a dissection is present. If the patient is taken emergently to the catheterization laboratory, aortic root angiography should be performed prior to coronary angiography.

### Bibliography

1. DeSanctis RW, Doroghazi RM, Austen WG, Buckley MJ. Aortic dissection. N Engl J Med. 1987;317:1060-7. PMID: 3309654

2. Ballal RS, Nanda NC, Gatewood R, D'Arcy B, Samdarshi TE, Holman WL, et al. Usefulness of transesophageal echocardiography in assessment of aortic dissection. Circulation. 1991;84:1903-14. PMID: 1934367

## Chest Pain Question 10
## Answer: D

**Educational Objective:** *Recognize the superiority of coronary artery bypass grafting over percutaneous transluminal coronary angioplasty in patients with diabetes mellitus.*

Patients with early positive results on exercise electrocardiography are more likely to have high-grade proximal obstructions in their coronary vessels. If a revascularization procedure is not performed, such patients are more likely to have adverse events, including myocardial infarction and death, within 1 year of diagnosis. This patient is receiving optimal medical treatment and has an adverse physiologic response to exercise; therefore, revascularization is warranted. Diabetes mellitus is a major risk factor not only for coronary artery disease, but also for restenosis in patients undergoing percutaneous transluminal coronary angioplasty (PTCA). In a large randomized trial and its accompanying nonrandomized registry, coronary artery bypass grafting was consistently shown to be superior to PTCA in patients with diabetes. How the use of stents and periprocedural platelet glycoprotein IIb/IIIa inhibition will affect these recommendations has not yet been determined in a large number of patients with diabetes. Thrombolysis is indicated only for patients who have acute coronary syndromes with ST-segment elevation.

### Bibliography

1. Detre KM, Guo P, Holubkov R, Califf RM, Sopko G, Bach R, et al. Coronary revascularization in diabetic patients: a comparison of the randomized and observational components of the Bypass Angioplasty Revascularization Investigation (BARI). Circulation. 1999;99:633-40. PMID: 9950660

2. Lincoff AM, Califf RM, Moliterno DJ, Ellis SG, Ducas J, Kramer JH, et al. Complementary clinical benefits of coronary-artery stenting and blockade of platelet glycoprotein IIb/IIIa receptors. Evaluation of Platelet IIb/IIIa Inhibition in Stenting Investigators. N Engl J Med. 1999;341:319-27. PMID: 10423466

3. Grundy SM, Benjamin IJ, Burke GL, Chait A, Eckel RH, Howard BV, et al. Diabetes and cardiovascular disease: a statement for healthcare professionals from the American Heart Association. Circulation. 1999;100:1134-46. PMID: 10477542

## Chest Pain Question 11
## Answer: B

**Educational Objective:** *Treat a descending aortic aneurysm dissection.*

Descending thoracic aortic aneurysms are most commonly found in the 6th decade in men and 7th decade for women. Many patients are asymptomatic when diagnosed. The asymptomatic patient is treated medically until the size of the aneurysm is 5 to 6 cm or symptoms present. Medical management includes aggressive blood pressure control, serial imaging for evaluation of size (diameter), and close follow up for symptom onset. β -Blockers have been shown to be especially useful in patients with Marfan syndrome.

Common symptoms of a descending thoracic aortic aneurysm include back, abdominal, chest or flank pains. Thromboembolic events can also be attributed to these aneurysms. Two life threatening complications are an aortoesophageal fistula, which presents with massive hemoptysis and shock, and rupture or a leak, which present with chest pain, left pleural effusion, and hypotension.

Prompt surgical intervention is warranted if size or symptoms indicate. A diuretic is not additionally helpful, unless needed for blood pressure control. Heparin and NSAIDs are of no use in this patient.

**Bibliography**

1. **Bickerstaff LK, Pairolero PC, Hollier LH, Melton LJ, Van Peenen HJ, Cherry KJ, et al.** Thoracic aortic aneurysms: a population-based study. Surgery. 1982;92:1103-8. PMID: 7147188
2. **Shores J, Berger KR, Murphy EA, Pyeritz RE.** Progression of aortic dilatation and the benefit of long-term beta-adrenergic blockade in Marfan's syndrome. N Engl J Med. 1994;330:1335-41. PMID: 8152445
3. **Griepp RB, Ergin MA, Lansman SL, Galla JD, Pogo G.** The natural history of thoracic aortic aneurysms. Semin Thorac Cardiovasc Surg. 1991;3:258-65. PMID: 1793761

## Chest Pain Question 12
## Answer: D

**Educational Objective:** *Recognize hypertrophic cardiomyopathy.*

In the patient described, the arterial pulse, heart murmurs, and electrocardiographic and echocardiographic findings are typical of hypertrophic cardiomyopathy with obstruction of the left ventricular outflow tract. A decrease in left ventricular compliance is also present, which leads to dyspnea. Of all the conditions listed as options for this question, hypertrophic cardiomyopathy is the only condition associated with a murmur that increases with Valsalva. Treatment should be aimed at decreasing the obstruction with β-adrenergic blockade. In general, drugs or maneuvers that decrease ventricular volume will increase the outflow tract obstruction, and those that increase volume will decrease the obstruction. Hence, digitalis and diuretics are not to be used in the initial therapy. Nitroglycerin is often hazardous to use in patients with this disease because the associated preload reduction results in diminished left ventricular volume and the outflow tract gradient increases. Anticoagulants would serve no useful purpose; neither venous thrombi nor emboli occur frequently, and it is not likely that coronary artery disease is present.

**Bibliography**

1. **Wigle ED, Rakowski H, Kimball BP, Williams WG.** Hypertrophic cardiomyopathy. Clinical spectrum and treatment. Circulation. 1995;92:680-92. PMID: 7671349

## Chest Pain Question 13
## Answer: D

**Educational Objective:** *Correctly diagnose variant (Prinzmetal's) angina.*

The syndrome of variant (Prinzmetal's) angina is caused by coronary artery vasospasm. It occurs in a younger patient more frequently than does atherosclerotic coronary artery disease and is associated with other vasospastic syndromes such as migraines. Attacks of variant angina tend to occur at rest between 2400 and 0800 hours, and a history of exertional pain is uncommon. Clinical features, however, do no reliably permit a diagnosis.

The electrocardiogram is of key diagnostic importance. ST-segment elevation is seen during pain in variant angina and rapidly resolves with the administration of vasodilatory drugs. In this setting, it is likely that the sublingual nitrate is acting as a direct coronary vasodilator.

The rapid resolution of the pain argues against myocardial infarction, and the focality of the ST-segment elevation and its resolution would not support a diagnosis of pericarditis. Esophageal spasm may improve rapidly with nitrates but is not associated with ST-segment elevation. Unstable angina would be unlikely to produce the transient ST-segment elevation seen in this patient.

**Bibliography**

1. **Mayer S, Hillis LD.** Prinzmetal's varient angina. Clin Cardiol. 1998;21:243-6. PMID: 9562933

## Chest Pain Question 14
## Answer: A

**Educational Objective:** *Evaluate the use of exercise testing in the diagnosis of coronary artery disease.*

Noninvasive stress testing for the diagnosis of coronary artery disease is most helpful when there is an intermediate pretest likelihood of disease. The middle-aged man with atypical angina falls in this category. A positive stress electrocardiogram (ECG) result in a patient with a low likelihood of disease, such as the 31-year-old woman, is most likely to be false positive. Patients with unstable angina, such as the 55-year-old man, should not have exercise testing because of the risk of myocardial infarction. Resting ST-segment changes, left ventricular hypertrophy, left bundle-branch block, and digitalis make exercise repolarization changes difficult to interpret. Therefore, if patients likely to have left ventricular hypertrophy need testing, such as the 69-year-old man, an exercise ECG would not be an appropriate study. If patients are symptomatic, an exercise imaging test (for example, thallium scintigraphy) would be appropriate. Stress testing is not likely to provide diagnostic information in asymptomatic patients following coronary angioplasty. Results do not correlate closely with the presence of restenosis.

**Bibliography**

1. **Cheitlin MD.** Finding the high-risk patient with coronary artery disease. JAMA. 1988;259:2271-7. PMID: 2965258

## Chest Pain Question 15
## Answer: D

**Educational Objective:** *Select the most appropriate long-term treatment for variant angina.*

The management of variant angina and "classic" angina differs significantly in some respects. Calcium antagonists are the drug of choice in the management of variant angina. Similar efficacy rates have been noted for nifedipine, diltiazem, and verapamil. Nonselective β-blockade (propranolol) may be detrimental, by causing blockade of the β$_2$ receptors in the coronary circulation. This results in unopposed α receptor-mediated vasoconstriction, which may prolong vasoconstriction in variant angina. Aspirin may worsen variant angina by inhibiting the synthesis of prostacyclin, a coronary vasodilator. Percutaneous transluminal coronary angioplasty (PTCA) is contraindicated in variant angina unless an obstructing lesion is also present. Angiotensin-converting enzyme (ACE) inhibitors (captopril) do not cause the necessary coronary artery vasodilation and therefore are not indicated.

**Bibliography**
1. **Mayer S, Hillis LD.**Prinzmetal's varient angina. Clin Cardiol. 1998;21:243-6. PMID: 9562933

## Chest Pain Question 16
## Answer: D

**Educational Objective:** *Manage patients with acute benign pericarditis.*

The symptoms, friction rub, and erythrocyte sedimentation rate indicate the presence of pericarditis. The electrocardiogram is often normal. There is no evidence of acute myocardial infarction. While pulmonary emboli can present with pleuritic chest pain, the three-component friction rub confirms the diagnosis of pericarditis. Normal findings on ECG, echocardiogram, and chest radiograph rule out myocarditis. Symptoms are likely to resolve with treatment with nonsteroidal anti-inflammatory agents.

**Bibliography**
1. **Permanyer-Miralda G, Sagrista-Sauleda J, Soler-Soler J.** Primary acute pericardial disease: a prospective series of 231 consecutive patients. Am J Cardiol. 1985;56:623-30. PMID: 4050698

## Chest Pain Question 17
## Answer: E

**Educational Objective:** *Prescribe the organic nitrate regimen most likely to avoid the development of nitrate tolerance.*

The time-released mononitrate preparation administered once daily results in a 10- to 14-hour nitrate-free interval and would be the optimal choice. Organic nitrates are safe and effective at relieving symptoms in coronary disease, although there is no convincing evidence that they improve survival. Although the mechanism remains controversial, several studies have shown that continuous delivery of nitrates to the vas-

cular system results in a loss of hemodynamic efficacy (nitrate tolerance) in as many as 85% of patients. Although drugs that replete sulfhydryl donors (methionine, captopril, acetylcysteine) temporarily restore sensitivity, only provision of a nitrate-free interval of sufficient duration has been clinically useful in maintaining nitrate efficacy. The vast majority of studies have found that a minimum of 10 hours free from nitrate delivery to the circulation is needed.

Orally administered nitrate preparations are released over periods of 1 to 2 hours (immediate-release) to 10 to 14 hours (sustained-release). The newer 5-mononitrates have an intrinsically longer elimination half-life due to slower metabolism and so remain in the circulation longer after delivery. The regimens described in Options A, B, C and D all fail to provide a sufficient time (2, 0, 4, and 2 hours, respectively) free of nitrate delivery to prevent tolerance.

**Bibliography**
1. **Parker JD, Parker JO.** Nitrate therapy for stable angina pectoris. N Engl J Med. 1998;338:520-31. PMID: 9468470

## Chest Pain Question 18
## Answer: A

**Educational Objective:** *Recognize myocardial pain in a patient with systemic lupus erythematosus caused premature atherosclerosis.*

A creatine kinase and/or troponin level should be obtained in this patient. The initial concern in this patient is whether the chest pain and electrocardiogram changes are caused by pericarditis or a myocardial process. The lack of positional and pleuritic components to the pain make pericarditis less likely. Cardiovascular disease owing to accelerated atherosclerosis is a major cause of death in some studies of systemic lupus erythematosus. Thus, if myocardial infarction is suspected, it is more likely to be caused by atherosclerosis than lupus vasculitis or myocarditis. She is less likely to have a pulmonary embolus, because antiphospholipid antibodies were not seen in the laboratory studies. Her lung examination was normal, so there is no concern that pulmonary fibrosis is present. No pericardial rub was heard, nor did the electrocardiogram suggest pericarditis, making an echocardiogram unhelpful. There is no history of reflux and no response to antacid, so esophageal manometry would not be the best choice.

**Bibliography**
1. **Petri M, Spence D, Bone LR, Hochberg MC.**Coronary artery disease risk factors in the Johns Hopkins Lupus Cohort: prevalence, recognition by patients, and preventive practices. Medicine (Baltimore). 1992;71:291-302. PMID: 1522805
2. **Urowitz MB, Bookman AA, Koehler BE, Gordon DA, Smythe HA, Ogryzlo MA.** The bimodal mortality pattern of systemic lupus erythematosus. Am J Med. 1976;60:221-5. PMID: 1251849

# Congestive Heart Failure

## Congestive Heart Failure Question 1
### Answer: B

**Educational Objective:** *Recognize the causes of decompensated heart failure.*

Determining the cause of this patient's cardiac decompensation is important. A repeat echocardiogram should be ordered first to assist in determining whether disease progression has occurred and is responsible for the decompensation. Ultrafast CT is reported to be a sensitive and noninvasive method to detect coronary calcifications. It is not, however, the first test of choice for this patient. Repeat noninvasive studies, for example, myocardial scintigraphy, remain an alternative later in this patient's course. Although the patient's symptoms on admission are related to decompensated heart failure, pulmonary infection must be ruled out. Respiratory infections may provoke an episode of decompensation. Dietary indiscretions should also be sought as an important contributing factor. There is no clinical evidence of digoxin toxicity, and obtaining a digoxin level at this time is less important. Nonetheless, after a 2-liter diuresis, it is important to rule out the presence of hypokalemia, which could predispose this patient to an arrhythmic event.

### Bibliography

1. **Opasich C, Febo O, Riccardi PG, Traversi E, Forni G, Pinna G, et al**. Concomitant factors of decompensation in chronic heart failure. Am J Cardiol. 1996;78:354-7. PMID: 8759821
2. **Bristow JD, Metcalfe J**.Physical signs in congestive heart failure. Prog Cardiovasc Dis. 1967;10:236-45. PMID: 4865413

## Congestive Heart Failure Question 2
### Answer: C

**Educational Objective:** *Know how to treat the side effects of β-blocker uptitration in a patient with heart failure.*

This patient has signs and symptoms of fluid overload with weight gain and increasing dyspnea. It is not unusual for a patient to develop some fatigue and volume overload early in the course of β-blocker administration and uptitration. Most of these symptoms occur at lower doses, are transient, and are easily treated. The real benefits of β-blocker therapy occur after 2 to 3 months of therapy. The administration of a diuretic will often relieve the volume overload and allow the patient to continue β-blocker therapy. Occasionally, the β-blocker dose may need to be reduced, but this should only occur after a diuretic has been tried. If the patient becomes hypotensive, temporary lowering of the dose of the angiotensin-converting enzyme inhibitor can be attempted with later resumption of the previous dose. Other techniques include a decrease in the diuretic dose and staggering of medications.

### Bibliography

1. **Sackner-Bernstein JD**.Use of carvedilol in chronic heart failure: challenges in therapeutic management. Prog Cardiovasc Dis. 1998;41(Suppl 1):53-8. PMID: 9715823
2. Effect of metoprolol CR/XL in chronic heart failure: Metoprolol CR/XL Randomised Intervention Trial in Congestive Heart Failure (MERIT-HF). Lancet. 1999;353:2001-7. PMID: 10376614

## Congestive Heart Failure Question 3
### Answer: D

**Educational Objective:** *Know how to assess volume status in a patient with heart failure.*

This patient has an elevated jugular venous pressure. Although his chest is clear and there is no edema, his central volume is high. He would therefore benefit from further diuresis. The angiotensin-converting enzyme inhibitor should also be increased to tolerance because of his adequate blood pressure and serum creatinine level. Although a β-blocker should eventually be added to this patient's regimen, the presence of fluid overload precludes β-blockade at this time. It is better to have the volume status stabilized and symptoms of orthopnea resolved with adequate diuresis prior to initiating β-blockade. The patient would also benefit from continued and extensive education concerning dietary sodium restriction, weight loss, and exercise. Diuretic doses can be adjusted as needed if the patient's volume remains stable.

### Bibliography

1. **Butman SM, Ewy GA, Standen JR, Kern KB, Hahn E**.Bedside cardiovascular examination in patients with severe chronic heart failure: importance of rest on inducible jugular venous distension. J Am Coll Cardiol. 1993;22:968-74. PMID: 8409071
2. **Gheorghiade M, Benatar D, Konstam MA, Stoukides CA, Bonow RO**. Pharmacotherapy for systolic dysfunction: a review of randomized clinical trials. Am J Cardiol. 1997;80:14H-27H. PMID: 9372994

## Congestive Heart Failure Question 4
### Answer: B

**Educational Objective:** *Understand the risk of recurrence of peripartum cardiomyopathy.*

Peripartum cardiomyopathy frequently recurs with subsequent pregnancies, but recurrence is unpredictable. Although the likelihood of such recurrence is greater in patients with persistently abnormal left ventricular dimensions and systolic function, recurrence has also been reported in women in whom left ventricular function is restored after the first episode. For these reasons, subsequent pregnancies should be discouraged in patients with peripartum cardiomyopathy who have persistent cardiac dysfunction. Women whose cardiac function has normalized after an episode of peripartum cardiomyopathy should be advised that subsequent pregnancies may not be risk free.

This patient, although asymptomatic, probably still has a mild degree of left ventricular systolic dysfunction because of her ejection fraction of 50% in the presence of moderate mitral regurgitation. There is no evidence that treatment with vasodilators will prevent recurrences of peripartum cardiomyopathy. In addition, angiotensin-converting enzyme inhibitors are contraindicated in pregnant patients because of potential fetal teratogenicity. Although high intake of salt has been implicated as a cause of peripartum cardiomyopathy in certain parts of Africa, there is no evidence that strict salt avoidance will reduce recurrences.

### Bibliography

1. **Ravikishore AG, Kaul UA, Sethi KK, Khalilullah M**. Peripartum cardiomyopathy: prognostic variables at initial evaluation. Int J Cardiol. 1991;32:377-80. PMID: 1838741
2. **Shotan A, Widerhorn J, Hurst A, Elkayam U**. Risks of angiotensin-converting enzyme inhibition during pregnancy: experimental and clinical evidence, potential mechanisms, and recommendations for use. Am J Med. 1994;96:451-3. PMID: 8192177

## Congestive Heart Failure Question 5
## Answer: B

**Educational Objective:** *Recognize the current epidemiology of heart failure in the United States.*

The prevalence of heart failure is increasing. The increase in the hospital discharge rates for patients with heart failure in recent years is due to various factors. Although heart failure may be diagnosed more often, the use of acute interventions to preserve myocardium is one of the reasons for the increased prevalence. Another reason is the aging of the population, since the incidence of heart failure increases with increasing age. The prevalence of hypertension has not changed, and the incidence of heart failure due to hypertension in the Framingham study did not change from 1950 to 1980 despite major advances in therapy. Treatment of hypertension may simply delay the onset of heart failure. There is no evidence to suggest an increase in the development of rheumatic valvular disease or cardiomyopathy in the United States.

### Bibliography

1. **Massie BM, Shah NB.** Evolving trends in the epidemiologic factors of heart failure: rationale for preventive strategies and comprehensive disease management. Am Heart J. 1997;133:703-12. PMID: 9200399

## Congestive Heart Failure Question 6
## Answer: A

**Educational Objective:** *Recognize that restenosis is a common cause of recurrent symptoms after angioplasty with or without stent placement.*

Stents are now used in approximately 70% of patients undergoing percutaneous transluminal coronary angioplasty in the United States. Stenting, along with the use of platelet glycoprotein IIb/IIIa inhibitors, has markedly reduced the incidence of acute thrombotic occlusion following angioplasty procedures. The incidence of restenosis has also been reduced by stenting, but restenosis still occurs in 8% to 15% of patients, based on various series. Restenosis is the most likely diagnosis for this patient, and she should undergo repeat coronary angiography. If the diagnosis is confirmed, coronary artery bypass surgery should be strongly considered because the success rate of opening an obstructed vessel that has already been stented is much lower than at the original procedure.

It is unlikely that she would have developed a ventricular aneurysm without an infarct. She was noted to have ischemia, but no mention of hypokinetic or irreversible ischemic area on her testing. Since she has known coronary artery disease, she could have developed a new coronary artery obstruction, but this is less likely. Gastroesophageal reflux is an unlikely cause of exertional dyspnea, and she has no risk factors for pulmonary embolism.

### Bibliography

1. **Kastrati A, Schomig A, Elezi S, Schuhlen H, Dirschinger J, Hadamitzky M, et al**. Predictive factors of restenosis after coronary stent placement. J Am Coll Cardiol. 1997;30:1428-36. PMID: 9362398
2. **Lincoff AM, Califf RM, Moliterno DJ, Ellis SG, Ducas J, Kramer JH, et al**. Complementary clinical benefits of coronary-artery stenting and blockade of platelet glycoprotein IIb/IIIa receptors. Evaluation of Platelet IIb/IIIa Inhibition in Stenting Investigators. N Engl J Med. 1999;341:319-27. PMID: 10423466

## Congestive Heart Failure Question 7
## Answer: A

**Educational Objective:** *Recognize risk factors for patients with heart failure and a poor prognosis.*

A pulmonary capillary wedge pressure of > 12 mm Hg and an elevated pulmonary artery systolic pressure of > 50 mm Hg as well as a reduction in cardiac output indicate a guarded outcome. Among metabolic parameters, hyponatremia continues to be regarded as a marker of a poor prognosis. To date, gender is not considered an index of a poor outcome. If appropriate, patients with a significant heart failure should be referred to a cardiac transplantation center for evaluation. The current survival of cardiac transplant patients at 1 year is 88%.

### Bibliography

1. **Cohn JN, Johnson GR, Shabetai R, Loeb H, Tristani F, Rector T, et al.** Ejection fraction, peak exercise oxygen consumption, cardiothoracic ratio, ventricular arrhythmias, and plasma norepinephrine as determinants of prognosis in heart failure. The V-HeFT VA Cooperative Studies Group. Circulation. 1993;87(Suppl):VI5-16. PMID: 8500240

## Congestive Heart Failure Question 8
## Answer: B

**Educational Objective:** *Recognize an ischemic cause in the differential diagnosis of acute heart failure with preserved systolic function.*

This patient has acute heart failure associated with pulmonary edema and preserved systolic function. Heart failure with preserved systolic function can account for as many as 30% to 40% of cases of heart failure, particularly in the older age group. Although aging of the myocardium can be associated with decreased cardiac compliance, acute heart failure is not the usual presentation. Since the incidence of coronary disease increases in women after menopause and is common in elderly patients, an ischemic cause must be excluded. The absence of chest pain is not a deterrent to pursuing an ischemic etiology. This patient has a murmur compatible with mitral valve insufficiency. Acute ischemia could worsen the mitral regurgitation and further exacerbate the episodes of acute dyspnea. Although dietary indiscretion can provoke excessive sodium and fluid retention, the symptoms usually occur gradually rather than acutely. Myocarditis is unlikely in the presence of preserved left ventricular function.

### Bibliography

1. **Litwin SE, Grossman W.** Diastolic dysfunction as a cause of heart failure. Am Coll Cardiol. 1993;22(Suppl A):49A-55A. PMID: 8376697

2. **Cowie MR, Wood DA, Coats AJ, Thompson SG, Poole-Wilson PA, Suresh V, Sutton GC.** Incidence and aetiology of heart failure; a population-based study. Eur Heart J. 1999;20:421-8. PMID: 10213345

3. **Chiamvimonvat V, Sternberg L.** Coronary artery disease in women. Can Fam Physician. 1998;44:2709-17. PMID: 9870124

## Congestive Heart Failure Question 9
## Answer: C

**Educational Objective:** *Know the best therapeutic regimen for a patient with heart failure, and preserved systolic function.*

There are no large studies reporting on use of medical therapy for patients with heart failure with preserved systolic

function. In general, however, the goals are to decrease the heart rate, maintain sinus rhythm if possible, reverse left ventricular hypertrophy, treat myocardial ischemia, and treat hypertension aggressively. Since angiotensin-converting enzyme (ACE) inhibitors have been shown to reverse left ventricular hypertrophy and are effective antihypertensive agents, the addition of an ACE inhibitor is reasonable. In at least one study of men with hypertension and left ventricular hypertrophy, a diuretic and an ACE inhibitor were better than other classes of drugs in reducing left ventricular hypertrophy. If ischemia is detected, nitrates are a reasonable additional alternative. There is no evidence that this patient has volume overload at this time, and furosemide is therefore not necessary. The history of moderately severe asthma makes the choice of a β-blocker undesirable. Although terazosin is an effective antihypertensive agent, it is not useful in reducing left ventricular hypertrophy.

### Bibliography

1. **Gottdiener JS, Reda DJ, Massie BM, Materson BJ, Williams DW, Anderson RJ.** Effect of single-drug therapy on reduction of left ventricular mass in mild to moderate hypertension: comparison of six antihypertensive agents. The Department of Veterans Affairs Cooperative Study Group on Antihypertensive Agents. Circulation. 1997;95:2007-14. PMID: 9133508

2. **Vasan RS, Levy D.** The role of hypertension in the pathogenesis of heart failure. A clinical mechanistic overview. Arch Intern Med. 1996;156:1789-96. PMID: 8790072

## Congestive Heart Failure Question 10
## Answer: A

**Educational Objective:** *Understand treatments associated with survival benefits in patients with congestive heart failure.*

In randomized controlled clinical trials, angiotensin-converting enzyme (ACE) inhibitors and angiotensin II receptor blockers have been shown to significantly reduce mortality rates in patients with congestive heart failure. These benefits were confirmed in a systematic review of available studies (odds ratio for mortality for patients on ACE inhibitors = 0.77). An additional study showed reductions in hospitalizations in patients with congestive heart failure who were treated with ACE inhibitors. Studies have demonstrated that ACE inhibitors are associated with a reduction in episodes of acute cardiac ischemia in patients with congestive heart failure.

Spironolactone was recently shown to be associated with significant decreases in mortality rates for patients with New York Heart Association class III and class IV congestive heart failure. Moreover, there was no evidence that spironolactone increased the incidence of clinically significant hyperkalemia.

β-Blockers have also been shown to reduce mortality rates in randomized controlled clinical trials. Although the use of digoxin may significantly reduce hospitalization rates and the need for other interventions in patients already receiving diuretics and ACE inhibitors, it has not been shown to confer a survival advantage in any large randomized controlled clinical trial. Some studies of other positive inotropic agents have shown increased mortality rates.

## Bibliography

1. **Lechat P, Packer M, Chalon S, Cucherat M, Arab T, Boissel JP**. Clinical effects of beta-adrenergic blockade in chronic heart failure: a meta-analysis of double-blind, placebo-controlled, randomized trials. Circulation. 1998;98:1184-91. PMID: 9743509
2. **Garg R, Yusuf S**. Overview of randomized trials of angiotensin-converting enzyme inhibitors on mortality and morbidity in patients with heart failure. Collaborative Group on ACE Inhibitor Trials. JAMA. 1995;273:1450-6. PMID: 7654275
3. The effect of digoxin on mortality and morbidity in patients with heart failure. The Digitalis Investigation Group. N Engl J Med. 1997;336:525-33. PMID: 9036306
4. **Pitt B, Zannad F, Remme WJ, Cody R, Castaigne A, Perez A**, et al.The effect of spironolactone on morbidity and mortality in patients with severe heart failure. Randomized Aldactone Evaluation Study Investigators. N Engl J Med. 1999;341:709-17. PMID: 10471456

## Congestive Heart Failure Question 11
## Answer: A

**Educational Objective:** *Recognize the benefits of angiotensin II receptor antagonists in patients with congestive heart failure.*

Studies have shown significant reductions in long-term mortality rates resulting from use of angiotensin II receptor blockers compared with placebo. However, studies have not shown significant reduction in the in-hospital mortality rate from administering angiotensin II receptor blockers. A study showed that losartan was associated with a significantly lower rate of the combined outcome of mortality and hospitalizations for congestive heart failure compared with captopril. Other studies comparing angiotensin II receptor blockers with angiointensin-converting enzyme (ACE) inhibitors have shown few clinically significant differences in most meaningful outcome variables, such as mortality, left ventricular ejection fraction, 6-minute walk test, and dyspnea.

## Bibliography

1. **Dickstein K, Chang P, Willenheimer R, Haunso S, Remes J, Hall C**, et al. Comparison of the effects of losartan and enalapril on clinical status and exercise performance in patients with moderate or severe chronic heart failure. J Am Coll Cardiol. 1995;26:438-45. PMID: 7608448
2. **Pitt B, Segal R, Martinez FA, Meurers G, Cowley AJ, Thomas I**, et al.Randomised trial of losartan versus captopril in patients over 65 with heart failure. Lancet. 1997;349:747-52. PMID: 9074572
3. **McKelvie RS, Yusuf S, Pericak D, Avezum A, Burns RJ, Probstfield J**, et al.Comparison of candesartan, enalapril, and their combination in congestive heart failure: randomized evaluation of strategies for left ventricular dysfunction (RESOLVD) pilot study. The RESOLVD Pilot Study Investigators. Circulation. 1999;100:1056-64. PMID: 10477530

## Congestive Heart Failure Question 12
## Answer: B

**Educational Objective:** *Recognize hemochromatosis, and know the best way to diagnose it.*

Hemochromatosis is a disorder in the regulation of iron storage that results in abnormal deposition of iron in many organ systems of the body. It is inherited through an abnormality on the HLA locus. It is a genetic disease that usually affects homozygotes. Clinically, patients will present with bronze discoloration of the skin and diabetes caused by iron deposition in the skin and the pancreas. This combination of findings gives hemochromatosis its eponym "bronze diabetes." Patients with hemochromatosis may present with arthritis due to cartilage damage secondary to iron deposition. This arthritis resembles osteoarthritis except that the metacarpophalangeal joints are frequently affected and, in about 50% of advanced cases, chondrocalcinosis is obvious on radiography. Hypogonadism may be due to deposition of iron in the testes or in the pituitary gland, which produces low testosterone and loss of libido. Abnormal iron storage can be found in the liver, leading to hepatic failure. Transferrin testing should be done to confirm the diagnosis of hemochromatosis.

Cardiac dysfunction can be a major manifestation of hemochromatosis. The deposition of iron in the heart will produce thickening of the cardiac wall and subsequent diastolic dysfunction. Eventually, systolic dysfunction will occur and contribute to congestive heart failure, which is a common cause of death in these patients. The typical electrocardiogram demonstrates low voltage, and the echocardiogram reveals a relatively small heart with thick walls. The main therapy for patients with congestive heart failure due to hemochromatosis is diuretic therapy. Vasodilators can often cause hypotension. Clinical improvement in cardiac function has been reported in patients who have been treated with phlebotomy or deferoxamine, which will decrease the tissue iron overload. Echocardiography is a useful tool for the assessment of ventricular structure and function and should be done in this patient with the first presentation of heart failure. It will not confirm the diagnosis of hemochromatosis, however. Coronary arteriography is not indicated at this point. The history is classic for the presentation of hemochromatosis, not for coronary artery disease.

Although hypothyroidism can present with some cardiac manifestations and can cause arthropathy, it would not account for the skin pigmentation and would be associated with "hung-up" deep tendon reflexes. Hyperpigmentation of the skin and hypotension are features of Addison's disease, which is associated with a decreased serum cortisol level. In Addison's disease, however, the skin is darker in areas of pressure, skin creases, and the areolas of the nipples. Arthritis is not a feature of Addison's disease.

**Bibliography**
1. **Bacon BR**. Hemochromatosis: diagnosis and management. Gastroenterology. 2001;120:718-25. PMID: 11179246

## Congestive Heart Failure Question 13
## Answer: C

**Educational Objective:**  *Recognize right heart failure and determine its cause.*

The edema, increased abdominal girth, and elevated venous pressure are evidence of right heart failure, and the setting of hypoxemia, erythrocytosis, and significant pulmonary disease forms adequate support for the diagnosis of cor pulmonale secondary to chronic obstructive pulmonary disease. The obesity and hypertension also raise the possibility of obstructive sleep apnea as a contributing factor, and pulmonary thromboembolic disease is a possible complication in a sedentary obese person with erythrocytosis. Treatment of cor pulmonale centers on management of the pulmonary abnormalities. Although the other diagnostic choices all may present with right heart failure and were in the differential diagnosis, they are less likely. Cardiac tamponade is not associated with a murmur or a third heart sound. Mitral regurgitation is not infrequently the cause of right heart failure, and this patient did have a systolic murmur, but the murmur in this patient increased with inspiration ("Carvallo's sign"), indicating tricuspid regurgitation. If mitral regurgitation were the cause of the right heart failure, cor pulmonale would be excluded by definition. Constrictive pericarditis is an uncommon clinical problem, often associated with atrial fibrillation, and unlikely to be associated with the murmur of tricuspid regurgitation. Pulmonic stenosis is associated with a systolic murmur that increases with inspiration, but is an infrequent clinical problem in this age group and would not explain the hypoxemia or erythrocytosis.

**Bibliography**
1. **MacNee W**. Pathophysiology of cor pulmonale in chronic obstructive pulmonary disease. Part one. Am J Respir Crit Care Med. 1994;150:833-52. PMID: 8087359
2. **Lembo NJ, Dell 'Italia LJ, Crawford MH, O'Rourke RA**. Bedside diagnosis of systolic murmurs. N Engl J Med. 1988:318;1572-8. PMID: 2897627

## Congestive Heart Failure Question 14
## Answer: C

**Educational Objective:**  *Recognize symptomatic mitral stenosis in a pregnant patient.*

This patient's history of new onset heart failure during pregnancy and physical exam findings that include an opening snap and diastolic murmur suggest mitral valve stenosis.

Pregnant patients with mild to moderate mitral stenosis can usually be managed medically through pregnancy and undergo delivery at term with low morbidity and mortality. Many pregnant patients developing atrial fibrillation during pregnancy have a marked improvement in symptoms when sinus rhythm is restored. When New York Heart Association class 3 or 4 symptoms persist despite reversion of sinus rhythm during pregnancy, balloon mitral commissurotomy can be done with a considerable increase in mitral valve orifice size and a decrease in pulmonary artery pressure.

The murmur of atrial septal defect is a high-pitched systolic murmur, not diastolic as in this patient. Patient ductus arteriosus produces both a systolic and diastolic murmur and therefore is unlikely in this patient. While the murmur of aortic regurgitation and tricuspid insufficiency are both diastolic murmurs, neither is associated with left atrial enlargement. Furthermore, the murmur of tricuspid stenosis increases with inspiration, but the murmur of mitral stenosis does not. The murmur of aortic regurgitation is not associated with an opening snap.

**Bibliography**
1. **Turi ZG, Reyes VP, Raju BS, Raju AR, Kumar DN, Rajagopal P, et al**. Percutaneous balloon versus surgical closed commissurotomy for mitral stenosis. A prospective, randomized trial. Circulation. 1991;83:1179-85. PMID: 2013139

## Congestive Heart Failure Question 15
## Answer: C

**Educational Objective:**  *Recognize heart failure caused by myocarditis.*

The most likely cause of the patient's atrial fibrillation and heart failure is myocarditis, which was caused by his viral illness. Indeed, the temporal relationship of his dysrhythmia to the upper respiratory illness is very compelling in this regard and should always be sought in such circumstances. The characteristics of myocarditis are often difficult to distinguish from those of coronary artery disease, especially in the older patient who also has traditional risk factors for the latter condition. Adding to the confusion is the well-established observation that acute myocarditis is not necessarily an entity that affects the myocardium globally, that is, it may present as a regional wall motion abnormality and thus even more closely mimic an acute myocardial infarction. It is also important to remember that when myocardial cells die, enzymes (that is, creatine phosphokinase [CPK]-MB and troponin) are released. There is nothing that makes this enzyme release specific for coronary artery disease, and therefore, such laboratory abnormalities must always be considered in the clinical context in which they occur. In this case, a myocardial infarction is not likely to be the cause of the patient's heart failure because the process was global rather than segmental in nature. Hypertensive heart disease is likewise excluded, as there is no evidence of left ventricular hypertrophy observed on either the electrocardiogram or the echocardiogram. The electrocardiogram shows atrial fibrillation with nonspecific ST-T wave changes. It does not demonstrate the ST-segment changes of acute myocardial infarction or the left ventricular hypertrophy that would be expected in long-term hypertension. The patient's elevated blood pressure is most likely a response to activation of the sympathetic nervous system caused by his heart failure. Significant valvular heart disease is also excluded by the results of the echocardiogram. Although a reduced cardiac output can soften the intensity of a cardiac murmur and thus lead to its underestimation, frequently other clues are present to facilitate the recognition of significant valvular heart disease (for example, left ventricular hypertrophy on examination or chest radiograph, a slowly rising carotid pulse). Finally, the echocardiogram also excludes the possibility of a pericardial effusion in this patient.

### Bibliography

1. Dec GW, Waldman H, Southern J, Fallon JT, Hutter AM, Palacios I. Viral myocarditis mimicking acute myocardial infarction. J Am Coll Cardiol. 1992;20:85-9. PMID: 1607543

## Congestive Heart Failure Question 16
## Answer: C

**Educational Objective:** *Recognize the features of cor pulmonale in a patient with the obesity-hypoventilation syndrome.*

The obesity-hypoventilation syndrome is an increasingly recognized cause of pulmonary hypertension and right heart failure (cor pulmonale). The presence of a chronic hypoxia and respiratory acidosis in the setting of obstructive sleep apnea is characteristic of this syndrome. Other clinical features include systemic hypertension and depression. As in this patient, 30% to 40% of patients with obesity-hypoventilation syndrome and obstructive sleep apnea are unable to tolerate continuous positive airway pressure (CPAP).

Any primary or secondary cause of pulmonary hypertension can lead to right heart failure. Acute pulmonary embolism can lead to right ventricular pressure overload and right heart failure, but pulmonary hypertension is not usually seen at this early stage, and a respiratory alkalosis would be expected. Chronic pulmonary thromboembolic disease is an underrecognized cause of pulmonary hypertension and can be identified upon demonstration of pulmonary arterial thrombus by ventilation-perfusion (V/Q) scanning, thin-section contrast-enhanced computed tomography (CT), and, if necessary, pulmonary arteriography. The diagnosis of primary pulmonary hypertension requires that no other potential cause of pulmonary hypertension be present.

Appetite-suppressant drugs, such as phen-fen, have been associated with a valvulopathy that typically involves the aortic and mitral valves, rather than the tricuspid valve. Pulmonary hypertension has been associated with these drugs, but it is rare.

### Bibliography

1. Weissman NJ, Tighe JF Jr, Gottdiener JS, Gwynne JT. An assessment of heart-valve abnormalities in obese patients taking dexfenfluramine, sustained-release dexfenfluramine, or placebo. Sustained-Release Dexfenfluramine Study Group. N Engl J Med. 1998;339:725-32. PMID: 9731088
2. Abenhaim L, Moride Y, Brenot F, Rich S, Benichou J, Kurz X, et al. Appetite-suppressant drugs and the risk of primary pulmonary hypertension. International Primary Pulmonary Hypertension Study Group. N Engl J Med. 1996;335:609-16. PMID: 8692238

## Congestive Heart Failure Question 17
## Answer: B

**Educational Objective:** *Recognize the usefulness of the serum-pleural fluid albumin gradient in differentiating true pleural exudate from pseudoexudate after diuresis.*

The patient has asymmetric subacute effusion that manifests in the context of a history of congestive heart failure. The medical history, findings of decompensated heart failure at examination, and presence of bilateral effusion allow a presumptive diagnosis of cardiogenic transudative effusion, and a therapeutic trial is instituted. Thoracentesis was appropriately undertaken at the reevaluation visit, because the effusion remained large and asymmetric despite improved control of heart failure.

Patients with congestive heart failure treated with diuretics can have conversion of pleural fluid values from clearly transudative values to borderline or even definite exudative values. Measuring serum and fluid albumin concentrations allows calculation of the serum-pleural fluid albumin gradient, which has been shown to be useful in separating truly exudative effusions from postdiuretic pseudoexudates. A serum-pleural fluid albumin gradient exceeding 1.2 g/dL suggests the presence of transudate.

Benign asbestos effusion is a diagnostic consideration, but this entity is highly exudative and must be diagnosed from a history of asbestos exposure; asbestos bodies rarely are found in pleural fluid. Pleural tuberculosis is an important diagnostic consideration, but tuberculous effusion is substantially more exudative than that in this case, and the diagnostic procedure of choice would be a pleural biopsy. The appearance of the fluid does not suggest chylothorax, so measurement of pleural fluid triglycerides to establish this diagnosis is unnecessary.

### Bibliography

1. Burgess LJ, Maritz F, Taljaard J. Comparative analysis of the biochemical parameters used to distinguish between pleural transudates and exudates. Chest. 1995;107:1604-9. PMID: 7781354
2. Heffner JE, Brown LK, Barbieri CA. Diagnostic value of tests that discriminate between exudative and transudative pleural effusions. Primary Study Investigators. Chest. 1997;111:970-80. PMID: 9106577

# Lipid Disorders

## Lipid Disorders Question 1
## Answer: D

**Educational Objective:** *Know the most appropriate treatment in a patient who has had a myocardial infarction and has a low high-density lipoprotein cholesterollevel.*

There are a number of proven strategies for reducing the risk of recurrent coronary events in patients who have had a myocardial infarction. These include β-blockers in almost all patients, angiotensin-converting enzyme inhibitors in selected patients, aspirin in most patients, exercise rehabilitation in most patients, and reducing low-density lipoprotein cholesterol (LDL-C) to achieve an LDL-C ≤ 100 mg/dL. There are also recent trial data regarding patients with low high-density lipoprotein cholesterol (HDL-C) and relatively normal LDL-C. This patient has a low HDL-C (< 45 mg/dL), and the recent clinical trial data can help guide his treatment. The Veterans Affairs HDL Intervention Trial (VA-HIT), reported in 1999, studied patients with coronary artery disease and an HDL-C level < 40 mg/dL and an LDL-C level < 140 mg/dL. The study found a 24% reduction in recurrent coronary and stroke events in patients treated with gemfibrozil. These data would appear applicable to the patient described here.

β-Blockers have proven benefit in post-MI patients. It is therefore advisable to continue this patient's β-blocker, despite the potential role of this drug in reducing HDL-C.

The Cholesterol and Recurrent Events (CARE) Trial, an American study of post–myocardial infarction (post-MI) patients, supported the value of lowering cholesterol in patients with "average" cholesterol levels. However, the CARE study did not show a benefit of further lowering of LDL-C in post-MI patients with baseline LDL-C levels of < 125 mg/dL. In fact, there are no clinical trial data yet available to support further lowering of LDL-C in post-MI patients with LDL-C levels < 125 mg/dL, and clearly none in patients with LDL-C levels already < 100 mg/dL. Administration of simvastatin is therefore inappropriate for his patient.

Additional reduction of the fat in this patient's diet is incorrect because he has already achieved his LDL-C goal and such a dietary change is likely to reduce his HDL-C even more.

An option that is not listed is the use of therapeutic doses of niacin. As reported in the Coronary Drug Project, niacin can raise HDL-C and lower triglycerides and has long-term mortality benefit in post-MI patients. Although niacin could be used in this patient as a single drug, it is usually less well tolerated than gemfibrozil and therefore would generally not be the drug of first choice.

### Bibliography

1. Randomized trial of cholesterol lowering in 4444 patients with coronary heart disease: the Scandinavian Simvastatin Survival Study (4S). Lancet. 1994;344:1383-5. PMID: 7968073
2. Baseline serum cholesterol and treatment effect in the Scandinavian Simvastatin Survival Study (4S). Lancet. 1995;345:1274-5. PMID: 7746058
3. **Smith SC Jr, Blair SN, Criqui MH, Fletcher GF, Fuster V, Gersh BJ, et al**. Preventing heart attack and death in patients with coronary disease. Circulation. 1995;92:2-4. PMID: 7788911
4. **Rubins HB, Robins SJ, Collins D, Fye CL, Anderson JW, Elam MB, et al**. Gemfibrozil for the secondary prevention of coronary heart disease in men with low levels of high-density lipoprotein cholesterol. Veterans Affairs High-Density Lipoprotein Cholesterol Intervention Trial Study Group. N Engl J Med. 1999;341:410-8. PMID: 10438259
5. **Sacks FM, Moye LA, Davis BR, Cole TG, Rouleau JL, Nash DT, Pfeffer MA, Braunwald E**. Relationship between plasma LDL concentrations during treatment with pravastatin and recurrent coronary events in the Cholesterol and Recurrent Events trial. Circulation. 1998;97:1446-52. PMID: 9576424

## Lipid Disorders Question 2
## Answer: C

**Educational Objective:** *Know the appropriate tests for cardiovascular risk assessment in the primary prevention setting.*

Numerous risk factors for atherosclerotic cardiovascular disease have been reported. High blood pressure, increased low-density lipoprotein-cholesterol, and cigarette smoking are the three best established risk factors. There is strong and increasing evidence that diabetes mellitus, especially type 2, confers a high risk for atherosclerotic disease and its complications. Patients with diabetes mellitus frequently have other cardiovascular disease risk factors, such as insulin resistance, hypertension, high triglyceride levels, low high-density lipoprotein cholesterol, hyperuricemia, and a prothrombotic state (this cluster of factors is often called the "metabolic syndrome"). The American Heart Association has designated diabetes mellitus as a major cardiovascular disease risk factor because of its high prevalence, its association with other risk factors (especially those in the "metabolic syndrome"), and its relation to overall increased cardiovascular risk. Patients with diabetes require careful assessment of all cardiovascular risk factors.

The American Diabetes Association recommends testing for possible diabetes in patients with other atherosclerotic risk factors, including a body mass index > 27. Fasting plasma glucose measurement and the oral glucose tolerance test are both suitable for diagnosing diabetes. However, the fasting glucose tolerance test is strongly preferred because it is easier and faster to perform, more convenient and acceptable to patients, and less expensive. Fasting is defined as no consumption of food or beverages other than water for at least 8 hours before testing. Therefore, in addition to a lipoprotein profile, as recommended by the National Cholesterol Education Program, a fasting plasma glucose test, as recommended by the American Diabetes Association, is also appropriate.

Determination of the ankle-brachial index is incorrect because this index has a very low prevalence of abnormality in younger patients and is recommended for risk assessment predominantly in patients over age 55 or 60.

In addition to the "traditional" risk factors discussed above, there has been great interest in a number of new "putative" risk factors. These include lipoprotein(a) concentration, low-density lipoprotein cholesterol particle size, apolipoprotein B concentration, total plasma homocysteine, and C-reactive protein, among others. None of these factors has been accepted as a routine measure for assessing coronary disease risk because of one or more problems with laboratory standardization, lack of consistency of scientific data regarding associations with coronary disease, or uncertainty about the independence of the factor in coronary risk determination.

**Bibliography**
1. **Ridker PM**. Evaluating novel cardiovascular risk factors: can we better predict heart attacks? Ann Intern Med. 1999;130:933-7. PMID: 10375342
2. **Coutinho M, Gerstein HC, Wang Y, Yusuf S**. The relationship between glucose and incident cardiovascular events. A metaregression analysis of published data from 20 studies of 95,783 individuals followed for 12.4 years. Diabetes Care. 1999;22:233-40. PMID: 10333939

## Lipid Disorders Question 3
## Answer: B

**Educational Objective:** *Determine risk for total cardiovascular disease in a patient with peripheral arterial disease.*

To prevent progression of peripheral arterial disease (PAD) and reduce the risk of major atherosclerotic events in other vascular beds (coronary and carotid vessels), medical management of PAD should include intensive risk factor reduction regardless of the severity of symptoms. This is true even in an asymptomatic patient with an ankle-brachial index of < 0.90. Smoking cessation, blood pressure and serum lipid control, and careful management of diabetes mellitus are indicated. Thus, in this patient, the most appropriate test is measurement of hemoglobin $A_{1c}$ to assess control of diabetes, in addition to measurement of serum lipids and the ankle-brachial index.

Glucose tolerance testing is not indicated in a patient with known diabetes mellitus. Risk factors for PAD are similar to those that predict atherosclerotic events in the coronary and cerebrovascular beds. Some risk factors, such as cigarette smoking, diabetes mellitus, high triglyceride levels, and low high-density lipoprotein cholesterol levels, appear to be even stronger determinants of PAD than of coronary artery disease. Among the newly recognized risk factors, apolipoprotein B, lipoprotein(a), homocysteine, fibrinogen, blood viscosity, and C-reactive protein have been associated with a risk of both PAD and coronary artery disease. However, there is no known way to reduce these risk factors. Therefore, measuring lipoprotein(a) will not further influence the management of this patient with established PAD.

Results of a treadmill exercise test are also unlikely to influence future management in this patient without clinical symptoms of coronary artery disease. In addition, the history states that this patient has limited walking capacity. Therefore, a treadmill exercise test is likely to have low sensitivity for coronary artery disease.

**Bibliography**
1. **Criqui MH, Denenberg JO, Langer RD, Fronek A**. The epidemiology of peripheral arterial disease: importance of identifying the population at risk. Vasc Med. 1997;2:221-6. PMID: 9546971
2. **Criqui MH, Langer RD, Fronek A, Feigelson HS, Klauber MR, McCann TJ, et al**. Mortality over a period of ten years in patients with peripheral arterial disease. N Engl J Med. 1992;326:381-6. PMID: 1729621
3. **Weitz JI, Byrne J, Clagett P, Forkouh ME, Porter JM, Sackett DL, et al**. Diagnosis and treatment of chronic arterial insufficiency of the lower extremities: A critical review. Circulation. 1996;94:3026-49. PMID: 8941154
4. **Pasternak RC, Grundy SM, Levy D, Thompson PD**. 27th Bethesda Conference: matching the intensity of risk factor management with the hazard for coronary disease events. Task Force 3. Spectrum of risk factors for coronary heart disease. J Am Coll Cardiol. 1996;27:978-90. PMID: 8609364

## Lipid Disorders Question 4
## Answer: D

**Educational Objective:** *Know how to initiate lipid-lowering diet therapy appropriate for a patient's level of risk according to the National Cholesterol Education Program treatment guidelines.*

This patient is asymptomatic and has no clinical complaints. She does have multiple risk factors for coronary artery disease. Her total cholesterol is above the desirable level, and her low-density lipoprotein cholesterol (LDL-C) of 166 mg/dL is "high risk." Her blood pressure is "high-normal," she is postmenopausal, and she smokes cigarettes. The most common causes of secondary hyperlipidemias (such as diabetes mellitus and hypothyroidism) are not present. Based on her lipid status and other risk factors for coronary artery disease, she is a candidate for LDL-C lowering therapy. Of course, smoking cessation and regular physical activity are also indicated.

According to the National Cholesterol Education Program treatment algorithm, the patient has 2 risk factors and an estimated 10-year risk assessment of approximately 8% based on the Framingham data, her target LDL-C should be <130 mg/dL. Her baseline LDL-C of 166 mg/dL is above the threshold where one would consider initiating intensive lifestyle modification (>130 mg/dL) AND drug treatment (≥160 mg/dL for persons with 10-year risk assessment of <10%). In this patient, diet alone cannot realistically achieve the LDL-C goal, and a Step I diet or Step II diet alone would not be sufficient to reach the LDL-C goal. Thus, drugs such as simavastatin are advised, in combination with diet and lifestyle modification, as *initial therapy* in this patient.

Hormone replacement therapy has no role in primary prevention. The Women's Health Initiative study was stopped prematurely because of an increased rate of breast cancer, myocardial infarctions, strokes, and blood clots in women taking estrogen with progesterone, compared with women taking placebo.

**Bibliography**

1. Executive summary of the third report of the national cholesterol education program (NCEP) expert panel on detection, evaluation, and treatment of high blood cholesterol in adults (Adult Treatment Panel III). JAMA. 2001;285:2486-97. PMID: 11368702

2. **Rossouw JE, Anderson GL, Prentice RL, LaCroix AZ, Kooperberg C, Stefanick ML, et al.** Risks and benefits of estrogen plus progestin in healthy postmenopausal women: principal results From the Women's Health Initiative randomized controlled trial. JAMA. 2002;288:321-33. PMID: 12117397

## Lipid Disorders Question 5
## Answer: A

**Educational Objective:** *Know low-density lipoprotein cholesterol treatment targets for a patient at high risk for development of coronary artery disease based on the presence of multiple cardiovascular risk factors.*

The National Cholesterol Education Program has set low-density lipoprotein cholesterol (LDL-C) goals that vary depending on the presence or absence of (mostly) nonlipid risk factors. A more intensive treatment goal is justified when the patient has a higher risk of coronary artery disease based on an overall cardiovascular risk estimate. The other risk factors include age (men ≤ 45 years, women ≤ 55 years or postmenopausal), hypertension (blood pressure > 140 mm Hg systolic or > 90 mm Hg diastolic), cigarette smoking, high-density lipoprotein cholesterol < 35 mg/dL, and family history of coronary artery disease at early age in first-degree relatives (male relatives < 55 years, female relatives < 65 years). Persons with diabetes mellitus has the same risk as a person with known coronary heart disease. The LDL-C goal is less than 100 mg/dL if risks include known coronary heart disease or diabetes mellitus. The LDL-C goal is less than 130 mg/dL if two or more risk factors are present, and the LDL-

C goal is less than 160 mg/dL if zero or one risk factor is present. This patient has several risk factors (age > 45 years, premature coronary artery disease in a first-degree relative, and blood pressure in the hypertensive range). He is also overweight (body mass index > 25), which predisposes him to additional risk for cardiovascular disease and diabetes mellitus. Therefore, the LDL-C goal for this patient is less than 130 mg/dL.

A total cholesterol goal of 220 mg/dL or less is incorrect for several reasons. Treatment goals are not based on total cholesterol, but, even so, a total cholesterol of 220 mg/dL is above the optimal level of 200 mg/dL that normally corresponds to an LDL-C of 130 mg/dL. A non–high density lipoprotein (non-HDL) cholesterol goal of 190 mg/dL is incorrect because there are no specific guidelines concerning non-HDL cholesterol levels. A triglyceride goal of 300 mg/dL is incorrect because the recommended triglyceride goal (a secondary goal in the National Cholesterol Education Program Guidelines) is less than 200 mg/dL.

**Bibliography**

1. Executive summary of the third report of the national cholesterol education program (NCEP) expert panel on detection, evaluation, and treatment of high blood cholesterol in adults (Adult Treatment Panel III). JAMA. 2001;285:2486-97. PMID: 11368702

2. **Grundy SM, Balady GJ, Criqui MH, Fletcher G, Greenland P, Hiratzka LF, et al.** Guide to primary prevention of cardiovascular diseases. A statement for healthcare professionals from the Task Force on Risk Reduction. American Heart Association Science Advisory and Coordinating Committee. Circulation. 1997;95:2329-31. PMID: 9142014

## Lipid Disorders Question 6
## Answer: A

**Educational Objective:** *Recognize the side effects of lipid-lowering drugs to avoid inappropriate drug choice.*

This patient has nearly equal elevation of total cholesterol and low-density lipoprotein cholesterol (LDL-C), high triglycerides, and low high-density lipoprotein cholesterol (HDL-C). The ideal drug would lower the patient's LDL-C, normalize the triglycerides, and raise the HDL-C. An acceptable drug would correct one or more of the abnormal blood lipid levels without exacerbating the lipid profile in any way. Cholestyramine is contraindicated in this patient because, although it can lower LDL-C, it can also elevate triglyceride levels, especially when these levels are already elevated at baseline.

The other drug choices are all acceptable. The best choice is probably niacin, since it lowers LDL-C, lowers triglyceride levels, and can also raise HDL-C. Gemfibrozil has similar actions but is typically much less potent in lowering LDL-C but is better tolerated. Lovastatin primarily lowers LDL-C, although they may raise HDL-C slightly and may lower triglyceride levels slightly. Some of the other statin preparations, most notably pravastatin, atorvastatin, and simvastatin, have beneficial effects on LDL-C, HDL-C, and triglycerides. These drugs are not listed but certainly could be considered reasonable treatment options for this patient.

**Bibliography**
1. **Knopp RH**. Drug treatment of lipid disorders. N Engl J Med. 1999;341;498-511. PMID: 10441607

### Lipid Disorders Question 7
### Answer: A

**Educational Objective:** *Understand the pathogenesis of type 2 diabetes mellitus and the critical importance of weight loss in the obese patient.*

Most of these abnormalities will improve if the patient could lose weight. With weight loss, his glucose levels will improve, his triglyceride levels will improve, and his low-density lipoprotein (LDL) cholesterol level may even improve somewhat. Furthermore, glucose reduction may also help his retinopathy and neuropathy. Thus, substantial effort should be given to trying dietary treatment in this patient as part of an intensive lifestyle modification regimen.

Whereas lovastatin may correct the lipid abnormalities, it will have little effect on glucose, weight, or blood pressure. Hydrochlorothiazide may actually worsen his glucose tolerance and increase his cholesterol levels. Increasing the glyburide dosage will likely have only a moderate effect on glucose levels if he does not lose weight. Insulin could improve his glucose levels, but such improvement will likely cause him to gain weight.

**Bibliography**
1. Executive Summary of the third report of the national cholesterol education program (NCEP) expert panel on detection, evaluation, and treatment of high blood cholesterol in adults (Adult Treatment Panel III). JAMA. 2001;285:2486-97. PMID: 11368702
2. **Henry RR, Wallace P, Olefsky JM**. Effects of weight loss on mechanisms of hyperglycemia in obese non-insulin-dependent diabetes mellitus. Diabetes. 1986;35:990-8. PMID: 3527829
3. **Lomasky SJ, D'Eramo G, Shamoon H, Fleischer N**. Relationship of insulin secretion and glycemic response to dietary intervention in non-insulin-dependent diabetes. Arch Intern Med. 1990;150:169-72. PMID: 2404478

### Lipid Disorders Question 8
### Answer: B

**Educational Objective:** *Know when to use cholesterol-lowering medication.*

This woman has no major cardiovascular risk factors except for an elevated low-density lipoprotein (LDL) cholesterol level, and she has no known coronary or peripheral vascular disease. She already follows a step II American Heart Association cholesterol-lowering diet, and further dietary restriction is not necessary. Although her cholesterol level is elevated, her LDL cholesterol is less than 190 mg/dL; therefore, it is not recommended that she be treated with medication. Her high-density lipoprotein (HDL) cholesterol level is also elevated, and this is a negative cardiovascular risk factor. However, her LDL cholesterol level is still higher than the goal of less than 160 mg/dL for her cardiovascular risk category, and she should therefore be encouraged to continue to follow her cholesterol-lowering diet.

If her LDL cholesterol level rises to over 190 mg/dL, she would be a candidate for drug therapy. Trying another hydroxymethylglutaryl coenzyme A (HMGCoA) reductase inhibitor might be useful, but there is currently no evidence that there is any difference in the risk of side effects among the different agents. Treatment with niacin would be another option if drug therapy is needed.

**Bibliography**
1. Executive Summary of the third report of the national cholesterol education program (NCEP) expert panel on detection, evaluation, and treatment of high blood cholesterol in adults (Adult Treatment Panel III). JAMA. 2001;285:2486-97. PMID: 11368702

### Lipid Disorders Question 9
### Answer: B

**Educational Objective:** *Know how to treat hypercholesterolemia properly.*

This patient with a marked elevation of total cholesterol and low-density lipoprotein (LDL) cholesterol (420 – 40 – 86/5 = 363 mg/dL) has familial hypercholesterolemia. Both her family history and physical examination are consistent with this diagnosis. Although changes in lifestyle will improve the condition, such patients invariably require medications for hypercholesterolemia. Of those options listed, only hydroxymethylglutaryl-CoA (HMGCoA) reductase inhibitors would be appropriate.

It is likely that this woman will require several cholesterol-lowering medications to achieve a satisfactory reduction of LDL concentration. Another approach is to begin treatment with niacin or bile acid–binding resins. In either case, after several months of treatment a second class of agents should be added.

After initiating diet there was a decrease in the high-density lipoprotein (HDL) cholesterol level. The HDL cholesterol level often decreases when a patient switches from a high-cholesterol, high-fat diet to a more healthy diet. LDL and total cholesterol levels also decrease. Similarly, populations with lower cholesterol who switch to lower-fat diets have lower levels of total, LDL, and HDL cholesterol and a lower prevalence of coronary artery disease. Thus, despite the concerns about the HDL cholesterol, lower-fat diets appear to be beneficial. For this reason, it is useful to have the patient focus on the positive benefits of lowered LDL cholesterol during the diet change.

Alcohol and gemfibrozil should not be recommended at this point. Although both increase HDL cholesterol levels, the patient's major medical problem is the marked elevation of her LDL cholesterol. Gemfibrozil will lower the LDL cholesterol level, but it is less effective than resin, niacin, or HMG-CoA reductase inhibitors.

### Bibliography

1.  **Cobb MM, Teitelbaum HS, Breslow JL**. Lovastatin efficacy in reducing low-density lipoprotein cholesterol levels on high- vs. low-fat diets. JAMA. 1991;265:997-1001. PMID: 1992214

## Lipid Disorders Question 10
## Answer: B

**Educational Objective:** *Recognize proper management of a patient with elevated fasting total serum cholesterol level.*

The National Cholesterol Education Project recommends that in all adults aged 20 years or older, a fasting lipoprotein profile (total cholesterol, low-density lipoprotein [LDL] cholesterol, high-density lipoprotein [HDL] cholesterol, and triglyceride) should be obtained once every 5 years. If the testing opportunity is nonfasting, only the values for total cholesterol and HDL cholesterol will be usable. In such a case, if total cholesterol is 200 mg/dL or HDL is <40 mg/dL, a follow-up lipoprotein profile is needed for appropriate management based on LDL. Values between 200 mg/dL and 239 mg/dL (borderline elevated) in the absence of established coronary heart disease, or two risk factors (one of which is male sex) should prompt dietary instruction and annual reassessment. The presence of risk factors, established coronary heart disease, presence of diabetes mellitus or a cholesterol level of 240 mg/dL or higher is an indication for fasting lipoprotein analysis. Additional fasting past 12 hours is unlikely to lower cholesterol levels further. Exercise or family testing may be appropriate parts of a risk modification program, but specific recommendations are not indicated until after a fasting lipoprotein analysis reveals abnormal cholesterol subfractions.

### Bibliography

1.  Executive summary of the third report of the national cholesterol education program (NCEP) expert panel on detection, evaluation, and treatment of high blood cholesterol in adults (Adult Treatment Panel III). JAMA. 2001;285:2486-97. PMID: 11368702

# Abdominal Pain

## Abdominal Pain Question 1
## Answer: B

**Educational Objective:** *Order the appropriate test in a patient with suspected symptomatic gallstones.*

This patient has symptoms that are characteristic of biliary pain, including right upper quadrant pain radiating to the scapula after eating. The best diagnostic test in this situation is ultrasonography, which has an accuracy of approximately 90% for cholelithiasis and is widely available, noninvasive, and relatively inexpensive. Computed tomography is less sensitive than ultrasonography in detecting cholelithiasis and is also more expensive and less readily available. Hepatoiminodiacetic acid (HIDA) scans are used to detect cystic duct obstruction and are not useful for detecting stones within the gallbladder itself. Oral cholecystography is not sufficiently accurate to use as a diagnostic test in this situation. Endoscopy is not useful for the diagnosis of biliary disease.

### Bibliography

1. **Kalloo AN, Kantsevoy SV.**Gallstones and biliary disease. Prim Care. 2001;28:591-606. PMID: 11483446

## Abdominal Pain Question 2
## Answer: B

**Educational Objective:** *Recognize acute pancreatitis, and choose the most appropriate diagnostic study to determine the cause.*

This young, previously healthy woman has a classic syndrome of acute pancreatitis manifested by epigastric pain radiating to the back, vomiting, and elevated pancreatic enzyme levels. The aim is to find a cause that can be treated to prevent subsequent attacks. Abdominal ultrasonography is indicated to look for gallstones, which are the most common cause of acute pancreatitis, and for choledocholithiasis. A plain abdominal radiographic series will be of little utility because a perforated viscus has been excluded by the absence of free peritoneal air on the upright chest radiograph. It is uncommon to find gallstones or pancreatic calcifications on plain radiographs. An abdominal computed tomographic (CT) scan will show pancreatic edema but is less sensitive for gallstones. Endoscopic retrograde cholangiopancreatography (ERCP) does not visualize the gallbladder well and is not indicated in the acute setting without signs of biliary obstruction or severe pancreatitis.

### Bibliography

1. **Steinberg W, Tenner S**. Acute pancreatitis. N Engl J Med. 1994;330:1198-210. UI: 94187814 PMID: 7811319

## Abdominal Pain Question 3
## Answer: B

**Educational Objective:** *Choose the best test to diagnose Helicobacter pylori infection.*

In a patient with suspected *Helicobacter pylori* infection, the best test for screening is an antibody test. Serum or whole-blood antibody tests for *H. pylori* are accurate, with a sensitivity of 80% to 95%, as well as inexpensive, making them the ideal screening test for *H. pylori* infection in an office-based setting. Spontaneous elimination of *H. pylori* is unusual; thus, a positive antibody test usually indicates active infection. The antibody test is not affected by concurrent use of $H_2$-receptor antagonists, proton pump inhibitors, or antibiotics.

Urea breath tests are perhaps the most accurate diagnostic tests, with sensitivities of 90% to 95%. These tests are noninvasive, office-based, and relatively inexpensive. However, the results of a urea breath test may be false-negative in as many as 30% of patients on concurrent proton pump inhibitor therapy and are even more likely to be false-negative in patients recently receiving antibiotics. However, the false-negative rate becomes <5% within 2 weeks of discontinuing proton pump inhibitor therapy and 4 or more weeks following discontinuation of antibiotic therapy. Thus, in a patient undergoing a urea breath test for detection of *H. pylori* infection, the proton pump inhibitor should be stopped 2 weeks prior to testing and antibiotics should be stopped 4 weeks prior to testing.

Endoscopic tests for *H. pylori* infection include biopsy for rapid urease test, histologic assessment, and/or culture. Although these tests are very accurate, with sensitivities and specificities of 90% to 95%, they are expensive in themselves, in part related to the concurrent costs of endoscopy.

### Bibliography

1. **Laine L, Estrada R, Trujillo M, Knigge K, Fennerty MB**. Effect of proton pump inhibitor therapy on diagnostic testing for Helicobacter pylori. Ann Intern Med. 1998;129:547-50. UI: 98420297 PMID: 9758575
2. **Megraud F**. How should Helicobacter pylori infection be diagnosed? Gastroenterology. 1997;113(6 Suppl):S93-8. PMID: 9394768

## Abdominal Pain Question 4
## Answer: A

**Educational Objective:** *Determine the appropriate management of a patient with asymptomatic gallstones.*

Asymptomatic gallstones should not be treated, because most remain asymptomatic and will not be associated with complicated biliary disease. The morbidity of treatment is greater than the morbidity of the asymptomatic stones over time. Elective cholecystectomy is reserved for the 15% of these patients who will ultimately develop symptomatic gallstone disease. Nonsurgical treatments with bile acids and/or lithotripsy are less effective than surgery for gallstone disease and are reserved for symptomatic stones in patients who either have refused surgery or are poor candidates for surgery because of comorbid medical illnesses. No dietary modification is effective in the management of gallstone disease.

### Bibliography

1. **Ransohoff DF, Gracie WA**. Treatment of gallstones. Ann Intern Med. 1993;119:606-19. PMID: 8363172

## Abdominal Pain Question 5
## Answer: E

**Educational Objective:** *Determine in which clinical situation eradication of Helicobacter pylori infection is associated with improved outcome.*

The only clinical situation in which eradication of *Helicobacter pylori* infection is unequivocally related to improved clinical outcome is in treatment of peptic ulcer disease. In patients with low-grade, gastric mucosa-associated lymphoid tissue (MALT) lymphoma, eradication of *H. pylori* results in tumor regression or disappearance in the majority of patients. Recurrence of gastric cancer in previously *H. pylori*-infected patients originally presenting with early gastric cancer may also be decreased. However, whether *H. pylori* elimination prevents gastric cancer has yet to be determined.

There are no studies indicating improved outcome or prevention of disease in asymptomatic individuals with or without a history of peptic ulcer disease and/or a family history of cancer. In patients with nonulcer dyspepsia, most studies show no improvement in symptoms following eradication of *H. pylori* infection. Gastroesophageal reflux disease (GERD) is not related to *H. pylori* infection, and recent data suggest that eradication of *H. pylori* may result in decreased responsiveness of patients with GERD to proton pump inhibitor therapy.

### Bibliography

1. **Talley NJ, Vakil N, Ballard ED 2nd, Fennerty MB**. Absence of benefit of eradicating Helicobacter pylori in patients with nonulcer dyspepsia. N Engl J Med. 1999;341:1106-11. PMID: 10511608
2. **Gillen D, Wirz AA, Neithercut WD, Ardill JES, et al**. Helicobacter pylori infection potentiates the inhibition of gastric acid secretion by omeprazole. Gut. 1999;44:468-75. PMID: 10075952

## Abdominal Pain Question 6
## Answer: D

**Educational Objective:** *Identify the appropriate evaluation of a patient with symptoms of gastroesophageal reflux disease who fails to respond to proton pump inhibitor therapy.*

This patient has symptoms suggestive of gastroesophageal reflux disease (GERD) unresponsive to escalating doses of proton pump inhibitor. None of the medications or supplements she is taking is known to have an effect on her symptoms. Twenty-four-hour esophageal pH recording on medication will help define whether the patient's symptoms are in fact due to GERD. Many such patients will have normal esophageal acid exposure and may have "functional heartburn." If 24-hour pH testing shows esophageal acid exposure is still elevated on 20 mg of omeprazole twice daily, the dose of proton pump inhibitor can be increased.

Patients in whom proton pump inhibitor therapy is unsuccessful may, in fact, be poor candidates for fundoplication. GERD may not be causing their symptoms. Increasing the dose of proton pump inhibitor at this point may still not relieve symptoms and is unlikely to better define the patient's problem(s). Upper endoscopy in this setting has a low yield, especially in a young woman.

### Bibliography

1. **Katzka DA, Paoletti V, Leite L, et al**. Prolonged ambulatory 24-hour pH monitoring in patients with persistent gastroesophageal reflux disease symptoms: testing while on therapy identifies the need for more aggressive anti-reflux therapy. Am J Gastroenterol. 1996;91:2110-3. PMID: 8855731

## Abdominal Pain Question 7
## Answer: A

**Educational Objective:** *Identify the principal causes of and appropriate evaluation for acute pancreatitis.*

This man with acute pancreatitis has no history of alcohol abuse, takes no medications, and has no signs of gallstone disease. Hypertriglyceridemia, usually greater than 1000 mg/dL, and hypercalcemia are recognized causes of acute pancreatitis and should be sought in the diagnostic approach. Abnormalities of cholesterol or glucose tolerance do not cause acute pancreatitis. The serum CA 19-9 is a nonspecific tumor marker that may be elevated in pancreatic cancer, but it is not helpful in the evaluation of acute pancreatitis.

### Bibliography

1. **Steinberg W, Tenner S**. Acute pancreatitis. N Engl J Med. 1994;330:1198-210. PMID: 7811319
2. **Toskes PP**. Hyperlipidemic pancreatitis. Gastroenterol Clin North Am. 1990;19:783-91. PMID: 2269517

## Abdominal Pain Question 8
## Answer: D

**Educational Objective:** *Recognize a typical case of foodborne infection caused by enterohemorrhagic Escherichia coli.*

The clinical scenario is typical for infection caused by enterohemorrhagic *Escherichia coli* (EHEC). Bloody diarrhea, abdominal cramping, and absence of fever are common, and the disease tends to occur in previously healthy people who consumed underheated ground beef. Untreated water is an important source of *Giardia lamblia* infection, which can also present with abdominal pain and loose stools but not with bloody diarrhea. A small ingestion of aspirin is not likely to cause significant abdominal distress or frank blood in the stool. There is a risk for enteric infection associated with swimming or bathing, but none of the EHEC infections is commonly associated with water activities. Chicken is an infrequent vehicle for EHEC, although it is an important source of *Campylobacter*, *Listeria*, and *Salmonella* species.

### Bibliography
1. **Su C, Brandt LJ**. Escherichia coli O157:H7 infection in humans. Ann Intern Med. 1995;123:698-714. PMID: 7574226

## Abdominal Pain Question 9
## Answer: D

**Educational Objective:** *Recognize and manage diverticulitis.*

This patient has progressive diverticular disease, now complicated by confirmed diverticulitis. He has developed an inflammatory mass between the sigmoid colon and bladder. There is a strong likelihood that he will develop recurring or progressive attacks with potential perforating or penetrating complications. Biopsy of the inflammatory mass would not be appropriate and may lead to fistulization. Likewise, instrumentation with a colonoscope and the introduction of air may cause perforation through an already weakened colonic wall. An urgent laparotomy in the setting of inflammation may require temporary diversion and a second operation. If the patient improves with nasogastric suction and antibiotics, scheduled or elective resection would greatly reduce the risk of inflammatory sequelae from current or subsequent attacks.

### Bibliography
1. **Stollman NH, Raskin JB**. Diverticular disease of the colon. J Clin Gastroenterol. 1999;29:241-52. PMID: 10509950

## Abdominal Pain Question 10
## Answer: C

**Educational Objective:** *Recognize the indications for treatment and know recommended therapy for Helicobacter pylori-associated active peptic ulcers.*

*Helicobacter pylori* gastritis is found in 90% to 100% of patients with duodenal ulcers and 70% to 90% of patients with gastric ulcers. Most other peptic ulcers are caused by NSAID therapy and, rarely, Zollinger-Ellison syndrome. The diagnosis of *H. pylori* infection may be based on invasive tests (which require endoscopy with a gastric mucosal biopsy for histologic assessment or urease activity) or noninvasive tests ($^{14}$C- or $^{13}$C-urea breath tests or serologic tests for IgG or IgA antibodies). In patients in whom an active duodenal or gastric ulcer is identified at endoscopy, antral biopsies should always be obtained for a urease test and histologic assessment. Because urease tests are relatively inexpensive and have a sensitivity of > 90%, the biopsy specimens need be sent for histologic assessment only if the urease test is negative. Single-agent therapy with bismuth, antibiotics, or omeprazole may suppress the activity of *H. pylori* infection but eradicates infection in < 30% of cases. Nevertheless, recent use of these agents may result in false-negative tests for *H. pylori*.

In this patient with recurrent duodenal ulcer disease, the most likely cause is *H. pylori* infection. The patient had no history of NSAID use, and the normal gastrin level excludes Zollinger-Ellison syndrome. Antral biopsies demonstrated chronic active gastritis, the principal cause of which is *H. pylori* infection.

An NIH Consensus Development Conference has recommended that all ulcer patients with *H. pylori* infection be treated with antimicrobial agents in addition to antisecretory drugs. These regimens have been shown to enhance the rate of acute ulcer healing and, more important, to reduce the ulcer recurrence rate to < 10%. Maintenance therapy with $H_2$-receptor antagonists should be reserved for patients in whom *H. pylori* cannot be eradicated and, for the time being, patients with a history of bleeding complications. Antacids and sucralfate may temporarily improve the symptoms but will not cure the patient. The role of surgery in peptic ulcer disease will be relegated increasingly to patients with ulcer complications such as gastric outlet obstruction, perforation, and bleeding that cannot be controlled with endoscopic hemostasis.

### Bibliography
1. **Graham DY, Lew GM, Malaty HM, Evans DG, Evans DJ Jr, Klein PD, et al**. Factors influencing the eradication of Helicobacter pylori with triple therapy. Gastroenterology. 1992;102:493-6. PMID: 1732120
2. NIH Consensus Conference. Helicobacter pylori in peptic ulcer disease. NIH Consensus Development Panel on Helicobacter pylori in Peptic Ulcer Disease. JAMA. 1994;272:65-9. PMID: 8007082

## Abdominal Pain Question 11
## Answer: C

**Educational Objective:** *Diagnose acute hematochezia, based on clinical findings.*

This 65-year-old man has a rather typical case of acute colonic ischemia. The patient, usually in the seventh decade of life or older, presents with a sudden onset of abdominal pain, most commonly located in the left lower quadrant. Within a short time, there is the passage of bright red blood per rectum, representing ischemic damage to the mucosa. Notably, no fever is present, and cardiac examination is normal. This disease most commonly affects the watershed area involving the splenic flexure, where anastomotic connections of the superior mesenteric and inferior mesenteric circulations supply blood.

Multiple polyps would not account for the patient's pain or elevated leukocyte count. The bleeding found with simple diverticular disease is virtually always painless. Although pseudomembranous colitis produced by *Clostridium difficile* infection rarely causes bleeding, it cannot be ruled out. However, the absence of fever and a diarrheal prodrome and previous antibiotics make this diagnosis much less likely. Bleeding from angiodysplasias may occur in patients in their 60s, but it is painless.

**Bibliography**

1. **Cappell MS**. Intestinal (mesenteric) vasculopathy. II. Ischemic colitis and chronic mesenteric ischemia. Gastroenterol Clin North Am. 1998;27:827-60. PMID: 9890115

## Abdominal Pain Question 12
## Answer: E

**Educational Objective:** *Recognize the need for abdominal angiogram in a patient with potential intestinal ischemia.*

This patient should have an abdominal angiogram. The patient has evidence of atherosclerotic disease, atrial fibrillation, and recent cardiac decompensation. Treatment with digoxin may increase the risk for intestinal ischemia. The differential diagnosis is between an embolic event and acute ischemia due to progressive disease of the mesenteric vessels. An angiogram should be diagnostic and assist the surgeons in defining an appropriate operation. The patient should be well hydrated before and after the dye load. Delaying the diagnostic examination could lead to infarction and perforation. Invasive endoscopic studies are contraindicated with progressive abdominal pain.

Pancreatitis and cholelithisis may produce midabdominal pain but are not associated with blood in the stool. Angiodysplasia is associated with gastrointestinal bleeding but not abdominal pain. While duodenal ulcer can produce abdominal pain and bleeding, the presence of leukocytosis and atrial fibrillation makes intestinal embolism much more likely.

**Bibliography**

1. **Cappell MS**. Intestinal (mesenteric) vasculopathy. II. Ischemic colitis and chronic mesenteric ischemia. Gastroenterol Clin North Am. 1998;27:827-60. PMID: 9890115

## Abdominal Pain Question 13
## Answer: E

**Educational Objective:** *Understand the clinical presentation of chronic pancreatitis.*

The diagnosis of chronic pancreatitis usually is suggested by history and confirmed by imaging studies or laboratory tests. The demonstration of diffuse, speckled calcification of the pancreas on a plain film of the abdomen is diagnostic of chronic pancreatitis. Although the sensitivity of this finding is only approximately 30%, a plain film of the abdomen should be the first diagnostic test because it is simple, not expensive, and specific.

Nephrolithiasis is not affected by meals. Her age makes ischemic colitis and diverticulitis unlikely causes of abdominal pain. With the scant information given, cholelithiasis is a possibility, but the alcohol history and pancreatic calcifications point more strongly to acute and chronic pancreatitis.

**Bibliography**

1. **Vlodov J, Tenner SM**. Acute and Chronic pancreatitis. Prim Care. 2001;28:607-28. PMID: 11483447

## Abdominal Pain Question 14
## Answer: E

**Educational Objective:** *Recognize nonulcer dyspepsia.*

The patient has nonulcer dyspepsia, a common constellation of vague epigastric symptoms consisting of intermittent epigastric distress without evidence of a systemic disease. Upper gastrointestinal endoscopy is usually normal in affected patients, as are other laboratory tests.

Further evaluation with abdominal computed tomography (CT) and/or endoscopic retrograde cholangiopancreatography (ERCP) is expensive, usually unrevealing, and not indicated in patients with nonulcer dyspepsia. The use of histamine $H_2$-receptor antagonists or $H^+/K^+$-ATPase inhibitors (for example, omeprazole) is generally ineffective and costly.

There is no consistent evidence that "triple therapy" (metronidazole, 250 mg four times a day; tetracycline, 500 mg four times a day; bismuth subsalicylate, 2 tablets four times a day; for 3 weeks) to eradicate *Helicobacter pylori* is efficacious in most patients with nonulcer dyspepsia. Reassurance, avoidance of NSAIDs, and symptomatic therapy with antacids are usually all that is required.

**Bibliography**

1. **Talley NJ**. The role of *Helicobacter pylori* in nonulcer dyspepsia. A debate—against. Gastroenterol Clin North Am. 1993;22:153-67. PMID: 8449564

2. **Johannessen T, Petersen H, Kristensen P, Kleveland P, Dybdahl J, Sandvik AK, et al**. The intensity and variability of symptoms in dyspepsia. Scand J Prim Health Care. 1993;11:50-5. PMID: 8484080

## Abdominal Pain Question 15
## Answer: C

**Educational Objective:**  *Recognize and screen for Zollinger-Ellison syndrome.*

Zollinger-Ellison syndrome (ZES), which is caused by hypergastrinemia due to gastrin-secreting tumors (gastrinomas), results in acid hypersecretion and peptic ulcer disease. The disease is rare, accounting for < 1% of cases of ulcer disease. More than 90% of patients with ZES have peptic ulcers. It was believed that ZES was associated with severe or multiple duodenal ulcers and/or ulcer complications, but most patients with ZES are indistinguishable clinically from other patients with ulcer disease. In fact, the most common presentation is a simple, single duodenal ulcer located in the bulb. A minority of patients have multiple ulcers or ulcers located in the more distal duodenum or jejunum. Gastric ulcers are unusual. Reflux esophagitis is common. Diarrhea and/or steatorrhea may be present in one third of patients and may be the sole manifestation in 7% of patients.

ZES should be considered in patients with recurrent peptic ulcer disease in whom there is no history of therapy with NSAIDs and no evidence of *Helicobacter pylori* infection. Furthermore, suspicion is warranted in any patient with an ulcer complication, ulcers distal to the duodenal bulb, ulcers refractory to routine therapy, rapid ulcer recurrences, or kidney stones. It should also be considered in patients with unexplained diarrhea or family histories suggesting peptic disease, parathyroid disease, or pituitary disease (MEN type 1).

The most sensitive and specific method for identifying ZES is demonstration of an increased fasting serum gastrin concentration (> 150 pg/mL). Hypergastrinemia due to other causes must be excluded. Antisecretory agents (especially omeprazole) may falsely elevate this test. Hypochlorhydria with increased intragastric pH is a much more common cause of hypergastrinemia than is gastrinoma. Therefore, gastric acid secretory studies should be performed in patients with fasting hypergastrinemia. In a patient with a serum gastrin of > 1000 pg/mL and acid hypersecretion, the diagnosis of ZES is established. An upper gastrointestinal series is unlikely to provide additional information to the endoscopy. A negative histological assessment makes *H.pylori* serology unnecessary. Colonoscopy has no role in the evaluation of peptic ulcer disease.

**Bibliography**

1. **Maton PN**. Review article: the management of Zollinger-Ellison syndrome. Aliment Pharmacol Ther. 1993;7:467-75. PMID: 7904187

2. **Pipeleers-Marichal M, Somers G, Willems G, Foulis A, Imrie C, Bishop AE, et al**. Gastrinomas in the duodenums of patients with multiple endocrine neoplasia type 1 and the Zollinger-Ellison syndrome. N Engl J Med. 1990;322:723-7. PMID: 1968616

3. **Fishbeyn VA, Norton JA, Benya RV, Pisegna JR, Venzon DJ, Metz DC, et al**. Assessment and prediction of long-term cure in patients with the Zollinger-Ellison syndrome: the best approach. Ann Intern Med. 1993;119:199-206. PMID: 8323088

## Abdominal Pain Question 16
## Answer: D

**Educational Objective:**  *Recognize gonorrhea on Gram stain.*

Gonorrhea causes a mucopurulent cervicitis that is characterized by an increased yellow or creamy vaginal discharge. Gynecologic examination will show an inflamed cervix that is very friable, with a purulent secretion emanating from the os. The Gram stain shows the intracellular gram-negative diplococci that are diagnostic of *Neisseria gonorrhoeae*. The patient should be screened for other sexually transmitted diseases and should be treated for Chlamydia infection also. Her partner or partners should also be screened and treated.

**Bibliography**

1. **Emmert DH, Kirchner JT**. Sexually transmitted diseases in women. Gonorrhea and syphilis. Postgrad Med. 2000;107:189-90,193-7. PMID: 10689416

## Abdominal Pain Question 17
## Answer: C

**Educational Objective:**  *Treat pelvic inflammatory disease associated with possible tubo-ovarian abscess.*

This adolescent patient presents with probable pelvic inflammatory disease complicated by a tubo-ovarian abscess. Several factors suggest that the case might be better managed by initial hospitalization and parenteral therapy, including the patient's young age, relatively severe degree of illness, and probable presence of a tubo-ovarian abscess. Outpatient management of pelvic inflammatory disease with cefoxitin-probenecid or ceftriaxone followed by 14 days of doxycycline can be utilized in milder cases without evidence of peritonitis, tubo-ovarian abscess, or vomiting. In hospitalized patients with possible pelvic peritonitis or tubo-ovarian abscess, the combination of gentamicin and clindamycin given parenterally until the patient improves would be an appropriate therapeutic regimen. Treatment regimens for pelvic inflammatory disease must, of necessity, be multidrug regimens to provide coverage against the multiplicity of pathogens that may be present, including *Neisseria gonorrhoeae, Chlamydia trachoma-*

*tis*, anaerobes, and aerobic gram-negative bacilli. Single-drug regimens, such as amoxicillin alone or third-generation cephalosporins alone, fail to provide complete coverage against the array of possible infecting pathogens and should not be used.

Although *Trichomonas vaginalis* was found in this patient, *Trichomonas* plays no direct role in upper genital tract infection. Simultaneous infection with multiple sexually transmitted disease pathogens is not uncommon. Although the trichomonal infection should be treated eventually, it is of no importance in the patient's current salpingitis episode and need not be treated urgently.

### Bibliography

1. **Workowski KA, Levine WC, Wasserheit JN**. U.S. Centers for Disease Control and Prevention guidelines for the treatment of sexually transmitted diseases: an opportunity to unify clinical and public health practice. Ann Intern Med. 2002;137:255-262. PMID: 12186516

# Gastrointestinal Bleeding

## Gastrointestinal Bleeding Question 1
## Answer: C

**Educational Objective:** *Follow-up rectal bleeding in an older patient.*

Age and first-time bleeding are risk factors for significant colonic disease associated with episodes of bright red blood in the stool. This patient who has a visible rectal fissure should still undergo colonoscopy based on the history of a first-time bleed 2 weeks before the visit. Barium enema with flexible sigmoidoscopy would be an acceptable alternative, but barium enema alone would not adequately assess the rectosigmoid. Stool occult blood tests are not sufficient evaluation in a patient with a history of a recent bleed. A CT scan of the abdomen is also not sufficient for further evaluation of this patient.

### Bibliography
1. **Helfand M, Marton KI, Zimmer-Gembeck MJ, Sox HC Jr.** History of visible rectal bleeding in a primary care population. Initial assessment and 10-year follow-up. JAMA. 1997;277:44-8. PMID: 8980209

## Gastrointestinal Bleeding Question 2
## Answer: A

**Educational Objective:** *Manage upper gastrointestinal bleeding in a patient with liver disease.*

This patient is most likely bleeding from esophageal varices. He has decompensated liver disease as manifested by ascites. Other potential sources of gastrointestinal bleeding include peptic ulcer disease, portal gastropathy, and Mallory-Weiss tear. Because of the high risk of continued active or recurrent bleeding and the high associated mortality rate, urgent endoscopy is appropriate. In actively bleeding varices, band ligation has a high success rate of stopping bleeding. If no other bleeding source is observed and large esophageal varices are present, band ligation offers a therapeutic approach with significantly fewer complications than sclerotherapy, and endoscopic therapy is as effective as surgical shunting for the management of variceal hemorrhage.

In this high-risk setting, it would not be appropriate to wait until morning to perform endoscopy. A transjugular intrahepatic portosystemic shunt (TIPS) may be considered if endoscopic therapy is unsuccessful. Portocaval shunt surgery is not indicated because lower risk options are available.

### Bibliography
1. **Laine L, Cook D**. Endoscopic ligation compared with sclerotherapy for treatment of esophageal variceal bleeding. A meta-analysis. Ann Intern Med. 1995;123:280-7. PMID: 7611595
2. **Cello JP, Grendell JH, Crass RA, Weber TE, Trunkey DD.** Endoscopic sclerotherapy versus portocaval shunt in patient with severe cirrhosis and acute variceal hemorrhage. Long-term follow-up. N Engl J Med. 1987;316:11-5. PMID: 3491317
3. **Sauer P, Theilmann L, Stremmel W, Benz C, Richter GM, Stiehl A.** Transjugular intrahepatic portosystemic stent shunt versus sclerotherapy plus propranolol for variceal rebleeding. Gastroenterology. 1997;113:1623-31. PMID: 9352865

## Gastrointestinal Bleeding Question 3
## Answer: E

**Educational Objective:** *Manage severe lower gastrointestinal bleeding.*

This patient has hemodynamically significant, active lower gastrointestinal bleeding. Colonoscopy performed urgently after colonic preparation is the most sensitive diagnostic test and is potentially therapeutic for angiomas, polyps, and possibly a specifically identified diverticulum.

Visceral angiography is a reasonable option if colonoscopy fails to reveal a source of bleeding and the patient continues to bleed actively. This interventional radiologic procedure may not be available at all facilities. A nuclear medicine scan may identify a general area of bleeding but not the specific source. Introduction of barium is inappropriate in an actively bleeding patient. The barium will interfere with both endoscopic and angiographic visualization of bleeding. Flexible sigmoidoscopy does not evaluate the entire colon for a bleeding source and is therefore an inadequate evaluation.

### Bibliography
1. **Jensen DM, Machicado GA, Jutabha R, Kovacs TOG**. Urgent colonoscopy for the diagnosis and treatment of severe diverticular hemorrhage. N Engl J Med. 2000;342:78-82. PMID: 10631275

## Gastrointestinal Bleeding Question 4
## Answer: A

**Educational Objective:** *Recognize volume depletion in gastrointestinal bleeding, and know the appropriate therapeutic response.*

This patient has hemodynamically significant and life-threatening gastrointestinal bleeding, as evidenced by orthostatic hypotension and volume depletion. The first and most important goal of treatment of volume-depleting gastrointestinal bleeding is volume restoration. The orthostatic hypotension and tachycardia demonstrated by this patient indicate the need for immediate establishment of intravenous access and volume replacement. Because most gastrointestinal bleeding stops spontaneously, the lifesaving intervention is usually volume replacement. Discontinuing NSAIDs is appropriate but is not the only step in treatment. A gastroenterology consultation is advisable because of the need for endoscopy to assess for stigmata of bleeding but would not be the first step in treatment. A volume-stable patient is ideal for endoscopy. Acid suppression with an $H_2$-receptor antagonist is commonly used in this setting but has not been shown to affect patient outcome. Treatment of a *H. pylori* infection is premature because a diagnosis has not been established. Emerging data suggest that major acid reduction improves the outcome of upper gastrointestinal bleeding.

### Bibliography

1. **Laine L, PetersonWL**. Bleeding peptic ulcer. N Engl J Med. 1994;331:717-27. PMID: 8058080
2. **Lin HJ, Lo WC, Lee FY, Perng CL, Tseng GY**. A prospective randomized comparative trial showing that omeprazole prevents rebleeding in patients with bleeding peptic ulcer after successful endoscopic therapy. Arch Intern Med. 1998;158:54-8. PMID: 9437379

## Gastrointestinal Bleeding Question 5
## Answer: A

**Educational Objective:** *Know the appropriate management for acute variceal hemorrhage.*

Octreotide is appropriate early treatment of patients with acute upper gastrointestinal bleeding suspected to be from gastroesophageal varices. Because of its favorable safety profile and evidence that octreotide may be effective in treatment of upper gastrointestinal bleeding of nonvariceal origin, intravenous infusion may be initiated at the time of initial contact and before endoscopic confirmation of a variceal bleeding source.

Because intravenous vasopressin has a high rate of adverse events and limited efficacy, its use is not recommended. Intravenous nitroglycerin also has limited efficacy in this setting. Balloon tamponade is a temporizing measure with a high incidence of accompanying adverse events and should be reserved for the small number of patients with refractory acute hemorrhage as a bridge to more definitive treatment. The transjugular intrahepatic portosystemic shunt (TIPS) should be reserved for patients with ongoing acute or recurrent variceal hemorrhage that persists despite endoscopic and pharmacologic therapy. TIPS is optimally utilized in patients with advanced hepatic dysfunction as a bridge to liver transplantation. Recent data support prophylactic use of antibiotics in cirrhotic patients with acute upper gastrointestinal hemorrhage, particularly in those with ascites.

### Bibliography

1. **Cello JP**. Endoscopic management of esophageal variceal hemorrhage: injection, banding, glue, octreotide, or a combination? Semin Gastrointest Dis. 1997;8:179-87. PMID: 9360282
2. **Bernard B, Grange JD, Khac EN, Amiot X, Opolon P, Poynard T**. Antibiotic prophylaxis for the prevention of bacterial infections in cirrhotic patients with gastrointestinal bleeding: a meta-analysis. Hepatology. 1999;29:1655-61. PMID: 10347104

## Gastrointestinal Bleeding Question 6
## Answer: D

**Educational Objective:** *Understand the importance of endoscopic findings in predicting outcome and understand the indications for endoscopic therapy in patients with gastrointestinal bleeding.*

This patient has a nonbleeding visible vessel associated with a high risk of recurrent bleeding. The visible vessel should be treated with injection of dilute epinephrine and/or coaptive coagulation using a thermal energy probe. If the ulcer were bleeding, endoscopic therapy would also be appropriate. Meta-analysis has demonstrated that endoscopic therapy for nonbleeding visible vessels significantly reduces recurrent bleeding, the need for emergency surgery, and mortality.

Surgical intervention is appropriate only if endoscopic therapy is unsuccessful. The specific intervention is a function of the clinical status of the patient and the findings at surgery. Studies have not demonstrated efficacy of $H_2$-receptor antagonists in acute bleeding in this situation. New data suggests that major acid reduction may improve therapy in acute upper gastrointestinal bleeding, but endoscopic injection and/or thermal coagulation therapy remains the preferred intervention. Intravenous vasopressin is inappropriate because of ischemic complications due to generalized vasoconstriction.

### Bibliography

1. Consensus conference: Therapeutic endoscopy and bleeding ulcers. JAMA. 1989;262:1369-72. PMID: 2668576
2. **Cook DJ, Guyatt GH, Salena RJ, Laine LA**. Endoscopic therapy for acute non-variceal upper gastrointestinal bleeding: a meta-analysis. Gastroenterology. 1992;102:139-48. PMID: 1530782

## Gastrointestinal Bleeding Question 7
## Answer: C

**Educational Objective:** *Determine the appropriate therapy for a patient with an ulcer who is Helicobacter pylori-positive and uses nonsteroidal anti-inflammatory drugs (NSAIDs).*

The management of the patient who develops an ulcer while taking nonsteroidal anti-inflammatory drugs (NSAIDs) and who is *Helicobacter pylori*-positive is problematic, as it is impossible to determine whether the ulcer is secondary to

NSAID use, *H. pylori* infection, or both. Thus, the ulcer must be treated as if both factors were causative.

The treatment of an *H. pylori*-positive ulcer is eradication of the infection, whereas the treatment of an NSAID-associated ulcer is to discontinue NSAID use. Thus, this patient should have his *H. pylori* infection treated and his NSAID therapy discontinued. Treating only one potential source of ulceration, that is, NSAID therapy or *H. pylori* infection, is unacceptable, and substitution of a cyclo-oxygenase-2 (COX-2)-specific NSAID, such as celecoxib or rofecoxib, for ibuprofen, although associated with a lower ulcer risk, has not been proven to avoid complicated ulcer disease (that is, bleeding).

Misoprostol is not indicated because NSAIDs should be stopped in this patient.

### Bibliography

1. **Soll AH**. Consensus conference. Medical treatment of peptic ulcer disease. Practice guidelines. Practice Parameters Committee of the American College of Gastroenterology. JAMA. 1996;275:622-9. PMID: 8594244

2. **Soll AH, Weinstein WM, Kurata J, McCarthy D**. Nonsteroidal anti-inflammatory drugs and peptic ulcer disease. Ann Intern Med. 1991;114:307-19. PMID: 1987878

## Gastrointestinal Bleeding Question 8
## Answer: B

**Educational Objective:** *Select the most appropriate emergent management for bleeding esophageal varices.*

The most appropriate next procedure is insertion of a balloon-tamponade tube and inflation of the gastric balloon. This patient is in extremis from probable recurrent esophageal variceal bleeding despite his earlier sclerotherapy, and he requires urgent stabilization. Balloon tamponade will control variceal bleeding in 90% of patients. Inflation of the gastric balloon alone and subsequent tamponade at the gastro-esophageal junction will stop bleeding in most patients due to pressure on feeding venous radicles that course along the cardia to the distal esophagus. Inflation of the esophageal tube is often unnecessary and is associated with excessive morbidity. Emergent surgical therapy is associated with at least a 50% mortality rate in patients with this condition. Intravenous vasopressin may decrease the bleeding rate, but it is unlikely to control severe hemorrhage and may result in intestinal ischemia in hypotensive patients. A transjugular intrahepatic portosystemic shunt (TIPS) may eventually be useful for this patient, but it is not appropriate in this urgent situation.

### Bibliography

1. **Terblanche J, Burroughs AK, Hobbs KE**. Controversies in the management of bleeding esophageal varices (1). N Engl J Med. 1989;320:1393-8. PMID: 2654633

2. **Terblanche J, Burroughs AK, Hobbs KE**. Controversies in the management of bleeding esophageal varices (2). N Engl J Med. 1989;320:1469-75. PMID: 2497348

3. **Infante-Rivard C, Esnaola S, Villeneuve J**. Role of endoscopic variceal sclerotherapy in the long-term management of variceal bleeding: a meta-analysis. Gastroenterology. 1989;96:1087-92. PMID: 2784398

## Gastrointestinal Bleeding Question 9
## Answer: B

**Educational Objective:** *Recognize that diverticular bleeding is the most common cause of lower gastrointestinal bleeding in older adults.*

Diverticular bleeding is the most common source of lower intestinal bleeding. Rectal bleeding may be evident in 10% to 30% of patients with diverticular disease, with severe blood loss in 3% to 5%. Recurrent bleeding is noted in 20% to 25% of patients. Most bleeding episodes cease spontaneously. Right-sided diverticula bleed more commonly. Clinical features include painless, rapid hematochezia and an urge to defecate, with or without signs of hypovolemia. Proctosigmoidoscopy should be the initial diagnostic test to exclude other nondiverticular causes. Occasionally, as in this patient, blood can be seen coming from the diverticulum or a red spot may be seen in a diverticulum, indicating the location of the bleeding. After appropriate colonic lavage, colonoscopy can identify a bleeding source in up to 75% of patients. Ischemic colitis would present with pain and bleeding, not painless bleeding. Colon cancer and ulcerative colitis would be unlikely considering this patient's normal colonoscopy three months ago. Diverticulitis is associated with fever and left side pain but not bleeding. Angiodysplasia can also produce a painless bleeding in older adults, but the results of the previous colonoscopy showing a pigmented spot on a diverticulum is more suggestive of diverticulosis.

### Bibliography

1. **Peura DA, Lanza FL, Gostout CJ, Foutch PG**. The American College of Gastroenterology Bleeding Registry: preliminary findings. Am J Gastroenterol. 1997;92:924-8. PMID: 9177503

2. **Foutch PG, Zimmerman K**. Diverticular bleeding and the pigmented protuberance (sentinel clot): clinical implications, histopathological correlation, and results of endoscopic intervention. Am J Gastroenterol. 1996;91:2589-93. PMID: 8946992

## Gastrointestinal Bleeding Question 10
## Answer: B

**Educational Objective:** *Recognize the telangiectasias associated with Osler-Weber-Rendu disease, and differentiate them from the telangiectasias of liver disease and petechiae.*

Telangiectasias of Osler-Weber-Rendu disease are sharply demarcated, flat, ruby-colored, 1- to 2-mm, punctum-like lesions. Although most telangiectasias are flat, some can be papular. Partial blanching occurs when pressure is applied. If the lesions are compressed with a glass slide, vascular pulsations can be seen, and, rarely, one or two branching vessels are also seen radiating from the central punctum. The palmar surfaces of the hands and fingers, nail beds, lips, ears, face, arms, and toes are most frequently affected. Sites of mucosal predilection are the tip and dorsum of the tongue and the anterior nasal septum.

Lesions mimicking those of Oslar-Weber-Rendu disease include the telangiectasias associated with liver disease and petechiae. Spider nevi of liver disease are fiery red, with a central punctum and *many* superficial branching vessels radiating outward from the center. An area of erythema surrounds the lesions. Spider nevi occur most commonly on the face and neck; less commonly on the shoulders, chest, back, arms, and hands; and only rarely below the umbilicus. Petechiae are pink-red to purple macules ranging in size from 0.5 to 2.0 mm. Petechiae do not blanch when compressed, are not palpable, and occur most frequently on the lower extremities. The telangiectasias are more strongly suggestive of the cause of the bleeding than is peptic ulcer disease.

## Bibliography

1. **Guttmacher AE, Marchuk DA, White RI Jr**. Hereditary hemorrhagic telangiectasia. N Engl J Med. 1995; 333: 918-24. PMID: 7666879

# Liver Disorders

## Liver Disorders Question 1
**Answer: D**

**Educational Objective:** *Manage a patient presenting with new-onset ascites.*

This patient has new-onset ascites due to portal hypertension. Diuretic therapy and dietary salt restriction should be instituted to prevent recurrence of ascites. In a minority of patients with mild fluid retention, dietary salt restriction alone is sufficient to mobilize ascites, but most patients require the addition of diuretic therapy. The traditional stepwise approach to diuretic treatment is initiation of an aldosterone antagonist, such as spironolactone, in increasing doses to a maximal dose (400 mg/day) as necessary, followed by addition of escalating doses of a loop diuretic in patients in whom the preceding treatment is unsuccessful. However, this stepwise approach often takes a long time, and many experts begin treatment with a combination of an aldosterone antagonist and a loop diuretic. In the setting of fluid retention due to cirrhosis, institution of therapy with a loop diuretic alone (Option C) is typically less effective than a potassium-sparing agent, is often complicated by hypokalemia, and should be avoided. Diet therapy is the cornerstone of ascites treatment: sodium restriction at the level of approximately 2 g/day is adequate without compromising the palatability of the diet too much. However, protein intake should not be restricted in patients with advanced liver disease, particularly in the setting of muscle wasting, unless problematic hepatic encephalopathy persists despite treatment with lactulose and/or antibiotics. Dietary free water restriction is indicated only in patients with hyponatremia (<130 meq/L). Initial, large-volume paracentesis is appropriate in patients who present with symptomatic, tense ascites that can often be successfully managed subsequently with dietary and diuretic therapy. Repeat, serial, large-volume paracentesis is reserved for the small number of patients with recurrent ascites that is refractory to medical management.

### Bibliography
1. **Runyon BA**. Care of patients with ascites. N Engl J Med. 1994;330:337-42 PMID: 8277955

## Liver Disorders Question 2
**Answer: A**

**Educational Objective:** *Identify the most appropriate prophylaxis for travelers to developing countries.*

This patient should receive immune serum globulin (ISG). She is traveling to a region of the world that is endemic for hepatitis A, and prophylaxis is indicated. Most of the populated areas of the world should be considered to be high prevalence relative to the United States. Prophylaxis is not required for travelers to low-prevalence areas such as Canada and northern or western Europe. Currently, there are two choices for prophylaxis against hepatitis A: ISG and hepatitis A vaccine. Rapid, passive transfer of immunity to hepatitis A is achieved with intramuscular injection of ISG. Although 0.02 mL/kg is the standard dose, current preparations of ISG may have low titers of antibody to hepatitis A virus (anti-HAV), and larger doses (0.06 mL/kg) may be required to confer immunity. Vaccination actively stimulates antibody production in more than 95% of patients, but development of antibody is delayed and may not be protective against HAV infection within the first month after vaccination. This patient is planning to travel in 2 weeks, and ISG would be the most effective prophylaxis. Hepatitis A vaccine should be given to all travelers to endemic regions when there is sufficient time to allow development of antibody in response to vaccine or for travelers who plan repeated trips to the region.

In the absence of high-risk behavior, such as illicit substance abuse or homosexual activity, the risk of acquiring hepatitis B is not significantly increased. It is not necessary to test the traveler for hepatitis B and prophylactically treat with either hepatitis B immune globulin (HBIG) or hepatitis B vaccine.

### Bibliography
1. **Fujiyama S, Iino S, Odoh K, Kuzuhara S, Watanabe H, Tanaka M, et al**. Time course of hepatitis A virus antibody titer after active and passive immunization. Hepatology. 1992;15:983-8. PMID: 1317343
2. **Lemon SM, Thomas DL**. Vaccines to prevent viral hepatitis. N Engl J Med. 1997;336:196-204. PMID: 8988900

## Liver Disorders Question 3
## Answer: E

**Educational Objective:** *Identify which contacts of a patient with active hepatitis B should be treated with hepatitis B immune globulin (HBIG).*

Hepatitis B immune globulin (HBIG) therapy is indicated for close personal, sexual, or household contacts of a person infected with hepatitis B virus. HBIG is not indicated for individuals who have only casual contact with the infected patient (options A through D). The serum of an infected patient may contain greater than $10^9$ viral copies per milliliter of blood, rendering it highly contagious. The increased risk in household contacts may be related to inadvertent exposure to contaminated blood through sharing of personal-care instruments, such as toothbrushes or razor blades. A dormitory roommate has a risk of acquiring hepatitis B that is similar to household contacts, and prophylaxis is recommended.

### Bibliography
1. **Lee W**. Hepatitis B virus infection. N Engl J Med. 1997;337:1733-45. PMID: 9392700
2. **Mitsui T, Iwano K, Suzuki S, Yamazaki C, Masuko K, Tsuda F, et al.** Combined hepatitis B immune globulin and vaccine for postexposure prophylaxis of accidental hepatitis B virus infection in hemodialysis staff members: comparison with immune globulin without vaccine in historical controls. Hepatology. 1989;10:324-7. PMID: 2527191

## Liver Disorders Question 4
## Answer: A

**Educational Objective:** *Provide primary prophylaxis for variceal hemorrhage in a patient with liver disease.*

The American College of Gastroenterology recommends that all patients with cirrhosis who have not had a bleeding episode and who have no contraindications to β-blockade should be screened by endoscopy to detect the presence of gastroesophageal varices. If large esophageal varices are detected, patients should be treated with nonselective β-blockers. Several large, randomized, controlled trials of nonselective β-blockers in patients with esophageal varices have demonstrated their superiority over placebo in preventing initial variceal hemorrhage, particularly in patients with large varices.

Recent reports suggest that cirrhotic patients who have large varices with signs of thinning but who have not experienced previous variceal bleeding may benefit from prophylactic endoscopic band ligation. However, these studies should be confirmed by larger, multicenter trials before this approach is generally adopted. There is inadequate evidence to support combined endoscopic therapy (sclerotherapy plus band ligation) in this setting. Isosorbide mononitrate is not the initial choice for primary prophylaxis of variceal bleeding because one large study suggests that it may be associated with greater long-term mortality than β-blockers. Dietary protein restriction should be instituted only in patients with advanced liver disease with problematic portosystemic encephalopathy that has been refractory to standard medical treatment.

### Bibliography
1. **Poynard T, Cales P, Pasta L, Ideo G, Pascal JP, Pagliaro L, Lebrec D**. Beta-adrenergic-antagonist drugs in the prevention of gastrointestinal bleeding in patients with cirrhosis and esophageal varices. An analysis of data and prognostic factors in 589 patients from four randomized clinical trials. Franco-Italian Multicenter Study Group. N Engl J Med. 1991;324:1532-8. PMID: 1674104
2. **Burroughs AK, Patch D**. Primary prevention of bleeding from esophageal varices. N Engl J Med. 1999;340:1033-5. PMID: 10099147

## Liver Disorders Question 5
## Answer: B

**Educational Objective:** *Identify and manage acute alcoholic hepatitis.*

This patient has classic features of acute alcoholic hepatitis: significant alcohol intake, often with acceleration of the amount of intake in the weeks prior to presentation, jaundice, fever, leukocytosis, and a tender, palpable liver. Liver enzyme levels are typically only modestly elevated with an aspartate aminotransferase:alanine aminotransferase (AST:ALT) ratio > 1. Alcoholic hepatitis may resolve spontaneously with abstinence from alcohol, hydration, and nutritional support. All patients who recover from alcoholic hepatitis must be referred for alcohol rehabilitation, although the success rate for this rehabilitation is less than 25%. Mortality rates for severe alcoholic hepatitis range from 10% to 40% and are due to the complications of progressive hepatic dysfunction: hepatorenal syndrome, ascites with spontaneous bacterial peritonitis, sepsis, or gastrointestinal hemorrhage.

Meta-analyses of existing trials indicate that glucocorticoid therapy is associated with significant improvement in survival in severe alcoholic hepatitis. Glucocorticoids are contraindicated in the subgroup of patients with spontaneous bacterial peritonitis or gastrointestinal bleeding. This patient has no evidence of infection or gastrointestinal bleeding; she is a candidate for glucocorticoid therapy.

Abdominal ultrasonography does not support the diagnosis of cholelithiasis. Spontaneous bacterial peritonitis is not supported by the paracentesis. Pyelonephritis or alcohol withdrawal cannot account for her ascites, jaundice, and mental confusion.

### Bibliography
1. **Lieber CS**. Alcohol and the liver: 1994 update. Gastroenterology. 1994;106:1085-105. PMID: 8143977
2. **Mathurin P, Duchatelle V, Ramond MJ, Degott C, Bedossa P, Erlinger S, et al.** Survival and prognostic factors in patients with severe alcoholic hepatitis treated with prednisolone. Gastroenterology. 1996;110:1847-53. PMID: 8964410

## Liver Disorders Question 6
## Answer: B

**Educational Objective:** *Distinguish causes of iron overload.*

Hemochromatosis is the most likely diagnosis based on this patient's ferritin level and is confirmed by the quantitative iron studies on liver biopsy. Most patients have percent iron saturation levels exceeding 80%, serum ferritin levels greater than 1000 µg/mL, and markedly increased liver iron concentrations. Iron overload due to chronic alcoholism and cirrhosis is sometimes difficult to differentiate from hemochromatosis. The distinction may be made by testing serum iron concentration and percent iron saturation of the patient's relatives or by quantitative iron assessment on liver biopsy. The amount of iron in the liver is often considerably less in patients with chronic alcoholism (usually not exceeding 10,000 µg of iron/g dry weight) than in patients with hemochromatosis. Studies testing for the hemochromatosis genes (for example, *Q86Y*) are very specific and provide a definitive diagnosis.

Hemochromatosis is a hereditary disease, strongly linked to HLA A-3, which leads to inappropriate iron absorption from the gut. Arthropathy, increased skin pigmentation, diabetes ("bronze diabetes"), and hepatomegaly are the most common clinical features. Increased pigmentation is noted over the face, extremities, in surgical scars, and on sun-exposed areas. Chondrocalcinosis, cardiomyopathy, and cirrhosis of the liver may occur as the disease progresses.

This patient's age and history, together with his normal mean corpuscular volume, preclude a diagnosis of thalassemia or the hereditary forms of sideroblastic anemia, which usually present with hypochromic anemia.

Wilson's disease may cause hepatic disease but is not associated with an iron overload syndrome. Kayser-Fleischer rings are noted on ophthalmologic examination. Hematologic abnormalities associated with Wilson's disease are rare and related to hemolysis from the release of unbound copper from the liver, a complication sometimes seen in the early stages of the disease. Serum copper levels and ceruloplasmin levels are normal in this patient.

**Bibliography**

1. **Felitti VJ, Beutler E**. New developments in hereditary hemochromatosis. Am J Med Sci. 1999;318:257-68. PMID: 10522553

## Liver Disorders Question 7
## Answer: C

**Educational Objective:** *Recognize primary biliary cirrhosis and the most efficacious way of diagnosing it.*

This is the classic description of primary biliary cirrhosis. Itching is the most common specific symptom of early primary biliary cirrhosis. Approximately 70% of affected patients have enlarged livers. The best screening test for suspected primary biliary cirrhosis is the antimitochondrial antibody test. It is positive in 95% of affected patients and has a 98% specificity if newer enzyme-linked immunosorbent assay (ELISA) tests are used. Endoscopic retrograde cholangiopancreatography (ERCP) is typically normal in patients with primary biliary cirrhosis. Its only role in the diagnosis of primary biliary cirrhosis is in the patient who presents with a similar syndrome but who has a negative antimitochondrial antibody test. ERCP would then be performed to look for other causes of disease, such as primary sclerosing cholangitis.

**Bibliography**

1. **Kaplan MM**. Primary biliary cirrhosis. N Engl J Med. 1987;316:521-8. PMID: 3543682
2. **Van de Water J, Cooper A, Surh CD, Coppel R, Danner D, Ansari A, et al**. Detection of autoantibodies to recombinant mitochondrial proteins in patients with primary biliary cirrhosis. N Engl J Med. 1989;320:1377-80. PMID: 2716784

## Liver Disorders Question 8
## Answer: C

**Educational Objective:** *Recognize autoimmune chronic hepatitis.*

The pattern of the liver function tests suggests some type of hepatitis. The fact that the patient has been symptomatic for more than 6 months is consistent with chronic hepatitis. A diagnosis of autoimmune chronic hepatitis, one of the most treatable types of liver disease, is strongly suggested by the striking elevation of globulins. The appropriate test to diagnose chronic hepatitis and to determine its severity is percutaneous liver biopsy. Endoscopic retrograde cholangiopancreatography (ERCP) is not helpful in these patients. An hepatoiminodiacetic acid (HIDA) scan is useful in the diagnosis of acute cholecystitis, but not in hepatitis. Technetium liver-spleen scan will not give a definite diagnosis, nor will magnetic resonance imaging of the abdomen.

The appropriate initial treatment of autoimmune chronic hepatitis is prednisone. Controlled trials have repeatedly shown rapid efficacy in improving symptoms, abnormal blood tests, and histologic findings in the liver.

**Bibliography**

1. **Tassoni JP Jr, Kaplan MM**. Rapidly progressive liver failure in a 65-year-old woman. Gastroenterology. 1991;100:1462-8. PMID: 2013390
2. **Johnson PJ, McFarlane IG, Eddleston AL**. The natural course and heterogenicity of autoimmune-type chronic active hepatitis. Semin Liver Dis. 1991;11:187-96. PMID: 1925643
3. **Maddrey WC, Combes B**. Therapeutic concepts for the management of idiopathic autoimmune chronic hepatitis. Semin Liver Dis. 1991;11:248-55. PMID: 1925650

## Liver Disorders Question 9
## Answer: D

**Educational Objective:** *Diagnose the cause of jaundice in a patient with ulcerative colitis.*

The most likely diagnosis in a young person with ulcerative colitis, cholestatic jaundice, and a negative hepatitis panel and abdominal ultrasonography is primary sclerosing cholangitis. This lesion is characterized by multiple intrahepatic and/or extrahepatic strictures of the biliary tract on cholangiography and gives the biliary radicles within the liver a "pruned tree" appearance. Because the ducts are scarred and thickened, there is usually no detectable dilatation on ultrasonography or computed tomography. Owing to the stricturing and biliary duct destruction, patients usually present with painless jaundice. The jaundice is of the cholestatic variety and can be associated with itching. The mechanism for the occurrence of primary sclerosing cholangitis in this setting is unknown but may be autoimmune in nature. A liver biopsy in this setting would show changes ranging from nonspecific pericholangitis with bile duct proliferation to fibrosis of the biliary ducts consistent with primary sclerosing cholangitis. Although sulfasalazine can cause hemolytic anemia, the bilirubin level, being mostly direct rather than indirect, does not suggest an active hemolytic process. The negative hepatitis panel rules out hepatitis as a cause of his jaundice. The normal ultrasound examination makes cholelithiasis and an obstructing pancreatic cancer unlikely.

### Bibliography
1. **Farrant JM, Hayllar KM, Wilkinson ML, Karani J, Portmann BC, Westaby D, et al**. Natural history and prognostic variables in primary sclerosing cholangitis. Gastroenterology. 1991;100:1710-7. PMID: 1850376
2. **Mihas AA, Murad TM, Hirshowitz BI**. Sclerosing cholangitis associated with ulcerative colitis. Light and electron microscopy studies. Am J Gastroenterol. 1978;70:614-9. PMID: 742613
3. **Wiesner RH, LaRusso NF**. Clinicopathologic features of the syndrome of primary sclerosing cholangitis. Gastroenterology. 1980;79:200-6. PMID: 7399227

## Liver Disorders Question 10
## Answer: C

**Educational Objective:** *Identify the optimal management of patients with fulminant hepatic failure.*

Fulminant hepatic failure (FHF) is defined by the development of acute liver failure with hepatic encephalopathy within 8 weeks of the onset of symptoms with jaundice. Subfulminant hepatic failure develops from 8 to 12 weeks of the onset of illness. The usual cause of FHF is viral hepatitis; other causes include drug-induced hepatitis, toxic or chemical liver injury, and less common causes such as vascular events, Wilson's disease, massive hepatic metastases, and primary nonfunction after liver transplantation.

The prognosis of FHF depends on certain factors: the tempo of disease progression (a subfulminant course is associated with a worse prognosis than a fulminant pattern) and laboratory tests (prothrombin time, total serum bilirubin, pH, and serum creatinine).

Principles of management of FHF include accurate recognition of tempo and cause; early detection and treatment of complications, particularly metabolic acidosis, renal failure, cerebral edema, and infection; and early transfer to a liver transplantation center, with consideration of transplantation in patients with a poor prognosis.

This patient should therefore be transferred to a liver transplantation center, even though he does not have the prognostic factors indicating a need for transplantation. His course may deteriorate over the next several days, and he should be in a center able to move quickly to transplantation. In patients with grade II or greater hepatic encephalopathy, care in the intensive care unit improves survival.

Management of such patients includes protein-restricted diet, lactulose, intravenous glucose, $H_2$-receptor antagonist, regular assessment of neurologic status by neurologic checks or intracranial pressure monitoring at grade III or IV encephalopathy, endotracheal intubation at grade III or IV encephalopathy, and placement of central line, arterial line, nasogastric tube, and urinary bladder catheter for monitoring. An increase in intracranial pressure is treated with mannitol. Infection is common, and daily cultures of blood, sputum, and urine are obtained; fungal prophylaxis may be appropriate.

### Bibliography
1. **Katelaris PH, Jones DB**. Fulminant hepatic failure. Med Clin North Am. 1989;73:955-70. PMID: 2657269
2. **Williams R, Gimson AE**. Intensive liver care and management of acute hepatic failure. Dig Dis Sci. 1991;36:820-6. PMID: 1903343

## Liver Disorders Question 11
## Answer: B

**Educational Objective:** *Distinguish among the causes of mildly elevated liver function tests.*

It is not uncommon to see mildly elevated liver enzymes in clinical practice. Viruses and alcoholism are the two most common causes; however, fatty infiltration of the liver sometimes occurs with obesity, starvation, diabetes mellitus, corticosteroids, and total parenteral nutrition. In this patient, it is likely that diabetes and obesity are the causes of her nonalcoholic steatohepatitis. Management includes controlling weight and blood glucose levels. Alcoholic steatosis might also be considered, but the patient would have to drink much more than she does. Because the patient has no gallstones or ductal dilatation on ultrasonography and no history of right upper quadrant pain, chronic cholecystitis is unlikely. The alkaline phosphatase level is not very high, and antimitochondrial antibodies are negative, so that biliary cirrhosis is also not a correct option. Autoimmune hepatitis tends to have a clinical presentation similar to that of viral hepatitis. Globulins are almost always elevated, and circulating autoantibodies (antinuclear antibodies [ANA], smooth muscle, rheumatoid factor) are quite common.

### Bibliography

1. **Bacon BR, Farahvash MJ, Janney CG, Neuschwander-Tetri BA.** Nonalcoholic steatohepatitis: an expanded clinical entity. Gastroenterology. 1994;107:1103-9. PMID: 7523217

2. **Caturelli E, Costarelli L, Giordano M, Fusilli S, Squillante MM, et al.** Hypoechoic lesions in fatty liver. Quantitative study by histomorphometry. Gastroenterology. 1991;100:1678-82. PMID: 2019373

## Liver Disorders Question 12
## Answer: A

**Educational Objective:** *Recognize that Wilson's disease may manifest itself as seronegative chronic hepatitis, and know that penicillamine is the therapy of choice.*

The diagnosis of Wilson's disease should always be considered in a young patient with chronic hepatitis and negative viral studies, especially in those with a family history of liver disease. The diagnosis is suggested by finding a low serum copper level, a low serum ceruloplasmin level, and high 24-hour urinary copper level, but the diagnosis is confirmed by measuring the amount of copper in a liver biopsy. Confirmation of Wilson's disease is mandatory before treatment. Penicillamine is the treatment of choice. In those who cannot take penicillamine, trientine and zinc have been helpful.

The absence of increased iron on liver biopsy rules out hemochromatosis. Viral hepatitis is excluded by the negative viral serologies. The negative ANA result argues against autoimmune hepatitis. The liver biopsy is not consistent with primary biliary cirrhosis.

### Bibliography

1. **Sternlieb I, Scheinberg IH.** Chronic hepatitis as a first manifestation of Wilson's disease. Ann Intern Med. 1972;76:59-64. PMID: 5021554

2. **Sternlieb I.** The outlook for the diagnosis of Wilson's disease. J Hepatol. 1993;17:263-4. PMID: 8315256

3. **Schilsky ML.** Identification of the Wilson's disease gene: clues for disease pathogenesis and the potential for molecular diagnosis. Hepatology. 1994;20:529-33. PMID: 8045514

## Liver Disorders Question 13
## Answer: C

**Educational Objective:** *Recognize inadvertent acetaminophen hepatotoxicity in alcoholic patients.*

Acetaminophen is a widely used and generally safe analgesic. It is a component of many over-the-counter preparations. The hepatotoxic potential of acetaminophen taken as an overdose is well-recognized.

The enhanced toxicity of acetaminophen taken within or only moderately above the recommended usual therapeutic doses in alcoholic patients, however, is less well-appreciated. In one study of 25 alcoholics with hepatotoxicity from moderate doses of acetaminophen, the mean daily dose was 6.4 g, with some alcoholics having liver injury at doses less than 3.0 g per day.

Important features that allow early recognition of this syndrome are marked elevation of aminotransferases, with serum aspartate aminotransferase (AST) typically greater than twice serum alanine aminotransferase (ALT); variable, often striking, prolongation of prothrombin time; and low or normal acetaminophen blood concentrations. The mechanism of acetaminophen hepatotoxicity in chronic alcoholics results from increased activity of the P-450 mixed function oxidase system (P-450IIE1), which produces a toxic intermediate of acetaminophen and reduces intracellular concentration of glutathione to scavenge this toxic intermediate.

Peak AST concentrations are significantly lower in patients with acute viral hepatitis and alcoholic hepatitis, with median values of 650 U/L and 120 U/L, respectively, compared with a median AST of 6888 U/L in alcohol-enhanced acetaminophen hepatotoxicity. The concentration of AST alone excludes either of these conditions as the primary explanation for the 42-year-old attorney's liver illness.

In Reye's syndrome, the AST is elevated to the low to middle hundreds or low thousands; the prothrombin time is prolonged; the serum bilirubin is usually normal or near normal; and the serum ammonia is usually markedly elevated. Although Reye's syndrome is most common in children, well-described cases in adults are reported. It is generally preceded by a viral illness, and aspirin use is common.

Ischemic injury to the liver is typically associated with shock or congestive heart failure. It may be associated with transient marked rise of aminotransferases in the range of acetaminophen hepatotoxicity. This patient had no predisposing cause for ischemic injury to the liver, and heart and lung examinations were normal.

### Bibliography

1. **Kumar S, Rex DK.** Failure of physicians to recognize acetaminophen hepatotoxicity in chronic alcoholics. Arch Intern Med. 1991;151:1189-91. PMID: 2043020

2. **Maddrey WC.** Hepatic effects of acetaminophen. Enhanced toxicity in alcoholics. J Clin Gastroenterol. 1987;9:180-5. PMID: 3553308

## Liver Disorders Question 14
## Answer: B

**Educational Objective:** *Recognize ascending cholangitis.*

This patient clearly has acute ascending cholangitis due to common bile duct stones. Prospective, controlled trials have shown that endoscopic retrograde cholangiopancreatography (ERCP) with papillotomy and either removal of a common duct stone or placement of a stent are more effective therapy than emergency surgery. The morbidity and mortality rates are lower and the success rates higher with emergency endoscopic treatment than with surgery. Similar controlled trials have shown that emergency endoscopy in the critically ill patient with gallstone pancreatitis is better than conservative therapy, such as antibiotics and supportive care.

The duration and severity of this patient's illness are not consistent with viral hepatitis or hepatic abscess. Jaundice would not be present in gallstone ileus or pancreatic pseudocyst.

### Bibliography

1. **Johnston DE, Kaplan MM**. Pathogenesis and treatment of gallstones. N Engl J Med. 1993;328:412-21. PMID: 8421460
2. **Lai EC, Mok FP, Tan ES, Lo CM, Fan ST, You KT, et al**. Endoscopic biliary drainage for severe acute cholangitis. N Engl J Med. 1992;326:1582-6. PMID: 1584258

## Liver Disorders Question 15
## Answer: A

**Educational Objective:** *Recognize the HELLP syndrome in association with severe preeclampsia.*

This patient has HELLP syndrome (**h**emolysis, **e**levated **l**iver enzymes, and **l**ow **p**latelet count). Many consider this syndrome, which occurs more frequently in white women and multiparas, an advanced condition associated with preeclampsia. Many patients have very high blood pressures (greater than 160/110 mm Hg), but some have blood pressures less than 140/90 mm Hg. Some obstetricians recommend screening all preeclamptic patients, especially those with abdominal pain, for this syndrome. Abdominal pain occurs in 90% of women with HELLP syndrome. Although experts disagree about rapid delivery, all agree that hospitalization and emergency treatment for the preeclampsia are mandatory. Microangiopathic hemolytic anemia is the hallmark of the HELLP syndrome. Disseminated intravascular coagulation (DIC) is rare in this syndrome. Prothrombin time, partial thromboplastin time, and fibrinogen levels are usually normal. Platelet transfusion and corticosteroids are of no proven benefit. Abnormalities peak 1 to 2 days postpartum and rapidly improve after 72 hours. Plasma exchange may be helpful in those whose laboratory values do not improve after 72 hours.

Acute fatty liver of pregnancy is associated with moderate liver enzyme elevations and a prolonged prothrombin time. DIC is common in this condition. Cholestasis of pregnancy is not associated with hemolysis or elevations of aspartate aminotransferase (AST), alanine aminotransferase (ALT), or lactate dehydrogenase (LDH). Hemolytic-uremic syndrome is characterized by microangiopathic changes associated with thrombocytopenia and acute renal failure. It is more commonly seen in children but has been reported occasionally in women in the postpartum period or in those taking oral contraceptives. Although immune thrombocytopenic purpura (ITP) is not uncommon in pregnancy and may be associated with immune hemolysis (Evans's syndrome), it is not usually associated with liver chemistry abnormalities. Furthermore, microangiopathy is, in essence, never a component of ITP, and its presence in a thrombocytopenic patient points to another diagnosis.

### Bibliography

1. **Weinstein L**. Syndrome of hemolysis, elevated liver enzymes and low platelet count: a severe consequence of hypertension in pregnancy. Am J Obstet Gynecol. 1982;142:159-67. PMID: 7055180
2. **Martin JN Jr, Blake PG, Perry KG Jr, McCaul JF, Hess LW, Martin RW**. The natural history of HELLP syndrome: patterns of disease progression and regression. Am J Obstet Gynecol. 1991;164:1500-13. PMID: 2048596

## Liver Disorders Question 16
## Answer: E

**Educational Objective:** *Treat spontaneous bacterial peritonitis.*

This patient likely has spontaneous (primary) bacterial peritonitis. A neutrophil count greater than 250/μL in ascitic fluid is so suggestive of peritonitis that antibiotic therapy should be started immediately without waiting for the culture results. The organisms responsible for this infection (primary peritonitis or spontaneous bacterial peritonitis) are aerobic enteric organisms such as *Escherichia coli*, enterococci, or *Klebsiella*. When culture results are available, modifications in antibiotics can be made. The response to therapy is usually prompt, so even in a person with negative ascitic fluid cultures, it is possible to tell when treatment is failing. Mortality from spontaneous bacterial peritonitis ranges from 30% to 78%, but this largely reflects the advanced liver disease and other comorbid conditions that accompany primary peritonitis. If evidence of encephalopathy is present after treatment of infection, lactulose could be useful. Ultrasonography can help determine the presence of ascitic fluid, blockage of bile, or the presence and size of masses such as abscesses. In this instance, however, there is nothing new to be learned from this test because the overwhelming likelihood is that the acute problem is infectious in nature. Problems of intractable ascites can be challenging, but diuretics are largely given for improvement of comfort and appearance or for secondary problems, such as pulmonary vascular congestion. Nothing about this patient suggests a reversible process for which diuretics would be expected to bring about improvement.

### Bibliography

1. **Bataller R, Gines P, Arroyo V.** Practical recommendations for the treatment of ascites and its complications. Drugs. 1997;54:571-80. PMID: 9339961
2. **Guarner C, Soriano G.** Spontaneous bacterial peritonitis. Semin Liver Dis. 1997;17:203-17. PMID: 9308125

### Bibliography

1. **Fregia A, Jensen DM**. Evaluation of abnormal liver tests. Compr Ther. 1994;20:50-4. PMID: 8137620
2. **Herrera JL**. Serologic diagnosis of viral hepatitis. South Med J. 1994;87:677-84. PMID: 7517578

## Liver Disorders Question 17
## Answer: D

**Educational Objective:** *Recognize the presentation of a mononucleosis syndrome, especially when caused by cytomegalovirus.*

This patient's illness is consistent clinically with an infectious mononucleosis-like syndrome. The laboratory studies reveal absolute and relative lymphocytosis with numerous atypical forms. Atypical lymphocytosis may be seen transiently in several viral illnesses, including hepatitis A, primary infection with HIV, and adenovirus infections. Acute symptomatic toxoplasmosis may also produce atypical lymphocytosis. In this patient, the hepatic transaminase elevations are characteristic but not diagnostic of infectious mononucleosis. However, the heterophil antigen test (monospot test) is negative, which may occur in 15% to 20% of cases of Epstein-Barr virus mononucleosis. Therefore, antibody titers for Epstein-Barr virus were ordered and found to be negative, essentially excluding Epstein-Barr virus as the cause. Most cases of heterophil-negative mononucleosis are caused by cytomegalovirus, which would be the most likely cause of this patient's illness. In general, lymphadenopathy and splenomegaly are milder in cytomegalovirus than Epstein-Barr virus mononucleosis, and exudative pharyngitis is rarely seen.

### Bibliography

1. **Cohen JI, Corey GR.** Cytomegalovirus infection in the normal host. Medicine (Baltimore) 1985;64:100-14. PMID: 2983175

## Liver Disorders Question 18
## Answer: D

**Educational Objective:** *Assess status after exposure to hepatitis B.*

A patient in the acute phase of hepatitis B virus (HBV) infection is always positive for IgM anti-HBc (IgM antibodies to the hepatitis B core antigen). In chronic HBV infection, the hepatitis B surface antigen (HbsAg) always remains positive. In people recovering from acute HBV infection, total anti-HBc is positive along with antibody to hepatitis B surface antigen (anti-HBs). Individuals who have received proper immunization for HBV are positive only for anti-HBs.

# Anemia

## Anemia Question 1
### Answer: B

**Educational Objective:** *Recognize the presentation of pernicious anemia in an elderly patient.*

The patient most likely has vitamin $B_{12}$ deficiency, based on the degree of macrocytosis and neurologic findings. An elevated serum lactate dehydrogenase level, due to intramarrow cell death from ineffective erythropoiesis, is consistent with this diagnosis.

Severe macrocytosis (mean corpuscular volume > 120 fL) is often associated with vitamin $B_{12}$ deficiency or folate deficiency (megaloblastic anemia), usually seen in conjunction with "oval" macrocytes. The presence of frequent hypersegmented neutrophils (> 5 segments) is strongly suggestive of vitamin $B_{12}$ or folate deficiency.

Bone marrow morphology in patients with vitamin $B_{12}$ or folate deficiency is referred to as "megaloblastic" and is characterized by the presence of large cells with immature nuclear chromatin but maturing erythrocyte cytoplasm (nuclear-cytoplasmic dissociation). Anemia accompanies this process; hence the term "ineffective erythropoiesis." The intramarrow death of megaloblastic cells causes the serum lactate dehydrogenase level to rise. If a patient has a low serum vitamin $B_{12}$ or folate level, a bone marrow examination is probably unnecessary. However, the physician should determine the cause of the deficiency. If a patient has a normal serum vitamin $B_{12}$ or folate level, a bone marrow examination is frequently helpful to exclude myelodysplastic syndromes or other infiltrative marrow disorders.

Folate deficiency can induce megaloblastosis within weeks to months, whereas vitamin $B_{12}$ deficiency requires years to cause megaloblastosis since stores of vitamin $B_{12}$ persist for years in the liver and other tissues. In patients with vitamin $B_{12}$ or folate deficiency, parenteral or oral repletion of vitamin $B_{12}$ or folate reverses some morphologic abnormalities within hours. Serum folate levels fluctuate quickly with changes in dietary consumption. Low erythrocyte folate levels often reflect prior nutritional depletion. In patients who are hospitalized and are begun on regular diets, the erythrocyte folate test may provide a better assessment of tissue folate levels than determination of the serum folate level. The erythrocyte folate test often requires a special laboratory, and results often are not quickly available.

In patients with megaloblastic anemias, erythrocyte production is diminished and a "corrected" reticulocyte count is inappropriately low for the degree of anemia. This patient had a corrected reticulocyte count of 1% (inappropriately low for a hemoglobin level of 9.4 g/dL).

In addition to changes in the blood, the epithelial cells in patients with megaloblastic anemias may become atrophic and cause a smooth tongue and cheilosis. Posterior column dysfunction, particularly in patients with vitamin $B_{12}$ deficiency, may lead to changes in vibratory or position sense, causing ataxia. Signs of dementia may appear. However, neurologic dysfunction is very uncommon in adults with folate deficiency.

Alcoholic cerebellar degeneration results in ataxia but not position loss. Although liver metastases are possible in a patient with a history of colon cancer, their presence would not account for the neurological findings in this patient. Brain metastases would most likely produce focal neurological findings and also would not account for the blood findings.

### Bibliography

1. **Toh BH, van Driel IR, Gleeson PA**. Pernicious anemia. N Engl J Med. 1997;337:1441-8. PMID: 9358143
2. **Carmel R.** Cobalamin, the stomach, and aging. Am J Clin Nutr. 1997;66:750-9. PMID: 9322548

## Anemia Question 2
### Answer: C

**Educational Objective:** *Recognize combined iron deficiency in the setting of anemia of chronic disease.*

The patient most likely has a microcytic anemia secondary to iron deficiency from aspirin- and ibuprofen-induced gastrointestinal blood loss. Microcytosis may also be found in some patients with chronic diseases such as systemic lupus erythematosus (although the anemia of chronic disease is more often normochromic, normocytic). Systemic lupus erythematosus has caused a significant inflammatory reaction in this patient, based on her clinical presentation and confirmed in part by her markedly elevated erythrocyte sedimentation rate.

Both the serum iron and serum total iron-binding capacity (TIBC) are decreased. However, the diagnosis of a superimposed iron deficiency is suggested by her use of nonsteroidal anti-inflammatory drugs and by the presence of occult blood in her stools. A serum ferritin level of 32(g/mL, although "normal" in the setting of an inflammatory disease, would be considered lower than expected and therefore consistent with iron deficiency.

The iron indices in option A are consistent with "pure" iron deficiency anemia, with a low serum iron level, increased serum TIBC, and decreased serum ferritin level. The indices in option B are consistent with an inflammatory disease, with a low serum iron level, low serum TIBC, and elevated serum ferritin level. The indices in option D are consistent with iron overload or sideroblastic anemia.

### Bibliography

1. **Jurado RL**. Iron, infections, and anemia of inflammation. Clin Infect Dis. 1997;25:888-95. PMID: 9356804

## Anemia Question 3
## Answer: D

**Educational Objective:** *Identify the association between thymoma and autoimmune diseases, including pure red cell aplasia.*

Each of the listed neoplasms may present as an anterior mediastinal mass and may be associated with anemia of chronic disease. However, pure red cell aplasia (which this patient has) is often associated with a benign or invasive thymoma. Approximately 5% to 15% of thymomas occur in patients with pure red cell aplasia. Other thymoma-associated autoimmune disorders include myasthenia gravis, systemic lupus erythematosus, thrombocytopenia, and, rarely, malabsorption states. A careful search by CT or MRI is always warranted in patients with newly diagnosed or relapsing red cell aplasia or myasthenia.

The other listed entities are also included in the differential diagnosis for an anterior mediastinal mass. Germ cell tumors have not been associated with pure red cell aplasia, and Hodgkin's disease, non-Hodgkin's lymphoma, and thyroid carcinoma are rarely associated with this disorder. Chronic lymphocytic leukemia is also commonly associated with red cell aplasia and may present with variable degrees of lymphadenopathy but not with an isolated anterior mediastinal mass, as in the patient discussed here.

### Bibliography

1. **Morgenthaler TI, Brown LR, Colby TV, Harper CM Jr, Coles DT**. Thymoma. Mayo Clinic Proc. 1993;68:1110-23. PMID: 8231276

## Anemia Question 4
## Answer: B

**Educational Objective:** *Understand the differential diagnosis of anemia and reticulocytopenia in a patient with sickle cell anemia.*

Patients with hemolytic disorders may occasionally present with reticulocytopenia and an "aplastic crisis." This patient has sickle cell anemia with parvovirus infection, which is causing an aplastic crisis. Parvovirus may infect patients with hemolytic anemias (for example, patients with hereditary spherocytosis, sickle cell disease, or thalassemia). In children with sickle cell anemia, over 80% of aplastic crises may be attributed

to parvovirus infections. In adults, the usual presenting features are rash, arthritis, and anemia. The "slapped cheek" syndrome is rarely a presenting feature. There is usually a complete suppression of erythropoiesis to a reticulocyte level of 0%. The bone marrow shows giant dysplastic (megaloblastoid) erythroblasts, occasionally with viral inclusions. The diagnosis is usually made by demonstrating IgM antibodies to the virus. IgG antibodies appear later during the course of the infection and persist. Parvovirus in the blood may be detected by the polymerase chain reaction, which is the definitive diagnostic method. Occasionally, other blood components such as leukocytes and platelets are affected and result in mild to moderate pancytopenia.

The diagnosis of paroxysmal nocturnal hemoglobinuria (PNH) should be considered in patients with bone marrow failure or aplasia, unusual location of thromboses, and unexplained hemolysis. The anemia may be severe, and patients with PNH typically have reticulocytopenia. There is no characteristic finding on bone marrow examination, although the bone marrow of patients with PNH may demonstrate myelodysplastic changes. The diagnosis is based on demonstration of exquisite sensitivity to complement-mediated lysis by the sucrose lysis test or the acidified serum lysis test (Ham's test).

Glucose-6-phosphate dehydrogenase (G6PD) deficiency is another cause of hemolysis that occasionally is associated with reticulocytopenia. In patients with G6PD deficiency, erythrocytes are subject to oxidative stresses. Hemoglobin becomes oxidized and precipitates within the erythrocytes, which then undergo destruction by the reticuloendothelial system. G6PD deficiency is an autosomal recessive disorder that predominantly affects males. After a hemolytic episode, qualitative assays may be normal because only erythrocytes that are resistant to G6PD remain. The African variant of G6PD is associated with a mild form of hemolysis, whereas the Mediterranean variant is usually severe. Causes include infectious stresses, drugs such as quinidine and sulfonamides, or, in the Mediterranean variant, favism (consumption of fava beans). Therapy requires avoiding certain medications and supportive care in crisis situations.

In contrast to this patient's presentation, patients with aplastic anemia have pancytopenia with severe anemia, reticulocytopenia, thrombocytopenia, and granulocytopenia. In patients with severe aplastic anemia, the bone marrow examination shows less than 5% cellularity with only residual lymphocytes and plasma cells. The abnormal cells described above that are attributable to parvovirus infection are not seen.

### Bibliography

1. **Pagliuca A, Hussain M, Layton DM**. Human parvovirus infection in sickle cell disease. Lancet. 1993;342:49. PMID: 8100315

## Anemia Question 5
## Answer: B

**Educational Objective:** *Understand the differential diagnosis of macrocytosis.*

This patient has a megaloblastic anemia based on her macrocytic indices and peripheral blood smear findings of hypersegmented neutrophils. Based on her clinical history, pernicious anemia is the most likely diagnosis.

In adult patients, pernicious anemia often presents with minimal symptoms. Mild weakness or fatigue of gradual onset is common. Patients appear relatively well. The pallor of anemia is combined with a slightly elevated serum bilirubin level, secondary to ineffective erythropoiesis, to produce a sallow, lemon-yellow skin color. The disease seems to occur disproportionately in blonde, blue-eyed persons who sometimes have premature graying or whitening of the hair. A smooth, depapillated tongue and cheilosis may be noted on the physical examination. The neurologic findings may be subtle or fully developed. Subacute combined degeneration of the spinal cord and brain may manifest as symmetric numbness and tingling of the extremities, impaired vibratory and position sense, and spastic ataxia. Slowed mentation, paranoia, and depression may occur. In order to cause dietary deficiency of vitamin $B_{12}$, liver stores of this vitamin must be depleted, a process that could take years. The diagnosis is made by finding a low serum vitamin $B_{12}$ level and the presence of intrinsic factor antibodies.

Myelodysplastic syndromes should be considered in the differential diagnosis of patients with macrocytic anemias. The peripheral blood smear sometimes shows hyposegmentation with pseudo Pelger Huët anomaly, in contrast to the hypersegmentation seen in pernicious anemia. Anemia in conjunction with hypothyroidism may be due to menorrhagia and iron deficiency anemia, or when associated with pernicious anemia, may be part of an autoimmune process that includes the presence of antithyroid antibodies and anti-intrinsic factor antibodies. This patient does not appear to have hypothyroidism.

Alcoholism and alcoholic liver disease or liver disease in general may cause anemia and other cytopenias. Although this patient relates regular alcohol intake, there is nothing in the peripheral blood smear (absence of target cells) that would imply liver disease. Congestive splenomegaly and sequestration may occur with cirrhosis. No splenomegaly was noted on this patient's physical examination. A complicating folic acid deficiency is possible if alcoholism impairs nutritional intake.

### Bibliography

1. **Toh BH, van Driel IR, Gleeson PA**. Pernicious anemia. N Engl J Med. 1997;337:1441-8. PMID: 9358143

## Anemia Question 6
## Answer: B

**Educational Objective:** *Recognize the possibility of acute chest syndrome, which should be treated initially with red blood cell exchange transfusion.*

Acute chest syndrome in patients with sickle cell anemia should be managed by exchange transfusion. Red blood cell exchange transfusions are done to increase the hemoglobin A to at least 50%. In adolescents and adults, pulmonary crises usually start with infarctions that may become secondarily infected. With time, multiple infarctions predominate, and pulmonary congestion and intrapulmonary shunting develop, leading to more hypoxia and sickling. Because of the increased blood volume resulting from red blood cell transfusions, it is not possible to increase the hemoglobin A to more than 50% without inducing volume overload. Erythropoietin administration has a limited role in patients with sickle cell disease. Erythropoietin has been used to accelerate recovery from aplastic crises in some patients. However, this patient has a brisk reticulocyte response, and it is likely that erythropoiesis is already under intense erythropoietin stimulation. Hydroxyurea may reduce the frequency of painful crises and acute chest syndrome but is not used in the acute treatment of the sickling process. The drug works by increasing hemoglobin F production, which helps prevent hemoglobin S polymerization and sickling.

### Bibliography

1. **Platt OS, Thorington BD, Brambilla DJ, Milner PF, Rosse WF, Vichinsky E, et al**. Pain in sickle cell disease. Rates and risk factors. N Engl J Med. 1991;325:11-6. PMID: 1710777
2. **Charache S, Dover GJ, Moore RD, Eckert S, Ballas SK, Koshy M, et al**. Hydroxyurea: effects on hemoglobin F production in patients with sickle cell anemia. Blood. 1992;79:2555-65. PMID: 1375104

## Anemia Question 7
## Answer: D

**Educational Objective:** *Recognize the diagnostic features of hereditary spherocytosis.*

The clinical history suggests an inherited blood disorder because her brother is also anemic. The splenomegaly and elevated reticulocyte count suggest a hemolytic disorder, since increased erythrocyte destruction frequently leads to splenic hyperplasia. A singular finding in patients with hereditary spherocytosis is that the mean corpuscular hemoglobin concentration (MCHC) is increased, exceeding the upper limit of normal (36 g/dL) in approximately 50% of patients. The high MCHC reflects mild cellular dehydration caused by a low content of $K^+$ that is not offset by the lesser rise in intracellular $Na^+$. Increased osmotic fragility occurs in any disorder in which cell volume is decreased, such as spherocytosis. A reduced MCHC and mean corpuscular volume are usually found in patients with iron deficiency anemia. Furthermore, reticulocytosis and splenomegaly are not presenting features of iron deficiency anemia. β-Thalassemia minor is a hereditary hemolytic anemia due to an imbalance of β-chain synthesis. All patients have a mean corpuscular volume of < 80 fL, and spherocytosis is not a morphologic feature. Autoimmune hemolytic anemia is characterized by hemolysis, splenomegaly, and a positive direct antiglobulin test, whereas this patient has a negative direct antiglobulin test.

### Bibliography

1. **Olivieri NF**. The beta-thalassemias. N Engl J Med. 1999;341:99-109. PMID: 10395635

2. **Engelfriet CP, Overbeeke MA, von dem Borne AE**. Autoimmune hemolytic anemia. Semin Hematol. 1992;29:3-12. PMID: 1570541

3. **Bolton-Maggs PH**. The diagnosis and management of hereditary spherocytosis. Baillieres Best Pract Clin Haematol. 2000; 13: 327-42. PMID: 11030038

## Anemia Question 8
## Answer: C

### Educational Objective: *Recognize and treat the HELLP syndrome.*

This presentation is characteristic of the HELLP syndrome (hemolysis, elevated liver enzymes, low platelets). Although this disorder occurs most commonly in the third trimester of pregnancy, up to 40% of cases may occur in the peripartum or immediate postpartum period. Patients generally present with malaise and right upper quadrant abdominal pain, which may occur in the absence of hypertension or significant proteinuria. Disseminated intravascular coagulation may occur in some patients, although it is rarely severe enough to affect the prothrombin time or activated partial thromboplastin time or cause a decrease in fibrinogen levels. The HELLP syndrome generally resolves after delivery, although some cases may continue for a week or more, particularly when the onset occurs after delivery. Nonrandomized studies involving small numbers of patients suggest that the use of glucocorticoids or plasmapheresis may shorten the duration of the postpartum HELLP syndrome. Generally, such treatment modalities are considered when the disease continues unabated for 7 days or more after delivery.

A diagnosis of preeclampsia requires hypertension and significant proteinuria, which this patient does not have. The postpartum hemolytic uremic syndrome is usually characterized by significant renal insufficiency, which is absent in this patient. Acute fatty liver of pregnancy usually occurs in the third trimester and is characterized by a severe coagulopathy with liver function studies that are more consistent with cholestasis.

### Bibliography

1. **McCrae KR, Cines DB**. Thrombotic microangiopathy during pregnancy. Semin Hematol. 1997;34:148-58. PMID: 9109217

2. **Martin JN Jr, Perry KG Jr, Blake PG, May WA, Moore A, Robinette L**. Better maternal outcomes are achieved with dexamethasone therapy for postpartum HELLP (hemolysis, elevated liver enzymes, and thrombocytopenia) syndrome. Am J Obstet Gynecol. 1997;177:1011-7. PMID: 9396884

## Anemia Question 9
## Answer: C

### Educational Objective: *Diagnose pancytopenia due to hypersplenism.*

Mild to moderately severe pancytopenia is often discovered incidentally and may be the first indication of otherwise occult cirrhosis, portal hypertension, and associated secondary hypersplenism. This patient has chronic cytopenias that are most likely due to hepatitis C induced cirrhosis (possibly acquired from blood transfusions), as evidenced by the presence of spider telangiectasias and a palpable enlarged spleen. Hypersplenism and increased splenic destruction or sequestration of blood elements may result from both splenic congestion and increased phagocytic activity. In addition, recent evidence suggests that decreased thrombopoietin levels in patients with cirrhosis may contribute to the frequently seen thrombocytopenia in these patients, as the liver is the major site of thrombopoietin production.

The chronicity of this patient's cytopenias and the elevated reticulocyte count rule against aplastic anemia, although viral hepatitis (especially hepatitis B) may be associated with bone marrow aplasia. HIV and certain antiretroviral drugs may also have marrow-suppressive effects. HIV infection, however, is less likely in this patient, given the clinical setting. Because she has an apparent HIV risk factor (remote blood transfusions), it would be prudent to test her for HIV.

It is always important to take a careful drug history in the evaluation of patients with cytopenias. Lisinopril has only rarely been associated with bone marrow suppression, and lisinopril was started in this patient after the onset of her cytopenias.

### Bibliography

1. **Shah SH, Hayes PC, Allan PL, Nicoll J, Finlayson ND**. Measurement of spleen size and its relation to hypersplenism and portal hemodynamics in portal hypertension due to hepatic cirrhosis. Am J Gastroenterol. 1996;91:2580-3. PMID: 8946990

2. **Kawasaki T, Takeshita A, Souda K, Kobayashi Y, Kikuyama M, Suzuki F, et al**. Serum thrombopoietin levels in patients with chronic hepatitis and liver cirrhosis. Am J Gastroenterol. 1999;94:1918-22. PMID: 10406260

## Anemia Question 10
## Answer: B

**Educational Objective:** *Identify the presentation of anemia related to lead poisoning.*

The patient has chronic lead intoxication that can be confirmed by measuring serum lead levels. He has a hypochromic, microcytic anemia with coarse basophilic stippling and reticulocytosis. He also has evidence of hemolytic anemia with increased serum lactate dehydrogenase and indirect bilirubin levels. His physical examination is remarkable for gingival "lead lines." Bone marrow examination shows erythroid hyperplasia and ringed sideroblasts. The anemia of lead poisoning fits this description. Sideroblastic anemia with hypochromic indices is typical. Hemolysis is common, and basophilic stippling, blue staining polyribosomal aggregates with mitochondrial fragments in the erythrocytes, is frequently seen. Lead inhibits pyrimidine 5′-nucleotidase which normally clears ribosomal fragments. Occupational exposures to lead are relatively uncommon today. However, workers who produce batteries or are exposed to paint, particularly those who remove leaded paint from old buildings, are at greatest risk if they are not protected from inhalation of paint particles during the sanding process. Other manifestations of lead toxicity in adults include peripheral neuropathy, abdominal colic, and saturnine gout (effects of lead on renal tubules that prevent the excretion of uric acid). Chelation therapy is indicated for patients with serum lead levels exceeding 70 µg/dL and should be continued until lead levels fall below 40 µg/dL. Agents such as EDTA or dimercaprol may also be effective.

This patient is unlikely to have iron deficiency since his reticulocytes are increased. In addition, basophilic stippling usually is not seen in patients with iron deficiency.

Thalassemia is associated with a microcytic anemia, reticulocytosis, and basophilic stippling. However, a normal complete blood count 4 years ago rules out this possibility. Therefore, quantitative studies to measure hemoglobin $A_2$ are not necessary.

Autoimmune hemolytic anemia should be excluded by performing a direct antiglobulin test in any patient who has evidence of hemolysis on a peripheral blood smear. However, the "lead lines" on this patient's gingivae are classic for lead poisoning, and autoimmune hemolytic anemia therefore is less likely.

Alcoholism may cause a transient sideroblastic anemia, which resolves with cessation of alcohol intake. Folic acid deficiency may complicate alcoholism but usually presents with macrocytosis.

### Bibliography

1. **Browder AA, Joselow MM, Louria DB.** The problem of lead poisoning. Medicine (Baltimore). 1973;52:121-39. PMID: 4633081

## Anemia Question 11
## Answer: C

**Educational Objective:** *Recognize that transfusion is not necessary even when a hemoglobin value is in the anemic range.*

In many patients with anemia, administration of hematinics such as iron may be the only therapy needed to correct the anemia over a period of time. Since this patient lost blood during surgery and has been a regular blood donor, he may need iron supplementation to improve erythropoiesis. Therefore, a short course of oral iron replacement therapy may be indicated. A repeat reticulocyte count should be obtained to document a response. Intravenous iron replacement may be indicated in some patients who are severely iron deficient or are unable to take oral iron. However, since intravenous iron administration can be associated with anaphylactic or systemic inflammatory reactions, its use is not justified in this patient.

Numerous mechanisms exist to maintain oxygen delivery. In the past, the hemoglobin measurement was the sole determinant of whether a patient should receive transfusions. Generally, it was considered acceptable to transfuse packed red blood cells when the hemoglobin level was less than 10.0 g/dL. Transfusions were thought to improve wound healing and reduce the risk of possible hypoxic complications. However, it has since been learned that wound healing is not enhanced by transfusions. In addition, studies show that a shift to anaerobic metabolism does not occur in healthy individuals until hemoglobin level drops to 7.5 g/dL or less. This patient is asymptomatic and has no history of complicating cardiovascular disease. Therefore, there is little indication for transfusions.

Although the patient is moderately anemic, his reticulocyte count is inappropriately low. Postoperatively, the reticulocyte response may be depressed because of various causes, especially infection. However, this patient has no sign of infection.

### Bibliography

1. **McFarland JG.** Perioperative blood transfusions: indications and options. Chest. 1999;115:113S-121S. PMID: 10331343
2. **Carson JL, Duff A, Berlin JA, Lawrence VA, Poses RM, Huber EC, et al.** Perioperative blood transfusion and postoperative mortality. JAMA. 1998;279:199-205. PMID: 9438739

## Anemia Question 12
## Answer: D

**Educational Objective:** *Recognize refractory anemia with ringed sideroblasts and prescribe appropriate therapy.*

Refractory anemia with ringed sideroblasts is one of the five morphologic subtypes of myelodysplastic syndromes as defined in the French-American-British (FAB) classification. It is characterized by slowly progressive anemia, variable degrees of leukopenia and thrombocytopenia, dimorphic erythrocyte morphology on peripheral blood smears, and a hypercellular bone marrow with dysplastic erythroid hyperplasia and ineffective hemopoiesis. The hallmark ringed sideroblasts are easily identified by Prussian blue stain for iron. The "ring" distribution is due to iron loading of mitochondria, which have a perinuclear distribution in erythroblasts.

The progressive anemia makes most patients transfusion dependent, especially because elderly patients are most often affected and because vascular or pulmonary disease frequently coexists.

Leukemic transformation occurs in $\leq 15\%$ of patients who have refractory anemia with ringed sideroblasts. Transformation is most likely in the subset of patients with complex clonal karyotypes or those with anomalies due to deletion of chromosome 5 or chromosome 7 associated with prior alkylating agent chemotherapy.

Occasional patients will respond to pyridoxine, and a 2- to 3-month trial of pyridoxine is warranted. Androgen therapy is ineffective. Erythropoietin therapy, even in high doses, benefits only about 10% of patients by increasing hemoglobin levels or decreasing transfusion requirements.

### Bibliography

1. **Heaney ML, Golde DW**. Myelodysplasia. N Engl J Med. 1999;340:1649-60. PMID: 10341278
2. **Hellström-Lindberg E**. Efficacy of erythropoietin in the myelodysplastic syndromes: a meta-analysis of 205 patients from 17 studies. Br J Haematol. 1995;89:67-71. PMID: 7833279

## Anemia Question 13
## Answer: A

**Educational Objective:** *Recognize that dilutional thrombocytopenia is the most frequent abnormality associated with massive transfusions.*

Approximately a 50% reduction in the platelet count occurs when transfusions of 1.5 to 2 times the blood volume are given over 4 to 8 hours. Blood stored for more that 2 to 3 days has essentially no platelets, which explains the thrombocytopenia. Fresh frozen plasma contains all of the clotting proteins in normal concentrations. This patient received one unit of fresh frozen plasma for each unit of transfused red blood cells, which resulted in no measurable alteration in the prothrombin time or activated partial thromboplastin time. Incompatible red blood cell transfusions can lead to the development of disseminated intravascular coagulation, which is characterized by thrombocytopenia. The other hallmarks of disseminated intravascular coagulation are absent in this patient, namely, he has a normal fibrinogen, prothrombin time, activated partial thromboplastin time, and negative d-dimers. Posttransfusion purpura is characterized by profound thrombocytopenia that develops 5 to 7 days after a transfusion. It occurs in patients who are negative for the PLA-1 human platelet antigen and have been transfused or pregnant in the past. Posttransfusion purpura almost always occurs in women.

Septic transfusion reactions can be associated with thrombocytopenia when either bacteremia or endotoxemia causes disseminated intravascular coagulation. This patient has no indication of either sepsis or disseminated intravascular coagulation.

### Bibliography

1. **McFarland JG**. Perioperative blood transfusions: indications and options. Chest. 1999;115:113S-121S. PMID: 10331343
2. **Ancliff PJ, Machin SJ**. Trigger factors for prophylactic platelet transfusion. Blood Rev. 1998;12:234-8. PMID: 9950093
3. **Carson JL, Duff A, Berlin JA, Lawrence VA, Poses RM, Huber EC, et al.** Perioperative blood transfusion and postoperative mortality. JAMA. 1998;279:199-205. PMID: 9438739

## Anemia Question 14
## Answer: B

**Educational Objective:** *Determine the etiology of microcytosis.*

The most likely cause of mild anemia with extreme microcytosis in a person of Mediterranean origin is the β-thalassemia trait. Assay of hemoglobin $A_2$ would show an increase in the level of this minor hemoglobin component. The peripheral smear would show microcytosis along with a large number of target cells. Target cells are not pathognomonic of thalassemia, however, and are seen in other conditions, such as hemoglobin C disease and lead intoxication. A glucose-6-phosphate dehydrogenase screen will be negative unless the patient has inherited this disorder by chance along with the β-thalassemia. The iron, total iron-binding capacity, and ferritin determinations would rule out iron deficiency, the most common cause of microcytosis and anemia, but would not provide a positive diagnosis. Furthermore, in this patient, the microcytosis is much more profound than the anemia. Iron deficiency that produces a mean corpuscular volume of 63 fL would generally be associated with a hematocrit in the 20% to 25% range.

### Bibliography

1. **Olivieri NF**. The beta-thalassemias. N Engl J Med. 1999;341:99-109. PMID: 10395635
2. **Davies SC, Wonke B**. The management of haemoglobinopathies. Baillieres Clin Haematol. 1991;4:361-89. PMID: 1912665

## Anemia Question 15
## Answer: A

**Educational Objective:** *Manage an older patient with low serum vitamin $B_{12}$ levels without other evidence of vitamin $B_{12}$ deficiency.*

Many older persons have low serum vitamin $B_{12}$ levels without other evidence of vitamin $B_{12}$ deficiency. It is not clear what follow-up is appropriate for these patients. Prescribing cobalamin and remeasuring vitamin $B_{12}$ levels in 1 month would be prudent and economical.

With a normal hemoglobin and peripheral blood smear, a bone marrow morphologic study has a low probability of revealing megaloblastosis. Even patients with obvious megaloblastic anemia due to cobalamin deficiency may have normal erythrocyte folate levels. In a nutritional survey of "healthy adults," many were found to have "low" erythrocyte folate levels. This test should not be used outside of a research protocol.

The significance of an elevated serum homocysteine level in the setting of a low serum vitamin $B_{12}$ level and normal blood morphology is unknown. The frequency of elevated serum homocysteine is remarkably high — much greater than the frequency of low serum folate or cobalamin. The use of pharmacologic doses of folate to lower serum homocysteine is being investigated as a possible prophylaxis of atherosclerosis.

In one study of a group of patients with low serum vitamin $B_{12}$ levels, the urine methylmalonic acid (MMA) was elevated only in patients with good clinical/hematologic evidence of cobalamin deficiency. Other surveys have found a surprisingly high frequency (40%) of elevated serum MMA in elderly patients with common geriatric disorders. At present, the significance of elevated serum MMA is unclear, and it should not be equated with intracellular cobalamin deficiency. Until additional, rigorously gathered data demonstrate the decision-enhancing utility of measuring the serum MMA in patients with a low serum vitamin $B_{12}$ level, a therapeutic trial with cobalamin is wise if the patient has any signs or symptoms that might be related to cobalamin deficiency.

### Bibliography

1. **Joosten E, van den Berg A, Riezler R, Naurath HJ, Lindenbaum J, Stabler SP, et al**. Metabolic evidence that deficiencies of vitamin $B_{12}$ (cobalamin), folate, and vitamin $B_6$ occur commonly in elderly people. Am J Clin Nutr. 1993;58:468-76. PMID: 8037789

2. **Matchar DB, Feussner JR, Millington DS, Wilkinson RH Jr, Watson DJ, Gale D**. Isotope-dilution assay for urinary methylmalonic acid in the diagnosis of vitamin $B_{12}$ deficiency. A prospective clinical evaluation. Ann Intern Med. 1987;106:707-10. PMID: 3551712

## Anemia Question 16
## Answer: A

**Educational Objective:** *Determine the etiology of extreme microcytosis in a patient with mild anemia.*

This patient most likely has α-thalassemia. With a relatively mild anemia and no significant physical abnormalities, the most reasonable course of action would be to follow the patient without intervention. Normally, four genes for the α-globin locus are present in the genetic complement, two on each of the chromosomes 16. Most frequently, α-thalassemia is caused by a deletion of one or more of the α-globin genes.

A single gene mutation produces a silent carrier state. Two-gene-deletion α-thalassemia produces a mild condition with moderate anemia, microcytosis, and target cells. A normal pattern with hemoglobin electrophoresis is seen in patients with two-gene-deletion α-thalassemia. This is almost certainly the condition that this patient has.

Deletion of three of the α-globin genes produces a more severe disorder called hemoglobin H disease. The production of α-globin is reduced to the point that large numbers of the β-globin chains coalesce abnormally to form $β_4$ tetramers. These tetramers bind oxygen very tightly, making them useless in the delivery of oxygen to tissues. Furthermore, the $β_4$ tetramers are relatively insoluble, forming protein aggregates called Heinz bodies. Patients with this condition have marked hemolysis and anemia, along with hepatosplenomegaly from the extramedullary hematopoiesis. The $β_4$ tetramers appear as an abnormal band called hemoglobin H with electrophoresis. Deletion of all four α-globin chains produces hydrops fetalis, which is usually fatal in utero. Single- or double-gene-deletion α-thalassemia is found in as many as 20% of persons in some regions of Southeast Asia. The two-gene deletion form of α-thalassemia can be confused easily with another hemoglobinopathy that is common to the region, hemoglobin E disease. Hemoglobin E would appear as a separate band on the electrophoresis, however. β-Thalassemia is associated with high levels of hemoglobin $A_2$ on the electrophoresis.

Patients with sickle cell anemia usually present early in life with severe hemolytic anemia and symptoms due to vasoocclusive disease. The MCV is normal to slightly low and hemoglobin electrophoresis demonstrates a large percentage of hemoglobin S with smaller amounts of hemoglobin F and $A_2$. The smear should show sickled cells.

Patients with hereditary spherocytosis will have spherocytes on the peripheral smear. The anemia is of variable severity.

The microcytic anemia in this patient superficially resembles the anemia produced by iron deficiency. The degree of microcytosis, however, is too profound for this level of anemia. Treating patients with thalassemia with iron is contraindicated because these patients have sufficient iron stores, as shown by the laboratory values in this patient.

The patient has no illness or signs of inflammation that might lead to anemia of chronic disease. The fact that the patient's iron studies are normal argues against anemia of chronic disease as well.

### Bibliography

1. **Davies SC, Wonke B**. The management of haemoglobinopathies. Baillieres Clin Haematol. 1991;4:361-89. PMID: 1912665

2. **Anderson HM, Ranney HM**. Southeast Asian immigrants: the new thalassemias in Americans. Semin Hematol. 1990;27:239-46. PMID: 2197727

3. **Liebhaber SA**. Alpha thalassemia. Hemoglobin. 1989;13:685-73. PMID: 2699473

## Anemia Question 17
## Answer: C

**Educational Objective:** *Differentiate between iron deficiency and thalassemia trait.*

The young woman has had recent onset of symptoms suggestive of anemia, and the blood count is much more suggestive of iron deficiency than of thalassemia trait. The most expedient way to establish whether iron deficiency is the cause of her symptoms and anemia is to measure the patient's serum ferritin level. The erythrocyte count is only 3.7 million, which is lower than would be expected for α-thalassemia trait. The elevated red cell distribution width favors iron deficiency over thalassemia trait. Therefore, hemoglobin electrophoresis or measuring blood counts of siblings is not recommended as an initial step.

Ultrasonography of the spleen is not useful in differentiating iron-deficiency anemia from thalassemia trait. The α/β globin chain synthesis rate ratio is not an appropriate initial step.

**Bibliography**
1. **Guyatt GH, Oxman AD, Ali M, Willan A, McIlroy W, Patterson C**. Laboratory diagnosis of iron-deficiency anemia: an overview. J Gen Intern Med. 1992;7:145-53. PMID: 1487761

## Anemia Question 18
## Answer: B

**Educational Objective:** *Generate a differential diagnosis for microangiopathic hemolytic anemia associated with thrombocytopenia, and recognize features specific for the hemolytic-uremic syndrome.*

The hemolytic-uremic syndrome (HUS) is very similar to thrombotic thrombocytopenic purpura (TTP). In HUS, as opposed to TTP, there is a clear association with a diarrheal illness due to verotoxin-producing enteric pathogens, and its clinical consequences tend to be more localized to the kidneys. There appears to be endothelial cell injury that initiates platelet thrombus formation (causing thrombocytopenia by consumption) associated with a microangiopathic hemolytic anemia. As opposed to disseminated intravascular coagulation, there is no activation of the soluble coagulation system in HUS/TTP, and therefore, the prothrombin time and activated partial thromboplastin time are normal. Both HUS and TTP are managed by plasmapheresis with plasma infusions. With this therapy, most patients survive, although mild chronic renal insufficiency usually follows. The hemolysis and thrombocytopenia are not due to autoantibodies, as is the case with Evans's syndrome. Both *Clostridium* bacteremia and babesiosis are associated with nonimmune hemolysis, but neither lead to microangiopathic erythrocyte features.

**Bibliography**
1. **Moake JL**. Haemolytic-uraemic syndrome: basic science. Lancet. 1994;343:393-7. PMID: 7905556

## Anemia Question 19
## Answer: A

**Educational Objective:** *Diagnose and manage a delayed hemolytic reaction.*

This patient has had a delayed hemolytic reaction. The high lactate dehydrogenase and disproportionately high indirect bilirubin level, along with a falling hematocrit and microspherocytes, strongly suggest this diagnosis. Most likely the patient was sensitized against minor erythrocyte antigens during her pregnancies, but the titers of these antibodies dropped to undetectable levels over time. The blood that was transfused for the bleeding ulcer contained these minor antigens, which led to a rapid build-up of antibodies as part of the anamnestic response. These new antibodies will be detectable on a new crossmatch.

Furosemide and fluids may protect the kidney from the deleterious effects of erythrocyte stroma released into the peripheral circulation. This intervention is not needed in this patient, however, because of the relatively slow rate of hemolysis. In contrast, an immediate hemolytic transfusion reaction, as occurs with the infusion of ABO-incompatible blood, is associated with fever, back pain, renal failure, hypotension, and, often, death. An osmotic fragility test would be positive because of the microspherocytes generated by the hemolytic reaction. This test would add nothing to the information gained by review of the peripheral blood smear. The utility of immunoglobulin blockade of reticuloendothelial cell function in patients with delayed hemolytic reactions is unknown. Because there is no evidence of refractory bleeding, a surgical consultation is not needed.

**Bibliography**
1. **Gloe D**. Common reactions to transfusions. Heart Lung. 1991;20:506-12. PMID: 1894531
2. **Contreras M, Mollison PL**. ABC of transfusion. Immunological complications of transfusion. BMJ. 1990;300:173-6. PMID: 2105802

## Anemia Question 20
## Answer: A

**Educational Objective:** *Recognize the microscopic findings of iron deficiency on a peripheral blood smear and know the clinical implications.*

The findings on the peripheral blood smear are suggestive of iron deficiency. The erythrocytes show hypochromia, anisocytosis, and poikilocytosis and are also likely to be microcytic. (This patient's mean corpuscular volume was 74 fL.) Although the thalassemias are associated with hypochromic, microcytic erythrocytes, it is unlikely that this patient has thalassemia intermedia. He may have thalassemia minor, but this disorder would not account for this degree of anemia. In addition, erythrocytes in thalassemia minor would be expected to show less hypochromia, anisocytosis, and poikilocytosis and usually more target cells. Hereditary spherocytosis is associated with spherocytes and an enlarged spleen and would be an unlikely presentation in a 65-year-old man. Sickle cell anemia would be associated with sickled cells on the peripheral blood smear.

If a confirmatory test (serum ferritin determination) supports the diagnosis of iron deficiency, a source of gastrointestinal blood loss should be sought, regardless of whether the stool is positive or negative for occult blood. A gastrointestinal lesion is far more likely than dietary inadequacies or malabsorption in an otherwise healthy adult.

**Bibliography**

1.  **Rasul I, Kandel GP**. An approach to iron-deficiency. Can J Gastroenterol. 2001;15:739-47. PMID: 11727004

## Anemia Question 21
## Answer: B

**Educational Objective:** *Recognize the appearance of the peripheral blood smear in thalassemia minor and know how to distinguish this disorder from iron deficiency.*

The peripheral blood smear shows cells that are hypochromic with numerous target cells. The degree of poikilocytosis and anisocytosis is only modest, compared with the striking hypochromia. In this clinical setting, the most likely diagnosis is thalassemia trait. Iron deficiency is possible, but a more striking variation in red blood cell size and shape would be expected with this degree of hypochromia. Iron deficiency would also be a less likely diagnosis in an asymptomatic, nonanemic young man. Other causes of hypochromia, especially sideroblastic anemia, are much less common.

Hereditary spherocytosis is characterized by small spherocytes, and sickle cell anemia is characterized by sickled cells on the peripheral blood smear.

**Bibliography**

1.  **Olivieri NF**. The beta-thalassemias. N Engl J Med. 1999;341:99-109. PMID: 10395635

## Anemia Question 22
## Answer: C

**Educational Objective:** *Recognize spherocytosis on a peripheral blood smear and know the differential diagnosis.*

The appearance of spherocytosis is the result of loss of red blood cell membrane and a decrease in the ratio of cell surface area to volume. This is generally the result of either an acquired hemolytic process or a hereditary condition with an abnormality of the red blood cell membrane, leading to the morphologic changes seen. The cause of an acquired hemolytic disorder is usually an immune process, in which the red blood cell membrane is coated with an antibody (usually a non-complement-fixing IgG) with subsequent splenic sequestration, loss of red blood cell membrane, and, ultimately, extravascular hemolysis. A direct Coombs test is likely to be diagnostic. Other mechanisms causing acquired hemolytic anemia (for example, microangiopathic processes, damage by a faulty heart valve) cause other changes in red blood cell appearance (fragmentation).

Most of the inherited hemolytic anemias cause specific changes in red blood cell appearance (for example, sickling, "bite cells" in glucose-6-phosphate dehydrogenase deficiency). In hereditary spherocytosis, which may not become manifest until later in life, the name of the disease describes the erythrocyte morphology. A family history and the osmotic fragility test are the main diagnostic tools, although the biochemical abnormality of the red blood cells is well characterized.

**Bibliography**

1.  **Bolton-Maggs PH**. The diagnosis and management of hereditary spherocytosis. Baillieres Best Pract Res Clin Haematol. 2000;13:327-42. PMID: 11030038

## Anemia Question 23
## Answer: D

**Educational Objective:** *Recognize the manifestations of homozygous sickle cell disease on the peripheral blood smear and know how to distinguish this disorder from other hemoglobin diseases.*

Although no history could be obtained, it is highly likely that this adolescent has homozygous sickle cell disease and has had occlusion of a major vessel in the distribution of the left middle cerebral artery. The peripheral blood smear shows characteristic sickle cells. Although the patient could possibly have a doubly heterozygous state, this is much less likely. If she had hemoglobin SC disease, her smear would be expected to show target cells and occasional "fat" or "clam shell" sickle cells rather than the thin, elongated forms seen in this smear. Sickle cell β-thalassemia would be expected to show microcytosis (this patient's mean corpuscle volume was 87 fL) and many target cells on the blood smear. Iron deficiency anemia, thalassemia, and spherocytosis are not associated with elongated sickled cells.

Strokes due to occlusion of a large vessel are not uncommon in patients with sickle cell disease and are an indication for chronic blood transfusion therapy to maintain the peripheral blood hemoglobin S level below 50%.

**Bibliography**

1. **Steinberg MH**. Management of sickle cell disease. N Engl J Med. 1999;340:1021-30. PMID: 10099145

## Anemia Question 24
## Answer: D

**Educational Objective:** *Recognize the value of the peripheral blood smear in distinguishing among the various causes in a patient with macrocytic anemia.*

Examination of a blood smear from a patient with macrocytic anemia should significantly narrow the differential diagnosis. This smear shows anisocytosis, poikilocytosis, macro-ovalocytes, and hypersegmented polymorphonuclear leukocytes. These changes are suggestive of a megaloblastic anemia caused by either folic acid deficiency or vitamin $B_{12}$ deficiency. In either case, the serum lactate dehydrogenase level will be markedly elevated. Additional details of the history and physical examination (dietary and medication history, neurologic symptoms and signs, and glossitis) should be sought. Determining the serum levels of folate, vitamin $B_{12}$ and, in some cases, the red blood cell folate, should be definitive.

Other causes of macrocytosis have different findings on the peripheral blood smear. Liver disease with macrocytic anemia should show either minimal changes or abundant target cells. Aplastic anemia, paroxysmal nocturnal hemoglobinuria, and hypothyroidism (which is less likely to cause pancytopenia) should show fewer erythrocyte abnormalities and normal neutrophils. Because reticulocytes have a high mean corpuscular volume, significant reticulocytosis responsive to hemolysis or blood loss may also produce a macrocytic anemia. The presence of polychromatophilia would be the clue in establishing the diagnosis.

**Bibliography**

1. **Toh BH, van Driel IR, Gleeson PA**. Pernicious anemia. N Engl J Med. 1997;337:1441-8. PMID: 9358143

# Cancer

## Cancer Question 1
**Answer: E**

**Educational Objective:** *Evaluate and manage a discrete breast lump.*

This patient illustrates the need for aggressive evaluation of her discrete, solid breast mass. Any middle-aged woman with a discrete breast mass should be referred to a surgeon for biopsy regardless of the presence of benign characteristics on physical examination or a negative mammogram. The risk of malignancy increases with age, leading to the axiom that any discrete mass detected on physical breast examination in a woman aged 50 years or older should be considered to be malignant until proven otherwise. Although certain characteristics are associated with benign lesions (for example, masses that are round, mobile, and soft), a review of malignant masses found a significant portion to be regular (41%) and mobile (61%). Therefore, clinical characteristics cannot be relied upon to predict the pathologic nature of a discrete mass. If this were a younger woman with multiple, round, tender lumps or if cysts were identified on ultrasound, a return in 6 weeks for examination during a different part of the menstrual cycle or an attempt at aspiration would be appropriate. However, there is no evidence to support the presence of a cyst. Although a "negative triad" — benign characteristics on physical examination, negative cytology on fine-needle aspiration, and a negative mammogram — has been suggested as an adequate evaluation, studies have reported false-negative rates as high as 16% in the presence of a malignant mass. Risk factors for breast cancer are helpful in predicting the likelihood of a mass's being malignant, but 75% of women with newly diagnosed breast cancer have no identifiable risk factors. Mammograms are the most sensitive method for detecting breast cancer, but large trials have reported that 3% to 45% of breast cancers are detected by palpation in women with negative mammograms.

### Bibliography

1. **Baines CJ, Miller AB, Bassett AA**. Physical examination. Its role as a single screening modality in the Canadian National Breast Screening Study. Cancer. 1989;63:1816-22. PMID: 2702588

2. **Venet L, Strax P, Venet W, Shapiro S**. Adequacies and inadequacies of breast examinations by physicians in mass screening. Cancer. 1971;28:1546-51. PMID: 5127799

3. **Yelland A, Graham MD, Trott PA, Ford HT, Coombes RC, Gazet JC, et al**. Diagnosing breast carcinoma in young women. BMJ. 1991;302:618-20. PMID: 2012873

4. **Barton MB, Harris R, Fletcher SW**. Does this patient have breast cancer? The screening clinical breast examination: should it be done? How? JAMA. 1999;282:1270-80. PMID: 10517431

## Cancer Question 2
**Answer: C**

**Educational Objective:** *Understand the importance of childhood sunburns in the pathogenesis of melanoma.*

The development of skin cancer is most strongly correlated with exposure to the ultraviolet radiation in sunlight. Exposure to fluorescent light has never been proved to cause the development of melanoma. There is a prolonged lag period between the actual exposure to ultraviolet radiation and the development of melanoma. The types of exposure listed in the options, other than the multiple childhood sunburns, would be insufficient on their own to cause skin cancer.

Several aspects of the relationship between melanoma and ultraviolet radiation have been puzzling. Why do some patients develop a melanoma, whereas others develop a basal cell or squamous cell carcinoma? Why do the tumors occur on the trunk in some patients and on the head and neck of other patients? Why do skin cancers appear in the third or fourth decade in some patients and not until the seventh or eighth in other patients? A paradigm has been developed to help answer many of these questions. It appears that several variables play a role:

The genetic make-up of patients in terms of their response to ultraviolet radiation: complexion, ability to tan, tendency to burn.

The timing of the exposure to ultraviolet radiation: childhood or adulthood.

The intensity of the exposure: strong enough to result in a sunburn (redness, erythema) or less intense (suberythemal).

Frequency of the ultraviolet radiation exposure: chronic, such as that in outdoor workers, or intermittent, such as that occurring during weekend recreation or once-a-year vacations in sunny climates.

The skin areas exposed: the usually exposed skin of the face, neck, and lower arms or the intermittently exposed skin of the chest, back, and shoulders.

Finally, there are two predominant cells in the epidermis exposed to ultraviolet radiation: keratinocytes and melanocytes.

Actinic keratoses and squamous cell carcinoma are derived from the actively replicating keratinocytes that reside in the basal layer of the epidermis, just above the basement membrane separating the epidermis from the dermis. These tumors are believed to be caused by chronic exposure to ultraviolet radiation of skin that is usually exposed to the sun, including the head, neck, and upper extremities.

Melanomas are derived from the much less numerous melanocytes, which also reside in the basal layer of the epidermis. They provide the melanin pigment that gives persons their complexion and the ability to tan in response to sun exposure. These cells normally do not divide and reproduce themselves. Consequently, with heavy ultraviolet radiation exposure, such as sunburn, considerable DNA damage can be done. The DNA damage can promote the development of melanoma.

### Bibliography

1. **Gilchrest BA, Eller MS, Geller AC, Yaar M.** The pathogenesis of melanoma induced by ultraviolet radiation. N Engl J Med. 1999;340:1341-8. PMID: 10219070

## Cancer Question 3
## Answer: D

**Educational Objective:** *Recommend appropriate follow-up for colorectal polyps found at screening sigmoidoscopy.*

This asymptomatic, average-risk patient had a hyperplastic polyp found at screening sigmoidoscopy and a negative fecal occult blood test. Hyperplastic polyps are not associated with an increased risk of neoplasia, and routine screening is recommended. This includes yearly fecal occult blood tests on dietary and medication restrictions and flexible sigmoidoscopy every 3 to 5 years. If an adenomatous polyp is found on sigmoidoscopy, colonoscopy is recommended because 50% of such patients will have neoplasms beyond the reach of the sigmoidoscope. Barium enema is reserved for those patients who are unable undergo endoscopic evaluation.

### Bibliography

1. **Pignone M, Rich M, Teutsch SM, Berg AO, Lohr KN.** Screening for colorectal cancer in adults at average risk: a summary of the evidence for the U.S. Preventive Services Task Force. Ann Intern Med. 2002;137:132-41. PMID: 12118972

## Cancer Question 4
## Answer: C

**Educational Objective:** *Recommend appropriate evaluation of unexplained iron-deficiency anemia.*

This postmenopausal woman has iron-deficiency anemia, and the most common cause is colorectal cancer. Colonoscopy is the most appropriate test, because it has the best diagnostic accuracy and allows for biopsy or removal of lesions. Barium enema is less accurate, and colonoscopy is required for biopsy or therapy if abnormalities are detected. Barium enema should be reserved for the uncommon circumstance in which a patient cannot tolerate colonoscopy or colonoscopy is unsuccessful. Flexible sigmoidoscopy is inappropriate in that it evaluates only the distal third of the colon. Even if a lesion were detected by flexible sigmoidoscopy, colonoscopy would be required to look for synchronous neoplasms. Esophagogastroduodenoscopy

(EGD) may show ulcers or other sources of upper gastrointestinal tract bleeding and allows for a small bowel biopsy to look for celiac sprue as a cause. However, EGD should be reserved for patients with upper gastrointestinal tract symptoms or a negative colonoscopy. CT scanning does not address the issue of iron-deficiency anemia in this patient.

### Bibliography

1. **Rockey DC, Koch J, Cello JP, Sanders LL, McQuaid K.** Relative frequency of upper gastrointestinal and colonic lesions in patients with positive fecal occult blood tests. N Engl J Med. 1998;339:153-9. PMID: 9664091

## Cancer Question 5
## Answer: A

**Educational Objective:** *Evaluate a patient with a positive screening fecal occult blood test.*

Colonoscopy is the most appropriate test for persons with a positive fecal occult blood test. Polyps may be detected and removed, and early-stage cancers may be found. This approach results in a 33% decrease in colorectal cancer mortality. Barium enema is recommended only for patients who are unable to undergo colonoscopy, and sigmoidoscopy is inappropriate because it may miss 50% of lesions. Even one positive window constitutes a positive fecal occult blood test, and there is no need to repeat the test. Cancers and large polyps may bleed intermittently, and any single positive test requires full evaluation. Anoscopy alone has no role in the evaluation of this patient.

### Bibliography

1. **Pignone M, Rich M, Teutsch SM, Berg AO, Lohr KN.** Screening for colorectal cancer in adults at average risk: a summary of the evidence for the U.S. Preventive Services Task Force. Ann Intern Med. 2002;137:132-41. PMID: 12118972

## Cancer Question 6
## Answer: C

**Educational Objective:** *Recommend appropriate colorectal cancer surveillance for a person with a familial colorectal cancer syndrome.*

This patient should undergo colonoscopy immediately. He has a familial colorectal cancer syndrome. A family history of colon cancer at the ages noted in his relatives is more consistent with hereditary nonpolyposis colorectal cancer (HNPCC) than with familial adenomatous polyposis (FAP), in which cancer occurs earlier. This man meets the clinical criteria for HNPCC, which are (1) three first-degree relatives with colorectal cancer, (2) spanning two generations, and (3) with one relative diagnosed with colorectal cancer at younger than 50 years of age. HNPCC is a syndrome with an autosomal dominant inheritance that imparts defects in the mismatch repair genes that function to repair somatic mutations. Individuals with this syndrome are at high risk of developing colon cancer at a young age, with few, if any, predisposing adenomatous polyps. Cancers often occur in the right colon. Surveillance colonoscopy is recommended every 2 years to begin at age 25 years or 10 years younger than the youngest affected relative. After age 40 years, colonoscopy should be performed yearly. Various other cancers, including those of the breast and female genital tract, may occur. Genetic testing is available, and affected persons should be considered for referral to a center with genetic counseling and testing facilities. The results of fecal occult blood testing, sigmoidoscopy, or barium enema would not change the need for colonoscopy in these high-risk patients, and therefore, these tests are not indicated.

### Bibliography

1. **Burt RW**. Screening of patients with a positive family history of colorectal cancer. Gastrointest Endosc Clin North Am. 1997;7:65-79. PMID: 8995113

## Cancer Question 7
## Answer: D

**Educational Objective:** *Recommend appropriate follow-up for a patient who has undergone surgical resection of colon cancer.*

This patient has had a curative resection of a colon cancer with no metastases. Overall, there is about a 50% recurrence rate for patients after resection of colorectal cancer. Eighty percent of recurrences develop within 2 years of resection, and virtually all occur within 5 years of resection. Colonoscopy is recommended to look for metachronous adenomas and cancers 1 year after resection, 3 years later, and then at 5-year intervals. If adenomas are detected, the patient should be managed as a routine adenoma patient. Patients with a history of colon cancer are at increased risk for recurrence and should not be followed with the screening program recommended for asymptomatic, average-risk persons (option C). Most recurrences occur as metastases distant from the resection site, but CT and liver tests are insensitive and not recommended.

### Bibliography

1. **Bertagnolli MM, Mahmoud N, Daly JM**. Surgical aspects of colorectal carcinoma. Hematol Oncol Clin North Am. 1997;11:655-77. PMID: 9257150

## Cancer Question 8
## Answer: D

**Educational Objective:** *Understand when patients should undergo screening for BRCA1 or BRCA2 abnormalities.*

Assessing risk and recommending screening for breast cancer can be difficult. Early diagnosis and treatment associated with screening mammography reduce mortality by approximately 20% to 30% compared to mortality in women who develop breast cancer without having been screened. Furthermore, a recently reported, prospective, randomized clinical trial suggests that tamoxifen therapy prevents the emergence of new breast cancers. However, both of these strategies have costs, both economically and in terms of morbidity and toxicity for the patient. To apply screening and prevention efficiently, it is essential to understand who is at risk for the disease.

The most important risk factors for breast cancer are sex and age. Women over the age of 50 years account for 75% of all breast cancers diagnosed in the United States, and the risk of developing breast cancers in this group is nearly 200-fold higher than in young males, nearly 100-fold higher than in older males, and nearly 10-fold higher than in women ages 35 to 50. However, applying prevention and screening to all women over age 50 is not recommended because a substantial group of these women will not develop breast cancer. Recently, two genes, *BRCA1* and *BRCA2*, seem to suppress breast cancer when they function normally. Certain families have abnormalities in *BRCA1* and/or *BRCA2* (mutations, deletions) that are inherited and confer a high risk of developing breast cancer and other malignancies. These susceptibility genes are present in all (germline) cells in the body. Commercially available tests can be used to detect these genetic changes in easily obtained leukocyte or oral swab specimens.

However, *BRCA1* and *BRCA2* abnormalities are relatively infrequent in the general population and account for 5% to 10% of breast cancers. These tests are expensive, the effects of different mutations within the genes are unknown, the penetrance of the disease is unclear for different individuals that do have abnormalities, and it is unknown whether enhanced screening or preventive measures are effective. Therefore, the decision to use the test is very complex, and the tests are best performed by trained genetic counselors. The odds of having a genetic abnormality are low unless the patient has a family history of breast cancer at early ages, especially when ovarian cancers are prevalent as well. In the absence of this type of history, which this patient does not have, *BRCA1* and *BRCA2* testing is not appropriate.

### Bibliography

1. **Fisher B, Costantino JP, Wickerham DL, Redmond CK, Kavanah M, Cronin WM, et al**. Tamoxifen for prevention of breast cancer: report of the National Surgical Adjuvant Breast and Bowel Project P-1 Study. J Natl Cancer Inst. 1998;90:1371-88. PMID: 9747868
2. **Gail MH, Brinton LA, Byar DP, Corle DK, Green SB, Schairer C, Mulvihill JJ, et al**.Projecting individualized probabilities of developing breast cancer for white females who are being examined annually. J Natl Cancer Inst. 1989;81:1879-86. PMID: 2593165
3. **Kerlikowske K, Grady D, Rubin SM, Sandrock C, Ernster VL**. Efficacy of screening mammography. A meta-analysis. JAMA. 1995;273:149-54. PMID: 7799496

4. Nyström L, Rutqvist LE, Wall S, Lindgren A, Lindqvist M, Rydén S, et al. Breast cancer screening with mammography: overview of Swedish randomised trials. Lancet. 1993;341:973-8. PMID: 8096941

## Cancer Question 9
## Answer: D

**Educational Objective:** *Manage a patient with squamous cell cancer of the supraclavicular region.*

This patient has squamous cell cancer in the supraclavicular area without a detectable primary lesion. This is most likely a lung cancer because of the patient's smoking history and hemoptysis and the location of the supraclavicular lymph node. Therefore, the patient should be evaluated for lung cancer with sputum cytology, CT scan of the chest, and fiberoptic bronchoscopy. This evaluation is important because if this is squamous cell carcinoma of the lung, this patient can be treated with radiation therapy, which has approximately a 5% cure rate. Patients with head and neck cancers commonly present with enlarged mid to upper cervical lymph nodes and do not have hemoptysis. This patient's cancer histology is not adenocarcinoma, which occurs in breast cancer. Therefore, mammography, ultrasound examination, and MRI of the breast are not necessary.

### Bibliography
1. Lembersky BC, Thomas LC. Metastases of unknown primary site. Med Clin North Am. 1996;80:153-71. PMID: 8569295
2. Hainsworth JD, Greco FA. Treatment of patients with cancer of an unknown primary site. N Engl J Med. 1993;329:257-63. PMID: 8316270

## Cancer Question 10
## Answer: E

**Educational Objective:** *Recognize long-term consequences of curative therapy for testicular cancer, and learn how to integrate the information into follow-up care.*

Cisplatin, a heavy metal, can cause bilateral hearing deficits, generally in the 4- to 8-kHz range. However, this is outside the range of conversational tones, and hearing aids are rarely required at the doses used to cure testicular cancer. Moreover, simply asking the patient about any hearing problems would alert the physician to the rare patient who is impaired enough to consider hearing aids, and therefore periodic audiometry is not indicated.

The risk of treatment-related leukemia is primarily attributed to etoposide. The leukemia is usually myeloid and often has a characteristic 11q23 chromosomal translocation. Etoposide-induced leukemias generally occur earlier after therapy (usually within a few years) than alkylating-agent associated leukemias. Although the relative risk of leukemia after treatment with the bleomycin, etoposide, and cisplatin regimen is about 15% to 25%, the absolute risk is less than 0.5% at 5 years. This patient is already 20 years beyond his initial chemotherapy; therefore, his risk of developing leukemia is low. Moreover, there is no screening test known to lower leukemia mortality.

Treatment-related solid tumors in patients with testicular cancer are primarily related to radiation (cancers of the bladder, pancreas, and stomach). They occur with a latency period of 10 years or more. This patient did not have radiation as part of his management. Moreover, screening tests for bladder, pancreatic, and stomach cancer are not known to decrease mortality. Therefore, standard practice is to discuss with the patient the cancer screening tests recommended for the general population.

### Bibliography
1. Travis LB, Curtis RE, Storm H, Hall P, Holowaty E, Van Leeuwen FE, et al. Risk of second malignant neoplasms among long-term survivors of testicular cancer. J Natl Cancer Inst. 1997;89:1429-39. PMID: 9326912

## Cancer Question 11
## Answer: C

**Educational Objective:** *Recognize that adenocarcinoma of the lung is the most common diagnosis in patients who do not smoke cigarettes.*

This patient has an intrapulmonary spiculated mass with involvement of her mediastinal lymph nodes as demonstrated on CT scan of the chest and biopsy of the nodes during mediastinoscopy. Other common primary sites of adenocarcinoma, including the breast and gastrointestinal and genitourinary tracts, are normal. Therefore, despite the lack of a smoking history, this patient has an adenocarcinoma of the lung.

Although 85% of patients with lung cancer are smokers, 15% of affected patients have never smoked cigarettes. Adenocarcinoma of the lung is responsible for two thirds of the lung cancers in nonsmokers. However, 70% of adenocarcinomas occur in patients who smoke cigarettes, along with more than 95% of small cell lung cancers and 90% of squamous cell cancers and large cell cancers. Cigarette smoking increases the risk of adenocarcinoma of the lung five-fold, compared to 15-fold for small cell lung cancers and squamous cell carcinoma of the lung. Women who do not smoke cigarettes are twice as likely to develop lung cancer as men for unknown reasons.

### Bibliography
1. Zang EA, Wynder EL. Differences in cancer risk between men and women: examination of the evidence. J Natl Cancer Inst. 1996;88:183-92. PMID: 8632492
2. Wingo PA, Ries LA, Giovino GA, Miller DS, Rosenberg HM, Shopland DR, et al. Annual report to the nation on the status of cancer, 1973-1996, with a special section on lung cancer and tobacco smoking. J Natl Cancer Inst. 1999;91:675-90. PMID: 10218505

## Cancer Question 12
## Answer: A

**Educational Objective:** *Know that patients treated for breast cancer and who receive tamoxifen therapy are at higher risk for second malignancies.*

Patients who have had breast cancer may be at risk for a second malignancy because of inherent susceptibility or as a consequence of therapy. Several treatments may increase a patient's long-term risk for other malignancies.

Several studies in both the adjuvant and the prevention setting document that tamoxifen therapy doubles the risk for endometrial cancer over that of women who have not received tamoxifen therapy. This risk is probably related to dose and time of treatment. However, the absolute risk of developing endometrial cancer for most patients receiving tamoxifen therapy is less than 1%, and the baseline risk of this malignancy is only 0.1% to 0.3% in the general population. Therefore, the benefits of tamoxifen therapy outweigh the risks for most patients. Because the risk of developing endometrial cancer is low, because the disease usually is curable when detected, and because tamoxifen frequently induces benign endometrial changes that create false-positive results, routine endometrial screening by transvaginal ultrasound, endometrial biopsy, or dilatation and curettage is not recommended. Although some early reports suggested an increase in gastrointestinal malignancies in patients taking tamoxifen, subsequent studies have not confirmed these observations.

Other therapies can increase the risk of other malignancies. Radiation therapy to the chest wall increases the risk of lung cancer, especially in smokers, and the risk of chest wall sarcoma. Certain types of chemotherapy increase the risk of acute myeloid leukemia and/or myelodysplasia. However, this patient received none of these treatments.

Inherent increased risk for breast cancer is seen in women with family or personal histories of breast cancer. The relative risk of developing a contralateral breast cancer compared to the general population is approximately twofold. However, tamoxifen therapy decreases the relative risk of developing a new contralateral breast cancer by 50% when compared to women who have had previous breast cancer but who have not taken tamoxifen.

### Bibliography

1. Tamoxifen for early breast cancer: an overview of the randomised trials. Early Breast Cancer Trialist's Collaborative Group. Lancet. 1998;351:1451-67. PMID: 9605801

2. Fisher B, Costantino JP, Redmond CK, Fisher ER, Wickerham DL, Cronin WM. Endometrial cancer in tamoxifen-treated breast cancer patients: findings from the National Surgical Adjuvant Breast and Bowel Project (NSABP) B-14. J Natl Cancer Inst. 1994;86:527-37. PMID: 8133536

3. Fisher B, Rockette H, Fisher ER, Wickerham DL, Redmond C, Brown A. Leukemia in breast cancer patients following adjuvant chemotherapy or postoperative radiation: the NSABP experience. J Clin Oncol. 1985;3:1640-58. PMID: 3906049

4. Fornander T, Rutqvist LE, Cedermark B, Glas U, Mattsson A, Silfversward C, et al.Adjuvant tamoxifen in early breast cancer: occurrence of new primary cancers. Lancet. 1989;1:117-20. PMID: 2563046

## Cancer Question 13
## Answer: D

**Educational Objective:** *Evaluate a patient with small cell lung cancer.*

This patient presents with histologic evidence of small cell lung cancer and radiographic evidence of mediastinal lymph node involvement. Thirty-five percent of patients with small cell lung cancer have bone metastases at their initial evaluation, and this patient has an increased chance of bony involvement because he is symptomatic. Therefore, this patient should have a bone scan.

Brain metastases are present at the time of diagnosis in 10% of patients with small cell lung cancer, and one half of these patients have no central nervous system signs or symptoms. This patient has headaches and other evidence of metastatic disease and is more likely to have brain metastases than patients who do not have central nervous system symptoms and other metastasis. A patient with brain metastases should have radiation therapy to control the metastases.

Small cell lung cancer is typically disseminated at presentation. Less than 5% of patients are candidates for resection, and this patient has a 6-cm mediastinal mass and probable bone metastasis. Nearly all large (greater than 4 cm in diameter) mediastinal masses in patients with lung cancer are involved with cancer. Therefore, these patients are rarely referred to thoracic surgeons if they already are diagnosed with small cell lung cancer. Patients with small cell lung cancer capable of tolerating therapy should be referred to a medical oncologist for chemotherapy. Small cell lung cancer grows rapidly, and therefore, timely referral and communication with the medical oncologist is important. A radiation oncologist may be needed if the small cell lung cancer is confined to the chest because radiation therapy can prolong survival for these patients. However, this patient likely has disseminated disease. Patients with extensive-stage small cell lung cancer may require radiation therapy for local problems, including brain metastases, painful bony metastases or impending fracture, and spinal cord compression. It appears that this patient has rather straightforward, extensive-stage small cell lung cancer and will likely be managed by combination chemotherapy as the initial treatment.

### Bibliography

1. Dearing MP, Steinberg SM, Phelps R, Anderson MJ, Mulshine JL, Ihde DC, et al. Outcome of patients with small-cell lung cancer: effect of changes in staging procedures and imaging technology on prognostic factors over 14 years. J Clin Oncol. 1990;8:1042-9. PMID: 2161447

2. McLoud TC, Bourgouin PM, Greenberg RW, Kosiuk JP, Templeton PA, Shepard JA, et al. Bronchogenic carcinoma: analysis of staging in the mediastinum with CT by correlative lymph node mapping and sampling. Radiology. 1992;182:319-23. PMID: 1732943

3. Johnson BE. Management of small-cell lung cancer. Clin Chest Med. 1993;14:173-87. PMID: 8384962

## Cancer Question 14
## Answer: D

**Educational Objective:** *Recognize that persistent fever and cough in patients at risk for lung cancer can be caused by obstructive pneumonia.*

This patient has had fever for more than 1 week with signs and symptoms suggestive of pneumonia. The patient has partial resolution after 10 days of oral antibiotic treatment, but her fever, cough, and shortness of breath return. This patient with a strong smoking history is at high risk for lung cancer with persistent fever and pulmonary symptoms; therefore, further evaluation for a potential cause of the persistent fever is appropriate. In this patient a chest radiograph should look for evidence of persistent infiltrate or the appearance of a pulmonary mass as the infiltrate resolves and cytologic examination of the sputum.

This patient has a 60-pack-year smoking history and therefore has a 0.5% chance of developing lung cancer per year, or 30% overall. This patient stopped smoking cigarettes 3 years ago, but she is still at high risk for developing cancer. Although the risk of lung cancer begins to fall within 1 year after stopping smoking cigarettes, it takes 5 to 10 years after smoking cessation for the relative risk to reduce by 50% compared with a current smoker. Patients with lung cancer present with postobstructive pneumonia approximately 10% to 20% of the time. The most common cause of fever in patients with underlying cancer is caused by complications of the tumor rather than by the tumor itself. Postobstructive pneumonia is one of the most common causes of fever in patients with lung cancer. Given that this patient has a relatively strong chance of developing lung cancer, observing the patient for 1 month, treating the patient with another course of antibiotics, or obtaining pulmonary function tests will unnecessarily delay the diagnostic evaluation of this patient.

If a mass appears or if there is still a persistent infiltrate, a CT scan of the chest should be performed to look for a mass. If a mass is documented, the patient should then have fiberoptic bronchoscopy and suspicious lesion should be biopsied.

### Bibliography

1. Browder AA, Huff JW, Petersdorf RG. The significance of fever in neoplastic disease. Ann Intern Med. 1961;55:932-42.

2. Vaaler AK, Forrester JM, Lesar M, Edison M, Venzon D, Johnson BE. Obstructive atelectasis in patients with small cell lung cancer. Incidence and response to treatment. Chest. 1997;111:115-20. PMID: 8996004

## Cancer Question 15
## Answer: D

**Educational Objective:** *Evaluate patients at high risk for lung cancer with hemoptysis.*

The most common cause of hemoptysis is from a benign source, such as bronchitis, and bronchiectasis. Only 20% of patients with hemoptysis have lung cancer. However, this patient with hemoptysis has other factors that place him at high risk for lung cancer. He is older than 40 years, has smoked cigarettes for 50 years, and has had hemoptysis for longer than 1 week. Therefore, he has a greater than 40% chance of having lung cancer and needs an appropriate evaluation. A chest radiograph will detect abnormalities in 70% of patients with hemoptysis and in 90% of patients with lung cancer. In high risk patients, 90% sensitivity is not high enough.

In addition, patients with causes of hemoptysis other than lung cancer can benefit from imaging with a chest radiograph and CT scan of the chest. CT scan of the chest is five times more sensitive for detecting bronchiectasis in patients with hemoptysis than chest radiographs.

This patient at high risk for lung cancer also needs to have fiberoptic bronchoscopy. It is effective in localizing the bleeding site in 40% of the patients and can establish the cause 80% of the time. Fiberoptic bronchoscopy is also effective for obtaining biopsies of suspicious lesions detected by chest radiograph or CT scan of the chest. This can then lead to the appropriate management of the patient after a diagnosis is made.

The other options of observation, antibiotics, and chest radiograph and CT scan of the chest are inadequate because the bleeding site is not identified and lesions are not diagnosed. It is important to pursue the diagnosis with fiberoptic bronchoscopy in this patient with hemoptysis because of his high risk for lung cancer.

### Bibliography

1. Johnston H, Reisz G. Changing spectrum of hemoptysis. Underlying causes in 148 patients undergoing diagnostic flexible fiberoptic bronchoscopy. Arch Intern Med. 1989;149:1666-8. PMID: 2742442

2. Colice GL. Detecting lung cancer as a cause of hemoptysis in patients with a normal chest radiograph: bronchoscopy vs CT. Chest. 1997;111:877-84. PMID: 9106564

3. Hirshberg B, Biran I, Glazer M, Kramer MR. Hemoptysis: etiology, evaluation, and outcome in a tertiary referral hospital. Chest. 1997;112:440-4. PMID: 9266882

## Cancer Question 16
## Answer: D

**Educational Objective:** *Recognize the association between small cell carcinoma of the lung and hyponatremia.*

The patient presents with a cough, shortness of breath, heavy smoking history, hyponatremia, and lung cancer. Lung cancer is clinically divided into small cell lung cancer and non small cell lung cancer. The non small cell lung cancers are principally composed of adenocarcinoma, squamous cell carcinoma, adenosquamous carcinoma, and large cell carcinoma. Small cell lung carcinoma is responsible for approximately 20% of lung cancers.

Up to 15% of patients with small cell lung cancer present with hyponatremia, defined as serum sodium concentration less than 130 meq/L. This patient's hyponatremia is caused by ectopic production of arginine vasopressin, which is produced by the tumor and secreted into the bloodstream and then circulates through the bloodstream and binds to the V2 receptors in the kidney, causing them to retain free water. Most patients with malignant hyponatremia are asymptomatic, and their low serum sodium concentration is identified only by routine serum chemistry examination. Only 1% of patients with non small cell lung cancer present with hyponatremia. Therefore, the most likely histologic diagnosis in this case is small cell lung cancer.

### Bibliography

1. Gross AJ, Steinberg SM, Reilly JG, Bliss DP Jr, Brennan J, Le PT, et al. Atrial natriuretic factor and arginine vasopressin production in tumor cell lines from patients with lung cancer and their relationship to serum sodium. Cancer Res. 1993;53:67-74. PMID: 8380126
2. Johnson BE, Chute JP, Rushin J, Williams J, Le PT, Venzon D, et al. A prospective study of patients with lung cancer and hyponatremia of malignancy. Am J Respir Crit Care Med. 1997;156:1669-78. PMID: 9372692

## Cancer Question 17
## Answer: D

**Educational Objective:** *Recognize that radical mastectomy is no more effective than breast-preserving surgery together with adjuvant radiation therapy and/or chemotherapy in patients with stage II breast cancer.*

This patient has stage II breast cancer. Prospective, randomized clinical trials show that breast-preserving therapy is as effective as mastectomy. However, other studies show that excision without radiation results in an unacceptably high rate of recurrence. Several prospective, randomized clinical trials also establish the survival benefits of adjuvant chemotherapy, especially in young women with positive lymph nodes, and of adjuvant tamoxifen therapy, especially in patients with estrogen-receptor positive tumors. Therefore, no more surgery is needed, but all three other therapeutic recommendations are appropriate.

### Bibliography

1. Polychemotherapy for early breast cancer: an overview of the randomised trials. Early Breast Cancer Trialist's Collaborative Group. Lancet. 1998;352:930-42. PMID: 9752815
2. Tamoxifen for early breast cancer: an overview of the randomised trials. Early Breast Cancer Trialist's Collaborative Group. Lancet. 1998;351:1451-67. PMID: 9605801

## Cancer Question 18
## Answer: A

**Educational Objective:** *Manage surgically staged nonseminomatous testicular germ cell cancer.*

The relapse rate for pathologic stage 1 nonseminomatous germ cell cancer with no further therapy is about 15%. Virtually all patients who relapse while being carefully followed are cured by cisplatin-based combination chemotherapy. Thus, careful follow-up spares 85% of patients the toxicity of systemic therapy and achieves the same cure rate. In fact, there is growing evidence from multiple case series that the same cure rate can be achieved without retroperitoneal exploration to pathologically stage patients with disease clinically confined to the testicle.

Although there is a putative blood-testis barrier that could limit diffusion of chemotherapy into the testicle, synchronous cancers of the contralateral testis are rare. Patients may develop metachronous disease in the contralateral testis (about 2% to 5% over the next 25 years). However, this does not justify a biopsy in the contralateral testis. Contralateral cancer can occur years later, and most patients are cured at that time. For similar reasons, empiric radiation of the remaining testicle is not indicated and renders the patient permanently infertile.

### Bibliography

1. Weissbach L. Guidelines for the diagnosis and therapy of testicular cancer and new developments. Urol Int. 1999;63:46-56. PMID: 10592490

## Cancer Question 19
## Answer: D

**Educational Objective:** *Recognize the anatomic area of most frequent occurrence of melanoma in nonwhite persons.*

Although the incidence of melanoma is rising among white populations, nonwhite persons also develop melanoma. Among Asians and African Americans, melanoma occurs most often in the palms, soles, and mucous membranes. Based on the anatomic location of the melanoma, the prognosis of nonwhite patients with melanoma occurring in the palms, soles, and mucous membranes is worse compared with that for persons with melanomas arising elsewhere on the body. Patients with melanomas of the palms and soles have a 46% 8-year survival rate.

In white populations, the most common melanoma is the superficial spreading type, which occurs on the head, neck, back, torso, and upper and lower extremities, and it is associated with a pattern of intermittent sun exposure.

### Bibliography

1. Rogers GS, Kopf AW, Rigel DS, Freedman RJ, Levine JL, Levenstein M, et al. Effect of anatomical location on prognosis in patients with clinical stage I melanoma. Arch Dermatol. 1983;119:644-9. PMID: 6870318

2. **Holman CD, Armstrong BK**. Pigmentary traits, ethnic origin, benign nevi, and family history as risk factors for cutaneous malignant melanoma. J Natl Cancer Inst. 1984;72:257-66. PMID: 6582314
3. **Kopf AW, Kripke ML, Stern RS**. Sun and malignant melanoma. J Am Acad Dermatol. 1984;11:674-84. PMID: 6386902

## Cancer Question 20
## Answer: A

**Educational Objective:** *Recognize a melanoma and distinguish it from other skin lesions.*

A melanoma is asymmetric in shape and has irregular, scalloped, notched, or indistinct borders. It is black or dark brown or has variegate (multiple) coloration, including shades of black, red, and blue. The lesion may also have depigmented or white areas. A useful mnemonic to describe the appearance of these lesions is ABCD: asymmetry, border irregularity, color is dark or variegate, and diameter is often greater than 0.5 cm.

Lesions mimicking melanomas include benign melanocytic nevi, atypical nevi, and seborrheic keratoses. Benign melanocytic nevi can also be darkly pigmented, but the color is uniform and evenly distributed throughout the mole. Benign melanocytic nevi are symmetrically round or oval and have regular, discrete borders without notching or indentation. Atypical (dysplastic) nevi have many features of melanoma, including asymmetry, indiscrete borders, and irregular pigmentation. The only certain method to distinguish the two is by biopsy. Similar to melanomas, seborrheic keratoses can be dark brown or black, but have discrete borders, are elevated above the surface of the skin (giving them a "stuck-on" quality), and have a waxy or warty surface texture. A solar lentigo is a flat, round, evenly pigmented macule found in areas of chronic sun exposure. The pigmentation may range from light tan to dark brown but, in contrast to melanoma, is uniformly distributed.

**Bibliography**
1. **Koh HK**. Cutaneous melanoma. N Engl J Med. 1991;325:171-82. PMID: 1805813

## Cancer Question 21
## Answer: B

**Educational Objective:** *Recognize the clinical features of basal cell carcinoma.*

Basal cell carcinoma classically presents as a pink, pearly or translucent, dome-shaped papule with telangiectasias. The papule may have a central umbilication. The tendency is for slowly progressive growth. Basal cell carcinoma is most commonly found on sun-exposed areas, including the face, bald scalp, ears, neck, upper chest, and dorsal hands.

Lesions mimicking basal cell carcinoma include squamous cell carcinoma, interdermal nevus, sebaceous hyperplasia, and seborrheic keratosis. Squamous cell carcinoma tends to be red rather than pink, has a scale, erodes and bleeds easily, and grows rapidly. An interdermal nevus is likely to be present for long periods of time without change, may have brown pigmentation, is not translucent, does not have telangiectasias, and is not limited to sun-exposed areas of the body. Sebaceous hyperplasia is typically confined to the face (most commonly the forehead, nose, and cheeks), has a yellowish color, and, if the yellow sebaceous gland is compressed with a glass slide, the gland will appear as "petals of a flower" under the slide. Seborrheic keratosis may be pink but more often is yellow, brown, or even black. The lesion tends to be a flat-topped plaque rather than a domed-shaped papule and has a "waxy, stuck-on" appearance.

**Bibliography**
1. **Garner KL, Rodney WM**. Basal and squamous cell carcinomas. Prim Care. 2000;27:447-58. PMID: 10815054

## Cancer Question 22
## Answer: D

**Educational Objective:** *Choose the appropriate diagnostic evaluation for a patient with potentially resectable non small cell lung cancer.*

This patient has squamous cell carcinoma in the right middle lobe bronchus. She is relatively healthy otherwise. Computed tomography can be useful in the evaluation of patients with lung cancer; however, one must be very cautious in interpreting whether mediastinal lymph nodes are involved with regional spread of carcinoma. Many nodes smaller than 2 cm in diameter are hyperplastic but contain no malignancy. Nodes larger than 2 cm are more likely to contain metastatic tumor; however, even a small percentage of these are hyperplastic, enlarged, benign nodes. Therefore, the most appropriate action would be to evaluate the mediastinal nodes by mediastinoscopy. Should they be free of obvious metastases, the patient would be a good candidate for resection for potential cure. If, however, the nodes are positive, it would be very unlikely that surgery would offer any advantage as a single modality of therapy, and other forms of treatment would be indicated. The other options would not provide critical information necessary for her management and therefore would not be the appropriate next approach.

**Bibliography**
1. **Crino L, Cappuzzo F**. Present and future treatment of advanced non-small cell lung cancer. Semin Oncol. 2002;29:9-16. PMID: 12094333

# Back Pain

**Back Pain Question 1**
**Answer: A**

**Educational Objective:** *Recognize the signs and symptoms of cauda equina syndrome and identify appropriate initial evaluation.*

This patient's symptoms and neurologic deficits suggest cauda equina syndrome. Although massive midline herniation of an intervertebral disk is a possible cause, locally invasive intraspinal malignancy or metastatic disease should be suspected in older adults with cauda equina syndrome. The severe neurologic deficits in patients with cauda equina syndrome mandate urgent evaluation and consideration of surgery; bed rest or other forms of conservative therapy are inappropriate when this disorder is suspected. After a thorough physical examination, including rectal examination, neuroimaging of the spine is the most appropriate step.

MRI is valuable when patients have significant neurologic deficits such as cauda equina syndrome. CT of the lumbar spine, which usually costs less than half of MRI, provides superior anatomic imaging of the osseous structures of the spine and good resolution for disk herniation. However, CT scanning cannot image intraspinal tumors nor can it differentiate scar tissue from new disk herniation. Although expensive, MRI is the procedure of choice for spinal cord tumors, epidural abscess, and cord compression. Myelography is an invasive procedure that has been replaced by MRI or CT scan in many instances. A bone scan may reveal metastatic disease to the bone or osteomyelitis but may not clearly image intraspinal tumors. Spinal traction has no proven benefit for back pain and, in this case, will unnecessarily delay the diagnosis. Spinal manipulation is contraindicated in the presence of cauda equina syndrome.

**Bibliography**

1. **Borenstein DG**. A clinician's approach to acute low back pain. Am J Med. 1997;102:16S-22S. PMID: 9217555

**Back Pain Question 2**
**Answer: C**

**Educational Objective:** *Diagnose vertebral osteomyelitis.*

The clinician should be alert to the possibility of vertebral osteomyelitis in the patient with back pain and predisposing factors, such as urinary tract infection or manipulation of the urinary tract. Although venous return from the pelvis drains into the venous plexus of the vertebral column (Batson's plexus), most cases of pyogenic vertebral osteomyelitis are thought to be hematogeneous in origin, probably by an arterial route. The segmental arteries supplying the vertebrae usually bifurcate to supply two adjacent segments. Thus, vertebral osteomyelitis usually involves two vertebrae as well as the intervertebral disk.

In this patient, the history of intermittent night sweats and feverishness suggests intermittent fevers, which, along with new-onset back pain after a urinary tract infection, support the diagnosis of vertebral osteomyelitis. Although fever is not always present in patients with this condition, its absence on physical examination may have resulted from recent use of nonsteroidal anti-inflammatory drugs. The abdominal and femoral bruits suggest diffuse vascular disease. Although the patient may have an abdominal aortic aneurysm, this condition would not account for his history of fever or for lower thoracic back pain. Urinary tract symptoms are present and fever is usually absent in patients with chronic bacterial prostatitis. Likewise, fever is not a common manifestation of metastatic prostate cancer. Ankylosing spondylitis most commonly presents initially in young patients and is characterized by the insidious onset of lumbar back pain, often with associated muscle spasms and tenderness over the sacroiliac joints. While metastatic prostate cancer may present with back pain, the acute nature of the pain, the presence of night sweats and fever and a only mildly enlarged gland makes metastatic cancer unlikely.

**Bibliography**

1. **Strausbaugh LJ**. Vertebral osteomyelitis. How to differentiate it from other causes of back and neck pain. Postgrad Med. 1995;97:147-8,151-4. PMID: 7777442

**Back Pain Question 3**
**Answer: C**

**Educational Objective:** *Manage subacute low back pain in a patient without neurologic symptoms.*

In a recent randomized controlled trial, Andersson et al showed that spinal manipulation in patients with subacute back pain without neurologic findings is as effective as medical management and results in the use of fewer medications. There is no proven benefit to either a prolonged course of strict bed rest or to spinal traction. Neither radiographs of the back nor MRI scans of the lower spine are recommended as initial approaches in patients with low back pain in the absence of significant neurologic symptoms.

### Bibliography

1. **Andersson GB, Lucente T, Davis AM, Kappler RE, Lipton JA, Leurgans S**. A comparison of osteopathic spinal manipulation with standard care for patients with low back pain. N Engl J Med. 1999;341:1426-31. PMID: 10547405

2. **Malanga GA, Nadler SF**. Nonoperative treatment of low back pain. Mayo Clin Proc. 1999;74:1135-48. PMID: 10560603

## Back Pain Question 4
## Answer: A

**Educational Objective:** *Manage acute back pain in a patient with a history of cancer.*

This is a middle-aged woman with a history of breast cancer and intermittent back pain who now presents with another episode of acute low back pain. It is vital to remember that any acute exacerbation of a chronic condition or new pain in a patient with cancer carries the risk of being caused by a metastatic lesion or an extension of the cancer. This patient's pain is worse than usual, occurs when she moves but not at rest, and occurs with both flexion and extension, which can all be signs of bone disease. Although the neurologic examination shows only subtle changes, her new back pain must be treated as an emergency because it has a high pretest probability of representing a new metastasis to the spine with the potential for acute and rapid loss of neurologic function if not diagnosed and treated immediately. Given the nature of her pain and the location of pain over the spine, CT or MRI of the spine is essential.

While the patient should be admitted for observation and pain control, emergency imaging is the most important next option to provide accurate diagnosis and initiate early therapy. Consideration should also be given to a dose of glucocorticoids, which is thought to reduce the volume of the tumor and, therefore, the likelihood of spinal cord compression.

Plain radiographs are only useful if they show a lesion. If results of radiography are negative, the patient may have a tumor that is not seen and which extends into the spinal canal, especially if arthritic changes are already present. Usually, an MRI is required to further define the lesion even when the radiograph is normal.

Lumbar epidural injections may be appropriate in the treatment of an acute exacerbation of a chronic pain problem, but not in this patient with a history of cancer.

While bone scans are appropriate tests to identify sites of metastases, they are not accurate enough to identify spinal cord compression and would not be appropriate when acute neurological signs are present.

### Bibliography

1. **Borenstein DG**. A clinician's approach to acute low back pain. Am J Med. 1997;102:16S-22S. PMID: 9217555

## Back Pain Question 5
## Answer: B

**Educational Objective:** *Treat a patient with an osteoporotic fracture.*

Having sustained one fracture, this patient is at high risk for subsequent fractures, even without additional risk factors, and she is therefore a candidate for treatment. She would benefit from hormone replacement therapy to maintain bone mass, even though she has already experienced the most rapid period of postmenopausal bone loss. However, because she refuses hormone replacement therapy, alendronate is the best choice. A reasonable alternative therapy is raloxifene. She should also receive oral vitamin D and calcium supplements if her dietary intake of calcium is inadequate, but treatment with vitamin D and calcium will only slow the rate of bone loss, not restore bone mass. Physical therapy may provide symptomatic benefit, but weight training should be undertaken cautiously, if at all, in a patient at risk of additional osteoporotic fractures.

### Bibliography

1. **Miller PD**. Management of osteoporosis. Adv Intern Med. 1999;44:175-207. PMID: 9929709

2. **Pinkerton JV, Santen R**. Alternatives to the use of estrogen in postmenopausal women. Endocr Rev. 1999;20:308-20. PMID: 10368773

3. **Meunier PJ**. Evidence-based medicine and osteoporosis: a comparison of fracture risk reduction data from osteoporosis randomised clinical trials. Int J Clin Pract. 1999;53:122-9. PMID: 10344048

## Back Pain Question 6
## Answer: A

**Educational Objective:** *Recognize the typical changes of ankylosing spondylitis involving the sacroiliac joints and the lumbar spine.*

The anteroposterior view shows sclerosis and erosions of both sacroiliac joints, and the lateral view shows bridging of the intervertebral disc spaces by syndesmophytes. These are called marginal syndesmophytes because they cling to the margins of the vertebral bodies. The inflammatory spondyloarthropathies (ankylosing spondylitis and the spondyloarthropathies associated with inflammatory bowel disease, psoriasis, and Reiter's syndrome) are characterized by sacroiliitis and syndesmophyte formation. In ankylosing spondylitis and the spondyloarthropathy associated with inflammatory bowel disease, the sacroiliitis is symmetric and the syndesmophytes are marginal. In psoriatic arthritis and Reiter's syndrome, the sacroiliac involvement is often asymmetric. The syndesmophytes are nonmarginal and sometimes resemble osteophytes protruding from the bony margins of the vertebrae. In advanced ankylosing spondylitis, the sacroiliac joints and the lumbar spine become fused. Because the fused lumbar spine resembles a stalk of bamboo on radiographs, this lesion is sometimes referred to as a "bamboo spine." Ankylosing spondylitis affects men about three times more often than women and typically develops in early adulthood. In the United States, it is about three times more common in white Americans than in black Americans.

Herniated intervertebral discs are poorly visualized on plain radiographs and are best visualized with MRI. Compression fractures are manifested by wedge-shaped compression of one or several vertebral bodies. Findings in osteomyelitis include a ragged, moth eaten appearance of medullary bone with destruction of the vertebral structures. None of these diagnosis would be likely in a patient with a 12-year-history of back pain.

### Bibliography

1. **Khan MA.** Spondyloarthropathies. Curr Opin Rheumatol. 1999;11:233-4. PMID: 10411374

## Back Pain Question 7
## Answer: B

**Educational Objective:** *Recognize the emergent nature of symptoms of impending spinal cord compression in patients with metastatic prostate cancer.*

This patient has a known history of prostate cancer metastatic to bone and has been receiving androgen suppression treatment for his metastatic disease. The majority of patients relapse 12 to 18 months from the time of initiation of primary hormonal therapy. The first sign of systemic relapse from the androgen suppression is usually a rising prostate-specific antigen (PSA) level, followed by objective progression in the osseous structures or soft tissues, and then development of symptoms. The median survival for patients who develop symptomatic relapse is only 9 months. A particular concern in this population is the development of spinal cord compression.

The most common presenting symptom associated with impending spinal cord compression is localized back pain, often associated with motor weakness. These findings in this patient should be treated as a medical emergency, and the patient should receive high-dose steroids and have an immediate magnetic resonance imaging (MRI) scan of the spine or a myelogram.

The use of strontium 89 has been associated with palliation of pain in up to 75% of patients with prostate cancer metastatic to bone, but it takes 1 to 3 weeks to achieve symptomatic relief and does not prevent spinal cord compression. All of the other options are inappropriate in this emergency situation. After diagnosis, depending on the level of spinal cord compression, the patient should be referred to a radiation oncologist or neurosurgeon for definitive treatment. An early improvement in motor strength is a strong predictor of subsequent functional improvement. While bone scans reflect sites of metastasis, they do not provide adequate information about cord compression. Conservative therapy and analgesia should be used after cord compression has been ruled out.

### Bibliography

1. **Zelefsky MJ, Scher HI, Krol G, Portenoy RK, Leibel SA, Fuks ZY.** Spinal epidural tumor in patients with prostate cancer. Clinical and radiographic predictors of response to radiation therapy. Cancer. 1992;70:2319-25. PMID: 1394060
2. **Huddart RA, Rajan B, Law M, Meyer L, Dearnaley DP.** Spinal cord compression in prostate cancer: treatment outcome and prognostic factors. Radiother Oncol. 1997;44:229-36. PMID: 9380821

## Back Pain Question 8
## Answer: C

**Educational Objective:** *Recognize the clinical presentation of a tumor involving the lumbosacral spine and most likely within the dural sac.*

Tumors of the conus medullaris and cauda equina are notoriously difficult to diagnose, rare, and often insidious. There are seldom localized symptoms or focal neurologic signs until late in the course. Meningiomas, neurofibromas, ependymomas, and hemangioblastomas head the list of lesions; all are potentially surgically approachable and even curable.

Diagnosis begins with the history of low back pain at rest and night pain that causes the patient to pace. The history of sleeping in a chair is classic for cauda equina tumors, although the lesion is too rare to speak to the predictive value of the complaint. Any such night/rest pain should also raise the possibility of metastatic cancer, myeloma, or osteoid osteoma spinal infections. The prostate, lungs, and kidneys are the likeliest sources for metastases in this elderly man. The screening radiograph and bone scans may be helpful for excluding lesions that are destructive of bone or metastatic bone. The sensitivity of plain radiographs, however, is limited. The absence of clues on the screening studies of inflammatory or neoplastic disease should lead to further pursuit of disease of the cauda or conus with magnetic resonance imaging. Absence of fever, weight loss, or spinal tenderness on examination makes abscess unlikely. Normal exam and straight-leg raise also help exclude disc herniation. None of the options other than cauda equina tumor produce saddle anesthesia.

### Bibliography

1. **Cooper PR.** Outcome after operative treatment of intramedullary spinal cord tumors in adults: intermediate and long-term results in 51 patients. Neurosurgery. 1989;25:855-9. PMID: 2601814
2. **Borenstein DG.** A clinician's approach to acute low back pain. Am J Med. 1997;102:16S-22S. PMID: 9217555

## Back Pain Question 9
## Answer: D

**Educational Objective:** *Appreciate the clinical aspects of low bone density, regardless of age, and plan appropriate treatment.*

This patient has osteoporosis based on the dual-energy x-ray absorptiometry (DEXA) measurement despite her relative youth and absence of fractures. However, supplementation of her calcium intake is not sufficient to increase bone density and lessen future fracture risk. Among the Food and Drug Administration (FDA)-approved agents, alendronate, 10 mg daily, is the most appropriate choice. Sodium fluoride is not FDA-approved. Nasal-spray calcitonin is not labeled for use before or within 5 years of menopause. Alendronate, a bisphosphonate, is the strongest of the approved agents in increasing bone density and has significant effects on the femur as well as the spine. Aspirin has no utility in the treatment of osteoporosis. As the patient is still premenopausal, additional estrogen supplementation would be of no value.

### Bibliography

1. Who are candidates for prevention and treatment for osteoporosis? Osteoporos Int. 1997;7:1-6. PMID: 9102057

2. Raisz LG. The osteoporosis revolution. Ann Intern Med. 1997;126:458-62. PMID: 9072932

3. Ralston SH. Osteoporosis. BMJ. 1997;315:469-72. PMID: 9284669

## Back Pain Question 10
## Answer: E

**Educational Objective:** *Treat a patient early in the course of a herniated disc.*

This patient is early in the course of her back pain, and recovery can be expected in 1 or 2 weeks. The best treatment is to encourage activity with the help of analgesics. In young patients the absence of symptoms or signs suggesting infection or tumor, plain radiographs are of no use in evaluating acute low back pain. It is likely that they would be abnormal, even if the patient had no back pain. In one study, 64% of asymptomatic healthy volunteers between 20 and 70 years of age were found to have abnormalities (bulging of the disc, protrusion of the disc, and herniation of the disk being the most frequent findings) of the lumbar region of the spine when imaged by MRI. The frequency of abnormalities increased with age. An MRI would show the herniated disc and foraminal encroachment, but this expensive study should be reserved for patients in whom surgery is contemplated, and it should not be used as a screening test. Most herniated disks resolve with conservative treatment. There is no evidence that physical therapy hastens recovery, and some evidence suggests that bed rest hinders recovery.

### Bibliography

1. Malmivaara A, Hakkinen U, Aro T, Heinrichs ML, Koskenniemi L, Kuosma E, et al.The treatment of acute low back pain—bed rest, exercises, or ordinary activity? N Engl J Med. 1995;332:351-5. PMID: 7823996

2. Beurskens AJ, de Vet HC, Koke AJ, Regtop W, van der Heijden GJ, Lindeman E, Knipschild PG. Efficacy of traction for nonspecific low back pain. 12-week and 6-month results of a randomized clinical trial. Spine. 1997;22:2756-62. PMID: 9431610

3. Jensen MC, Brant-Zawadzki MN, Obuchowski N, Modic MT, Malkasian D, Ross JS. Magnetic resonance imaging of the lumbar spine in people without back pain. N Engl J Med. 1994;331:69-73. PMID: 8208267

## Back Pain Question 11
## Answer: B

**Educational Objective:** *Recognize inflammatory back pain and manage ankylosing spondyltis.*

His symptoms wake him at night and ameliorate with walking. These symptoms are characteristic of inflammatory back pain. The location of the pain deep in the gluteals suggests sacroiliac involvement. Ankylosing spondylitis most commonly presents in early adulthood with morning stiffness and lower back and gluteal pain. Up to half will have inflammation in the colon and 5-10% will have frank inflammatory bowel disease. Early disease may have normal range of motion, with progressive loss of lumbar flexion as the disease progresses.

Osteomyelitis, while insidious, is associated with fever, night sweats, and malaise and is uncommon in young men unless known to use IV drugs or have had a recent spinal tap. Lumbar strain would present acutely with decreased range of motion, tenderness of the paraspinal muscles and may be associated with trauma or overuse. While the pain of rheumatoid arthritis does improve with use, the joints most commonly involved are the small joints (especially of hands and wrists). Herniated discs will present most often with acute pain of a radicular nature, most commonly in the lower lumber dermatomes (L3-4, L4-5, L5-S1). Physical examination will be notable for a positive straight leg raise.

### Bibliography

1. Kerr HE, Sturrock RD.Clinical aspects, outcome assessment, disease course, and extra-articular features of spondyloarthropathies. Curr Opin Rheumatol. 1999;11:235-7. PMID: 10411375

**Back Pain Question 12**
**Answer: B**

**Educational Objective:** *Recognize the signs of spinal stenosis.*

Bony entrapment of lumbar roots from osteoarthritic disc degeneration is more common than herniation of the disc contents in patients older than 50 years of age. The symptoms of worsening pain with walking and relief with flexion, as in sitting or walking up hill, (pseudoclaudication) are characteristic of lumbar spinal stenosis. Ankylosing spondylitis and spondylolisthesis occur in patients who are much younger than age 66 years. Standing still for 1 to 2 minutes usually relieves pain from ischemic muscle (claudication), and the pulses in the feet are adequate. Spondylolisthesis might be one factor in spinal stenosis of the lumbar region, but most patients have other causes. Herniated disc is less likely given the negative straight leg raise. The reduced mobility in lumbar spine and advanced age increase the likelihood of degenerative arthritis in this patient.

**Bibliography**

1. **Katz JN, Dalgas M, Stucki G, Katz NP, Bayley J, Fossel AH, et al**. Degenerative lumbar spinal stenosis. Diagnostic value of the history and physical examination. Arthritis Rheum. 1995;38:1236-41. PMID: 7575718

2. **Fritz JM, Delitto A, Welch WC, Erhard RE**. Lumbar spinal stenosis: a review of current concepts in evaluation, management, and outcome measurements. Arch Phys Med Rehabil. 1998;79:700-8. PMID: 9630153

# Joint Disease

## Joint Disease Question 1
### Answer: C

**Educational Objective:** *Recognize that patients with hemoglobin SC disease have an increased frequency of aseptic necrosis of the humeral heads.*

Hemoglobin (Hb) SC disease resembles mild sickle cell anemia. Growth and development are normal, and life expectancy is only slightly decreased. However, patients with Hb SC disease may develop all of the vaso-occlusive complications that occur in patients with Hb SS anemia. Aseptic necrosis of the humeral head occurs more often in patients with Hb SC disease than in those with Hb SS anemia. The radiographic changes are characteristic of aseptic necrosis. Proliferative retinopathy also occurs frequently in patients with Hb SC disease. However, most patients with Hb SC disease do not develop acute chest syndrome, aplastic crises, stroke, or bone marrow infarction. Preservation of splenic function protects patients with Hb SC disease from overwhelming sepsis. Osteomyelitis does not frequently develop in patients with Hb SC disease.

### Bibliography

1. **Platt OS, Thorington BD, Brambilla DJ, Milner PF, Rosse WF, Vichinsky E, et al.** Pain in sickle cell disease. Rates and risk factors. N Engl J Med. 1991;325:11-6. PMID: 1710777
2. **Milner PF, Kraus AP, Sebes JI, Sleeper LA, Dukes KA, Embury SH, et al.** Sickle cell disease as a cause of osteonecrosis of the femoral head. N Engl J Med. 1991;325:1476-81. PMID: 1944426
3. **Zarkowsky HS, Gallagher D, Gill FM, Wang WC, Falletta JM, Lande WM, et al.** Bacteremia in sickle hemoglobinopathies. J Pediatr. 1986;109:579-85. PMID: 3531449

## Joint Disease Question 2
### Answer: E

**Educational Objective:** *Recognize the diagnostic criteria for acute rheumatic fever.*

The patient has two major criteria, carditis and subcutaneous nodules, for the diagnosis of acute rheumatic fever. Although the addition of other major criteria, such as choreoathetosis, erythema marginatum, or arthritis, strengthens the likelihood of the diagnosis, a definite diagnosis cannot be made without a positive throat culture for streptococci or a rise and fall in antistreptolysin-O titer. The presence of two or more of the Jones criteria can also be observed in other systemic diseases not due to streptococcal infection. A high erythrocyte sedimentation rate and first-degree atrioventricular block are findings that are not specific for acute rheumatic fever.

### Bibliography

1. **Ferrieri P**. Proceedings of the Jones Criteria workshop. Circulation. 2002;106:2521-3. PMID: 12417554
2. **Denny FW**. T. Duckett Jones and rheumatic fever in 1986. T. Duckett Jones Memorial Lecture. Circulation. 1987;76:963-70. PMID: 3311452
3. **Stollerman GH**. Rheumatogenic group A streptococci and the return of rheumatic fever. Adv Intern Med. 1990;35:1-25. PMID: 2405590

## Joint Disease Question 3
### Answer: A

**Educational Objective:** *Recognize Heberden's nodes of osteoarthritis, and distinguish it from other common forms of arthritis involving the hands.*

Heberden's nodes found in osteoarthritis are bony spurs at the dorsolateral and medial aspects of the distal interphalangeal joints that frequently result in flexor and lateral deviations of the distal phalanges. Heberden's nodes usually develop slowly over months to years, but in some patients the onset is rapid and associated with moderate to severe inflammatory changes.

Lesions mimicking osteoarthritis include rheumatoid arthritis, scleroderma, psoriatic arthritis, and gout. Rheumatoid arthritis is associated with swelling of the proximal interphalangeal and metacarpophalangeal joints. The distal interphalangeal joints are rarely involved. Scleroderma is characterized by puffy fingers; shiny, tense, and indurated skin; and absence of normal skin folds. The proximal interphalangeal joints can be inflamed, and flexion contractures are common. Numerous telangiectasias are present on the fingers, and vascular infarctions develop in the late stages. Patients with psoriatic arthritis have swelling and deformity of the distal interphalangeal joints. However, these findings are associated with nail and, usually, skin findings. The nail changes include discoloration, pitting, and lifting of the distal nail plate from the nail bed. The skin findings consist of a thick, silvery scale on a discrete red plaque. Gout can cause acute inflammation and swelling of a joint, but the distal interphalangeal joint is an uncommon site, especially for an initial attack.

### Bibliography

1. **Peat G, Croft P, Hay E**.Clinical assessment of the osteoarthritis patient. Best Pract Res Clin Rheumatol. 2001;15:527-44. PMID: 11567537

## Joint Disease Question 4
## Answer: A

**Educational Objective:** *Recognize the typical radiographic appearance of osteoarthritis of the hands and wrists.*

As is typical of osteoarthritis, the arthritic involvement shown in the radiograph is predominant in the first carpometacarpal joints, the proximal interphalangeal (PIP) joints, and the distal interphalangeal (DIP) joints and is characterized by joint space narrowing, sclerosis, and osteophyte formation. This patient's hand films show generalized osteopenia that is not increased about the involved joints, as would occur with rheumatoid arthritis. Patients with rheumatoid arthritis would be unlikely to have involvement of the DIP joints and the first carpometacarpal joints, and osteophyte formation would not occur in affected joints. Osteoarthritis may often cause obvious, firm enlargement of the DIP joints (Heberden's nodes) and the PIP joints (Bouchard's nodes); these nodes correspond to the areas of osteophyte formation. This patient has an inflammatory variant of osteoarthritis of the hands that is most common in middle-aged or elderly women and tends to run in families.

X-rays are not usually diagnostic during an initial attack of gout, but show only soft tissue swelling around the affected joint. In chronic gout, intrarticular or periarticular erosions can occur. These are round or oval in shape and have sclerotic margins.

The x-ray features of psoriatic arthritis include DIP erosive disease, which can evolve into terminal whittling of the interphalangeal joints and a "pencil in the cup" appearance.

**Bibliography**
1. **Swagerty DL Jr, Hellinger D**.Radiographic assessment of osteoarthritis. Am Fam Physician. 2001;64;279-86. PMID: 11476273

## Joint Disease Question 5
## Answer: A

**Educational Objective:** *Recognize the typical radiologic changes of rheumatoid arthritis involving the hands and wrists.*

The radiologic changes associated with rheumatoid arthritis are characteristically symmetric, as in this patient. As shown, the distal interphalangeal (DIP) joints are typically spared; the most severely affected areas are the carpal bones, metacarpophalangeal (MCP) joints, and proximal interphalangeal (PIP) joints. Associated findings include periarticular osteopenia (best appreciated in the MCP joints), soft-tissue swelling (best seen in the second and third PIP joints), widespread joint space narrowing, and marginal erosions (most prominent in the second MCP joints). Patients with advanced rheumatoid arthritis may develop ulnar deviation at the MCP

joints and both boutonnière deformities (flexion of the PIP joint and extension of the DIP joint) and swan-neck deformities (extension of the PIP joint and flexion of the DIP joint).

Rheumatoid arthritis has its peak incidence between the fourth and sixth decades of life and is about 2.5 times more common in women than in men. Morning stiffness in and around joints that lasts for more than 30 minutes is so typical of active rheumatoid arthritis that it is an important clue to the diagnosis.

The x-ray changes in osteoarthritis are prominent in the PIP and DIP joints and are characterized by joint space narrowing, sclerosis, and osteophyte formation.

X-rays are not usually diagnostic during an initial attack of gout, but show only soft tissue swelling around the affected joint. In chronic gout, intrarticular or periarticular erosions can occur. These are round or oval in shape and have sclerotic margins.

The x-ray features of psoriatic arthritis include DIP erosive disease, which can evolve into terminal whittling of the interphalangeal joints and a "pencil in the cup" appearance.

**Bibliography**
1. **Taouli B, Guermazi A, Sack KE, Genant HK**. Imaging of the hand and wrist in RA. Ann Rheum Dis. 2002;61:867-9. PMID: 12228153

## Joint Disease Question 6
## Answer: C

**Educational Objective:** *Recognize the clinical manifestations of Reiter's syndrome.*

Inflammatory oligoarticular arthritis in the setting of previous or intercurrent nongonococcal urethritis and/or conjunctivitis is characteristic of patients with Reiter's syndrome. It is important to recognize that the majority of patients with this disorder present with just one or two features of the clinical triad of urethritis, conjunctivitis, and inflammatory arthritis, with fewer than one third of patients developing all three manifestations during the course of the disease. Mucocutaneous manifestations of Reiter's syndrome that may aid in diagnosis include oral ulcers (which are typically painless), keratoderma of the soles, circinate balanitis, and nail dystrophy. Periostitis, Achilles tendinitis, and peri-insertional osteoporosis at ligamentous and tendinous attachment sites are enthesopathic features of Reiter's syndrome. As is the case with other seronegative spondyloarthropathies, increased titers of circulating rheumatoid factors are typically not present in patients with Reiter's syndrome; however, some patients may present with low titer of antinuclear antibodies.

Gout is unlikely because the synovial fluid is negative for crystals. The absence of rheumatoid factor, the asymmetrical involvement of the joints, and keratotic skin changes make rheumatoid arthritis unlikely. The highly inflammatory nature of the effusion and involvement of fingers and foot make osteonecrosis unlikely. Despite the low titer of antinuclear antibody, there are no other manifestations of systemic lupus erythematosus. In addition, the previous history of nongonococcal urethritis most strongly supports a diagnosis of Reiter's syndrome.

### Bibliography

1. **Arnett FC.** Seronegative spondyloarthropathies. Bull Rheum Dis. 1987;37:1-12. PMID: 3326644
2. **Willkens RF, Arnett FC, Bitter T, Calin A, Fisher L, Ford DK, et al.** Reiter's syndrome. Evaluation of preliminary criteria for definite disease. Arthritis Rheum. 1981;24:844-9. PMID: 7247978

## Joint Disease Question 7
### Answer: C

**Educational Objective:** *Recognize the clinical manifestations of late-stage Lyme disease.*

This patient has late-stage Lyme disease and the appropriate diagnostic test is enzyme-linked immunosorbent assay (ELISA) for antibody to *Borrelia burgdorferi*. The patient did not recall tick exposure and did not observe erythema chronicum migrans; however, approximately 20% to 40% of patients do not experience or observe the rash. Although erythema chronicum migrans is classically a huge, annular erythematous eruption, it is occasionally much more subtle and can escape detection. Inguinal adenopathy with constitutional symptoms is very nonspecific; however, it is the hallmark of early localized (stage I) Lyme disease. Disseminated infection (stage II) usually develops within days to weeks of inoculation and may be manifested by arthralgia, transient arthritis, central nervous system involvement (typically cranial neuropathies, meningoencephalitis, and radiculoneuropathies), and cardiac dysfunction (typically myopericarditis and atrioventricular block). At this point in time, ELISA for antibodies to *Borrelia burgdorferi* should be positive. Because this patient fits the clinical description of disseminated (stage II) Lyme disease with central nervous system involvement (meningitis), intravenous ceftriaxone would be the best therapy. Glucocorticoids may be administered in conjunction with antibiotics in some cases of refractory cardiac rhythm abnormalities.

The remaining options for this question are diagnostic tests in support of rheumatoid arthritis, systemic lupus erythematosus, ankylosing spondylosing, and acute rheumatic fever. None of these conditions evolves in a pattern similar to Lyme disease, and are all unlikely causes of the patient's symptoms.

### Bibliography

1. **Steere AC.** Lyme disease. N Engl J Med. 1989;321:586-96. PMID: 2668764

## Joint Disease Question 8
### Answer: B

**Educational Objective:** *Recognize the clinical presentation of gout.*

This patient clearly has tophaceous gout and is being crippled from the chronic arthritis and accumulation of tophi in and around his joints.

This patient does not have rheumatoid arthritis. Tophaceous gout can mimic the exact clinical appearance of rheumatoid arthritis, with symmetrical joint involvement, synovial thickening, and subcutaneous nodules. Arthrocentesis, serum uric acid level, or biopsy of a nodule is necessary to exclude tophaceous gout in a patient with suspected rheumatoid arthritis. Sometimes however, the chalky material extruding from the nodules is highly suggestive of gout.

Synovial thickening is not a feature of osteoarthritis or osteonecrosis, and, like systemic lupus erythomatosus, these conditions are not associated with multiple subcutaneous nodules.

### Bibliography

1. **Weselman KO, Agudelo CA.** Gout Basics. Bull Rheum Dis. 2001;50:1-3. PMID: 12092090

## Joint Disease Question 9
### Answer: D

**Educational Objective:** *Recognize hyperuricemia associated with cyclosporine therapy.*

Cyclosporine results in hyperuricemia in many transplant patients, some of whom develop clinical gout. Cyclosporine decreases the filtration of uric acid and interferes with the secretion of uric acid in the renal tubules. Some patients require therapy to lower serum uric acid. Allopurinol is usually the drug of choice among transplant physicians because of the fear of injuring the transplanted kidney with the increased uric acid excretion, which would occur with uricosuric agents. Prednisone is not usually a major cause of hyperuricemia, although it can induce a catabolic state.

Hyperoxalemia and hyperphosphatemia are very unusual in transplant patients unless the graft fails, and this patient's renal function is normal. Hypercalcemia with a normally functioning graft is unusual, but it could be induced with vitamin D supplementation. Moreover, the crystals shown on arthrocentesis are typical of monosodium urate crystals, not calcium oxalate, calcium pyrophosphate, or basic calcium phosphate.

### Bibliography

1. **Lin HY, Rocher LL, McQuillan MA, Schmaltz S, Palella TD, Fox IH.** Cyclosporin-induced hyperuricemia and gout. N Engl J Med. 1989;321:287-92. PMID: 2664517

## Joint Disease Question 10
## Answer: E

**Educational Objective:** *Make the diagnosis of lateral epicondylitis of the elbow ("tennis elbow").*

No further testing is necessary. This woman has lateral epicondylitis of the elbow, commonly referred to as "tennis elbow." This is a clinical diagnosis that depends on the complaint of localized pain made worse by wrist extension, point tenderness, and an absence of signs of limitation of motion or inflammation of the joints of the elbow. Lateral epicondylitis is common in middle-aged persons and is believed to be due to overuse of relatively weak forearm muscles. Only a small minority of cases of lateral epicondylitis can be attributed to playing tennis. Treatment of the disorder consists of application of ice, nonsteroidal anti-inflammatory drugs, local steroid injection, use of a forearm brace or isometric exercises to strengthen the forearm.

A rheumatoid factor is useful only when rheumatoid arthritis is suspected clinically. This woman's case has nothing to suggest rheumatoid arthritis, which typically presents with symmetric polyarthritis and morning stiffness. Because the patient has no evidence of a systemic collagen vascular disease (fever, skin lesions, arthritis, muscle weakness, neurologic disease, serositis, etc.), testing for antinuclear antibodies (ANA) is not appropriate. The erythrocyte sedimentation rate (ESR) is used as an index of inflammation, and the absence of local swelling, heat, or redness, along with the lack of systemic involvement, makes inflammation unlikely. A radiograph of the elbow is not indicated with no history of trauma, normal range of motion, and a picture consistent with the clinical diagnosis of lateral epicondylitis.

### Bibliography

1. **Foley AE**. Tennis elbow. Am Fam Physician. 1993;48:281-8. PMID: 8342481
2. **Kamien M**. A rational management of tennis elbow. Sports Med. 1990;9:173-91. PMID: 2180031

## Joint Disease Question 11
## Answer: B

**Educational Objective:** *Recognize hemochromatosis and recall its systemic complications.*

This patient has hemochromatosis, which can cause cirrhosis. The arthropathy of chondrocalcinosis may take many forms. It may be asymptomatic; it may resemble osteoarthritis with gradually increasing pain and deformity, differing only by its predilection for wrists and metacarpophalangeal joints; it may involve acute attacks of inflammation (pseudogout); or it may consist of a destructive arthropathy such as that seen in neuropathic joint disease. Chondrocalcinosis is most commonly idiopathic but may be associated with a number of metabolic diseases, including hyperparathyroidism and hemochromatosis. In this patient's case, the elevated iron saturation (serum iron/iron binding capacity > 55%) and the elevated plasma glucose are clues to the presence of hemochromatosis. Hemochromatosis is a hereditary condition characterized by excessive iron stores. It usually affects white men and presents between 40 and 60 years of age. Complaints of joint pain may be the initial sign of this condition. If untreated, hemochromatosis can cause diabetes, cirrhosis, hyperpigmentation of the skin, gonadal failure, and restrictive cardiomyopathy. The incidence of hepatocellular carcinoma is increased in patients with hemochromatosis and cirrhosis. All first-degree relatives of persons with hemochromatosis should be screened with serum ferritin concentration and fasting transferrin. In addition, because hemochromatosis is relatively common in white populations, many authorities recommend screening all white men with osteoarthritis.

Uveitis, nephrolithiasis, interstitial lung disease, and colitis are all seen in diseases that also feature arthritis but are not found in hemochromatosis.

### Bibliography

1. **Rull M**. Calcium crystal-associated diseases and miscellaneous crystals. Curr Opin Rheumatol. 1997;9:274-9. PMID: 9204266
2. **Edwards CQ, Kushner JP**. Screening for hemochromatosis. N Engl J Med. 1993;328:1616-20. PMID: 8110209

## Joint Disease Question 12
## Answer: B

**Educational Objective:** *Know the differential diagnosis of painful knee conditions.*

The anserine bursa, one of the 12 knee bursae, is interposed between the medial collateral ligament and the tendinous portions of the sartorius, gracilis, and semitendinous muscles, 3 to 4 cm below the tibial plateau. Of the 12 bursae, inflammation of the anserine bursa is said to be the most commonly found clinically and is often associated with osteoarthritis of the knees. Treatment consists of local corticosteroid injection and physiotherapy.

Pseudogout would show acute inflammatory arthritis and evidence of chondrocalcinosis on radiographic examination of the knee.

The knee would be an usual initial presentation of gout. It would present as an inflammatory arthritis, and the pain would be localized to the joint, not below the joint.

Osteochondritis dissecans would be seen on radiograph as a clearly demarcated sclerotic area of bone surrounded by radiolucency. The sclerotic area is located at an articular surface and may be completely detached from the surface, showing up as a loose body. Osteochondritis dissecans occurs most commonly at the distal femur of young men. It is thought to be a form of osteonecrosis.

Bibliography

1. **Reveille JD**. Soft-tissue rheumatism: diagnosis and treatment. Am J Med. 1997;102(1A):23S-29S. PMID: 9217556

## Joint Disease Question 13
## Answer: B

**Educational Objective:** *Correctly diagnose crystal-induced diseases.*

This elderly woman suffers from typical manifestations of the Milwaukee shoulder-knee syndrome. Milwaukee shoulder-knee syndrome is a form of basic calcium phosphate (BCP) disease (hydroxyapatite disease) characterized by destructive arthritis of the shoulder and knees and the presence of BCP crystals in synovial fluid. This syndrome is most common in elderly women. Tears of the rotator cuff often accompany this condition, and the movement of the humeral head superiorly toward the acromion strongly suggests rotator cuff pathology. Arthrocentesis should be performed and will reveal BCP crystals, which are usually amorphous and nonrefringent on polarized microscopy.

Frozen shoulder is associated with a tightening and thickening of the joint capsule (adhesive capsulitis) and with a decreased active and passive range of motion. Radiographs are usually normal. Causes of frozen shoulder include disuse, inflammatory conditions, trauma, and reflex sympathetic dystrophy, among others.

Calcium pyrophosphate dihydrate deposition (CPDD) disease may be associated with a generalized destructive form of osteoarthritis. Synovial fluid is characterized by weakly positively birefringent crystals in rods and rhomboids. The pattern of joint involvement and the absence of typical crystals make this diagnosis unlikely.

Tophaceous gout may induce a generalized destructive arthropathy, but tophaceous gout is unusual in women. Synovial fluid in gout would be characterized by sodium urate crystals that are needle-shaped and strongly negatively birefringent. Sodium urate crystals are not present in this patient's synovial fluids.

Reflex sympathetic dystrophy may induce a chronic pain syndrome characterized by a frozen shoulder and erosive changes after injury or immobilization. Reflex sympathetic dystrophy is not characterized by the presence of synovial fluid crystals.

Bibliography

1. **Fam AG**. Calcium pyrophosphate crystal deposition disease and other crystal deposition diseases. Curr Opin Rheumatol. 1992;4:574-82. PMID: 1503884
2. **Agudelo CA, Wise CM.** Crystal-associated arthritis in the elderly. Rheum Dis Clin North Am. 2000;26:527-46. PMID: 10989511

## Joint Disease Question 14
## Answer: A

**Educational Objective:** *Diagnose cervical spine instability in a patient with rheumatoid arthritis.*

The physician should immediately consider the possibility of cervical spine disease in any patient with long-standing rheumatoid arthritis who has lost the ability to walk. More than half of patients with rheumatoid arthritis for more than 10 years will show evidence of cervical spine involvement, and some of these patients may exhibit frank instability. This is particularly relevant to this patient's care because she will undergo general anesthesia requiring intubation. If the neck films do reveal instability of the cervical spine, she may require nasotracheal intubation or stabilization before her elective surgery (or at least special care during anesthesia).

Parenchymal lung involvement is common in patients with rheumatoid arthritis; however, preoperative pulmonary function testing is most appropriate for those patients with pulmonary symptoms or evidence of lung involvement on physical examination.

Uveitis and Sjögren's syndrome are complications of rheumatoid arthritis but do not pose a surgical risk, provided that adequate lubrication of the eyes is provided to patients with Sjögren's syndrome.

Bibliography

1. **Halla JT, Hardin JG, Vitek J, Alarcon GS**. Involvement of the cervical spine in rheumatoid arthritis. Arthritis Rheum. 1989;32:652-9. PMID: 2655607
2. **Nakano KK, Schoene WC, Baker RA, Dawson DM**. The cervical myelopathy associated with rheumatoid arthritis: analysis of 32 patients, with two postmortem cases. Ann Neurol. 1978;3:144-51. PMID: 655664

## Joint Disease Question 15
## Answer: D

**Educational Objective:** *Recognize the clinical manifestations of Sjögren's syndrome.*

Sjögren's syndrome is characterized by parotid enlargement, xerostomia, and rheumatoid arthritis.

Sjögren's syndrome is rare in men, with a female to male ratio of 10:1. Anti-Ro (anti-SSA) and anti-La (anti-SSB) autoantibodies are present in 60% to 70% of the patients. These autoantibodies are not specific for Sjögren's syndrome; they may also occur in a subsets of patients with systemic lupus erythematosus and in asymptomatic women.

The syndrome of dry eyes, parotid gland enlargement and arthritis is not found in systemic lupus erythematosus, lymphoma, or sarcoidosis.

Bibliography

1. **Manoussakis MN, Moutsopoulos HM**. Sjögren's Syndrome: current concepts. Adv Intern Med. 2001;47:191-217. PMID: 11795075

## Joint Disease Question 16
## Answer: D

**Educational Objective:** *Correctly manage a patient with gout.*

This man has a presumptive diagnosis of gout on the basis of gouty-like attacks involving the typical joints affected by gout and the presence of a significantly elevated serum uric acid. This diagnosis should be confirmed with an arthrocentesis and synovial fluid analysis when the joint is acutely swollen. Because he has had only one gouty attack per month, he would be considered to have acute gout, not intercritical gout or tophaceous gout. Because of the markedly elevated uric acid level, this patient would be at risk for the development of chronic tophaceous gout, and a 24-hour urine test for uric acid excretion should be done to determine if he is an over-producer or underexcretor. A 24-hour urine collection for calculation of the amount of uric acid excreted is necessary to determine if uricosuric agents or allopurinol may be necessary. A patient who is a significant overproducer (greater than 1000 mg uric acid/24 h) is at an increased risk for uric acid nephrolithiasis, and allopurinol therapy should be considered. For underexcretors, uricosuric agents are preferable.

Allopurinol is very effective for the chronic treatment of hyperuricemia and gout. Unfortunately, allopurinol can induce serious toxicities and even death. Allopurinol therapy should be reserved for overproducers (overexcretors) of uric acid, patients with uric acid nephrolithiasis, patients with uric acid nephropathy, and patients who cannot tolerate uricosuric agents.

Colchicine is very effective for the treatment of gout, but it can induce adverse reactions. Colchicine may be administered in high doses for an acute attack or in low doses to prevent gout recurrence. An excellent response to colchicine during an acute attack in a patient with hyperuricemia is good presumptive evidence for the presence of gout. This patient, however, does not require high-dose colchicine at the time of his visit. Low-dose prophylactic colchicine (0.5 to 0.6 mg twice daily) may prevent acute gouty attacks and would be an option for this patient but would not prevent uric acid kidney stones. Colchicine may also be effective in patients with pseudogout.

Arthrocentesis is necessary for the definitive diagnosis of gout. However, in asymptomatic joints without effusion, the yield of both fluid and crystals is considerably less.

Corticosteroid injections are not indicated in an asymptomatic joint.

The patient could be observed to determine if the attacks become more frequent. However, if he were a significant overproducer, he would be at risk of spontaneous obstruction and secondary infection from uric acid nephrolithiasis.

### Bibliography

1. **Terkeltaub RA**. Gout and mechanisms of crystal-induced inflammation. Curr Opin Rheumatol. 1993;5:510-6. PMID: 8357747

## Joint Disease Question 17
## Answer: A

**Educational Objective:** *Diagnose and treat disseminated gonococcal infection.*

Ceftriaxone should be begun for the presumptive diagnosis of disseminated gonococcal infection (DGI). Penicillin is no longer recommended because of the prevalence of penicillinase-producing *Neisseria gonorrhoeae*. Although the precise diagnosis cannot be made from the information given, there are a number of features suggesting that this patient has DGI. The apparent early tendinitis with subsequent monoarthritis or oligoarthritis is classic for DGI. Onset during menses is also typical, and a sparse vesiculopapular or pustular rash (often unnoticed by the patient) is often present.

Adult-onset Still's disease (which could be treated with high-dose aspirin) can cause a rash and fever as well as arthritis, but the fever is usually higher, the rash a salmon-colored (in Caucasians), maculopapular, evanescent eruption, and the joint involvement less prominent. Rheumatic fever (also treated with high-dose aspirin) is possible, but there is no history of preceding pharyngitis, and the rash does not sound like erythema marginatum, which is macular, circinate, and often most obvious on the trunk. Inflammatory bowel disease (for which sulfasalazine may be used) can be accompanied by arthritis and dermatologic changes, but she has no bowel complaints, and without further studies, it does not seem reasonable to make this diagnosis. Systemic lupus erythematosus and other inflammatory arthritides common in women of this age (which would respond to prednisone) might be considered, but the rash is not typical for lupus, no serologic testing has been done, and it is irresponsible to treat with prednisone until an infection has been considered. There is no reason to suspect a gluten-sensitive enteropathy in this patient, even one associated with dermatitis herpetiformis. Neither condition is associated with arthritis. The case presents little to suggest malabsorption, and the rash of dermatitis herpetiformis consists of a group of vesicles about 3 to 10 mm in diameter often associated with evidence of excoriation.

### Bibliography

1. **Scopelitis E, Martinez-Osuna P**. Gonococcal arthritis. Rheum Dis Clin North Am. 1993;19:363-77. PMID: 8502777
2. **Hawley HB**. Gonorrhea. Finding and treating a moving target. Postgrad Med. 1993;94:105-11. PMID: 8341619

## Joint Disease Question 18
## Answer: E

**Educational Objective:** *Diagnose giant cell arteritis.*

This patient has symptoms of polymyalgia rheumatica. Evidence on the physical examination (fever and arthritis) as well as laboratory evidence (elevated erythrocyte sedimentation rate) point to a generalized inflammatory process. Giant cell arteritis may be present in up to 30% of patients with polymyalgia rheumatica. The presence of jaw pain on chewing (jaw claudication) suggests the presence of giant cell arteritis. Patients with polymyalgia rheumatica who have jaw claudication, headaches, scalp tenderness, or visual symptoms have a greater likelihood of concomitant giant cell arteritis.

The onset of systemic lupus erythematosus in a 73-year-old person would be unusual and jaw claudication is not part of that disease. The muscle aching, stiffness, and weight loss are not seen in gout. Polyarteritis nodosa is an uncommon condition that usually presents with fever and weight loss. Usually a particular organ or organs may become involved and the resulting manifestations include skin rash, peripheral neuropathy, polyarthritis, or renal sediment abnormalities. Arthralgias and arthritis is usually asymmetric, episodic, and nondeforming. The patient's symptoms do not match this syndrome.

While patients with rheumatoid arthritis do present with proximal, symmetrical joint invlovment, the presence of jaw claudication and an erythrocyte sedimentation rate of over 100 mm/h make this diagnosis unlikely.

**Bibliography**

1. **Hunder GG, Bloch DA, Michel BA, Stevens MB, Arend WP, Calabrese LH, et al**. The American College of Rheumatology 1990 criteria for the classification of giant cell arteritis. Arthritis Rheum. 1990;33:1122-8. PMID: 2202311
2. **Salvarani C, Cantini F, Boiardi L, Hunder GG**. Polymyalgia rheumatica and giant-cell arteritis. N Engl J Med. 2002;347:261-71. PMID: 12140303

## Joint Disease Question 19
## Answer: C

**Educational Objective:** *Properly manage a patient with a septic joint that does not respond to appropriate antibiotic therapy.*

The management of septic arthritis requires the administration of an appropriate antibiotic and frequent drainage of fluid and debris from the joint. In most cases, the latter can be performed by closed drainage of the joint using a large-bore needle. The response to treatment should be monitored by serial assessment of the synovial fluid leukocyte count, reaccumulation of effusion, pain in the joint, and joint motion. Persistent pain and swelling associated with failure of the synovial fluid leukocyte count to decrease significantly during the initial week of treatment indicate a suboptimal therapeutic response. When symptoms have been present for a number of days before beginning treatment, loculated foci of infection within the joint may account for failure to respond to appropriate antibiotics and closed drainage. In such cases, arthroscopic debridement of the joint can expedite recovery and improve the functional outcome.

Changing to another antibiotic or increasing the dose of the current antibiotic is not indicated and would be ineffective without adequate joint drainage.

Continuing current therapy when that therapy has proved ineffective is inappropriate. A "wait-and-see" approach is ill advised in this setting.

**Bibliography**

1. **Esterhai JL Jr, Gelb I**. Adult septic arthritis. Orthop Clin North Am. 1991;22:503-14. PMID: 1852426
2. **Lane JG, Falahee MH, Wojtys EM, Hankins FM, Kaufer H**. Pyarthrosis of the knee. Treatment considerations. Clin Orthop. 1990;252:198-204. PMID: 2302885

## Joint Disease Question 20
## Answer: B

**Educational Objective:** *Differentiate between polymyalgia rheumatica and temporal arteritis.*

This patient has classic signs of polymyalgia rheumatica, with profound limb girdle stiffness, anemia, and an elevated erythrocyte sedimentation rate. He does not have symptoms of temporal arteritis such as visual loss, headache, scalp tenderness, jaw claudication, or cough, and there is no tenderness or beading of the temporal arteries. Although some patients with polymyalgia rheumatica develop temporal arteritis, this patient's current management should focus on polymyalgia rheumatica, and nonsteroidal anti-inflammatory drugs or low-dose prednisone may be beneficial. As a diagnostic test, however, marked improvement after a short course—sometimes 1 day of prednisone, 15 mg—is characteristic of polymyalgia rheumatica. Thus, treating this patient with prednisone is the best approach. Chest radiography may show a lung malignancy, but this is unlikely in patients who do not smoke. If NSAIDs were necessary, the cyclooxygenase-2 specific NSAIDs such as celecoxib or rofecoxib are safer in elderly patients, who have an increased risk of upper gastrointestinal bleeding.

**Bibliography**

1. **Salvarani C, Cantini F, Boiardi L, Hunder GG**.Polymyalgia rheumatica and giant-cell arteritis. N Engl J Med. 2002;347:261-71. PMID: 12140303

## Joint Disease Question 21
## Answer: B

**Educational Objective:** *Recognize the ramifications of hyperuricemia and the indications for its treatment.*

Although not unique to gout, podagra is a classic first feature of monosodium urate crystal disease (gout). Podagra can also be seen in calcium pyrophosphate dihydrate deposition disease (CPPD), trauma, and sarcoidosis, as well. Even though no fluid was aspirated, and there is no proof that this patient has gout, the history is compatible with that diagnosis. Multiple episodes of podagra suggest more attacks in the future are likely; therefore, prophylaxis is necessary.

Short-term nonsteroidal anti-inflammatory drugs (NSAIDs) could be prescribed for each flare, but this patient has stated that the attacks are agonizing, so that prevention rather than treatment is necessary. NSAIDs also predispose patients to ulcers and bleeding and may worsen his underlying renal dysfunction. Daily colchicine has been used in patients for prophylaxis, but it has fallen out of favor because of its remarkable potential toxicity to the bone marrow. In a patient with renal failure probenecid, a uricosuric agent, would be less effective prophylaxis. Thus, allopurinol should be used with titration so that a normal uric acid level can be reached. The usual dose needed is 300 mg/d, although this should be decreased in the presence of significant renal failure. It should be started well after the last attack has subsided and with NSAID coverage in order to avoid a drug-induced flare. When started during a flare or while the flare is resolving, polyarticular gout can be precipitated by the addition of allopurinol.

Patients with gout are predisposed to renal calculus formation, and the higher the urinary excretion of uric acid the greater, the likelihood of stone formation. In such patients, therapy with probenecid should not be used.

**Bibliography**

1. **Weselman KO, Agudelo CA.**Gout basics. Bull Rheum Dis. 2001;50:1-3. PMID: 12092090

## Joint Disease Question 22
## Answer: B

**Educational Objective:** *Appreciate the causes, proper evaluation, and potential long-term outcomes of ankle injuries.*

Examination of an acutely injured ankle can be difficult because of pain and swelling. A reasonable approach is to apply ice, use nonsteroidal anti-inflammatory drugs (NSAIDs) acutely, and proceed to bracing and weightbearing as soon as possible; this regimen minimizes disability related to the injury. In all likelihood, this woman has sprained her ankle. Ankle sprain is the most common sports injury, especially in basketball players, who may land on an opponent's foot or on the lateral aspect of their foot after jumping and excessively invert an ankle. This patient sprained her lateral ankle ligament complex. The prognosis of such injuries, if they are mild and not recurrent, is excellent, with no long-term instability.

Stress radiography and arthrography may be necessary to define the degree of injury, but they are not needed immediately unless there is a complete tear of one of the talofibular ligaments or the calcaneofibular ligament is torn. These more serious injuries should be suspected if there is ecchymosis, tenderness of the anterolateral ankle, an anterior drawer sign, or other evidence of instability of the ankle. Occasionally, anesthesia is needed in order to do these tests. At the time of the initial evaluation, anteroposterior, lateral, and mortise views of the ankle are necessary to evaluate possible distal fibula

and/or medial malleolus fractures. Likewise, fracture of the talar dome or tibial plafond can be evaluated by plain film.

There is no role for injection of glucocorticoids or casting and splinting at this time.

**Bibliography**

1. **Klenerman L.** The management of sprained ankle. J Bone Joint Surg Br. 1998 Jan;80:11-2. PMID: 9460944
2. **Rubin A, Sallis R.** Evaluation and diagnosis of ankle injuries. Am Fam Physician. 1996;54:1609-18. PMID: 8857783

## Joint Disease Question 23
## Answer: D

**Educational Objective:** *Appreciate the differential diagnosis of acute febrile migratory polyarthritis.*

This woman has a migratory polyarthritis of recent onset. Important diseases to consider in the differential diagnosis of this problem include gonococcal, HIV, *Borrelia burgdorferi*, and viral infections, subacute bacterial endocarditis, and acute rheumatic fever. Adolescent patients should be interviewed without their parents being present to obtain an accurate history that might contain information that the son or daughter does not want the parent to know. When the patient was interviewed without her mother being present, she later said that she was taking oral contraceptives and had at least three sexual partners in the 3 months preceding her visit. She also said that she is not always insistent that her partners use condoms.

In this woman's age group, gonococcal infection would be the most likely organism as the cause of an infectious arthritis. The skin lesions in this case most resemble those seen in the disseminated gonococcal infection syndrome. Their focal nature and evolution into pustules is classic for a satellite lesion in disseminated gonococcal infection. Most cases of disseminated gonococcal infection result from a recent sexual exposure, and in many women the primary gonococcal infection (oral, anal, or genital) may be asymptomatic. Anal, oral, and pharyngeal swabs should be done to culture for gonococcus. Thayer-Martin medium was designed for use in plating cervical specimens. It contains antibiotics to suppress overgrowth of the culture by vaginal flora; thus, it would not be the most appropriate medium for culture of synovial fluid or the material in a pustule, which has no normal flora. It is also not optimum for anal or throat swabs, but no other medium has been proved superior. When trying to grow gonococcus, it is important to plate all specimens rapidly and grow them at a high concentration of $CO_2$, usually by use of a candle jar. All patients with gonococcal infection should be screened for other venereal infections, especially HIV and syphilis. Treatment for possible *Chlamydia* should accompany intravenous ceftriaxone treatment of the arthritis in this patient.

*Neisseria meningitidis* can also cause a syndrome resembling disseminated gonococcal infection. In such patients, there may be a preceding or accompanying mild upper respiratory syndrome. Petechial lesions on the trunk, lower extremities, or mucosae suggest an alternative diagnosis.

Patients with an acute HIV infection can present with a migratory arthritis, and HIV serologies should be obtained. If further history reveals evidence of unprotected sexual activity, counseling may be warranted.

Subacute bacterial endocarditis can present as a polyarthritis, occasionally with necrotic skin lesions. Isolation of gonococcus from the blood in the disseminated gonococcal infection syndrome is unusual, and blood cultures are usually negative. In the absence of a history of risk factors for the development of bacterial endocarditis, this diagnosis remains distinctly unlikely, but should be excluded nonetheless, given the potential consequences of missing it.

Hepatitis B virus or C virus infection can cause vasculitis and acute migratory polyarthritis, but this occurs in the pre-icteric phase. The skin lesions are usually urticarial or maculopapular rather than pustular. The onset of joint pain is usually rapid and is generally symmetric, with a simultaneous or additive onset. Liver function tests may be mildly abnormal during the phase of joint inflammation, but these results may not be diagnostic of hepatitis virus infection. Antigenemia may be absent early in infection, but blood testing for the presence of hepatitis B and C virus infection might be helpful if gonococcus had not yet been isolated from a body fluid or a pustule.

Viral arthritis such as that seen in parvovirus infection, is more commonly bilaterally symmetric and presents in a pattern similar to rheumatoid arthritis. Arthralgia is more prominent than true inflammatory joint disease.

Acute rheumatic fever is associated with erythema marginatum rather than pustules and usually affects the large joints, especially the knees, ankles, elbows, and wrists, in a migratory pattern associated with an acute febrile illness. One third or more of patients do not have or recall an upper respiratory infection within the preceding month. Thus, this patient's syndrome is not strongly suggestive of acute rheumatic fever, but throat culture for streptococcus (as well as gonococcus) and an antistreptolysin-O assay would be reasonable if gonococcus is not isolated early in the evaluation.

The skin lesions seen in this case make Lyme arthritis much less likely. The pattern of joint disease in early Lyme disease is a migratory polyarthritis (seen in over 50% of patients with untreated early disease), but the large knee effusion, common in later manifestations of this infection, would be unusual in such an early stage of *Borrelia burgdorferi* infection. It would be appropriate to obtain serological studies to test for serum antibodies to *B. burgdorferi* in such a case.

Poststreptococcal reactive arthritis may represent an incomplete form of rheumatic fever. The joint inflammation is classically described as being additive, as opposed to the migratory pattern seen in the current case. The prognosis is excellent.

Safe sex techniques should be discussed with this patient before she leaves the office.

### Bibliography

1. **Pinals RS**. Polyarthritis and fever. N Engl J Med. 1994;330:769-74. PMID: 8107744

## Joint Disease Question 24
## Answer: D

**Educational Objective:** *Perform arthrocentesis in a patient taking anticoagulant agents when the synovial fluid findings are likely to influence management.*

This patient has an acute synovitis in the left knee superimposed on chronic osteoarthritis. The differential diagnosis includes hemarthrosis owing to anticoagulation, crystal-induced arthritis, septic arthritis, reactive arthritis, and traumatic arthritis, or internal derangement because of overuse. Synovial fluid analysis is the most direct approach to diagnosis and should not be avoided or postponed because the patient is taking an anticoagulant agent. There is often a concern that arthrocentesis may provoke or exacerbate intrarticular bleeding, but a recent study found that bleeding did not occur after aspirations in 25 patients taking warfarin. Another report of 28 patients confirmed these findings.

Treating without a diagnosis could result in unnecessary costs, exposure to medications that might have harmful effects, and delay in initiating the appropriate treatment. If the patient has septic arthritis, there would be increased risk of irreversible joint damage. MRI may reveal a torn meniscus or fracture and might be indicated if the joint fluid is non inflammatory.

### Bibliography

1. **Baker DG, Schumacher HR Jr.** Acute monoarthritis. N Engl J Med. 1993;329:1013-20. PMID: 8366902
2. **Thumboo J, O'Duffy JD.** A prospective study of the safety of joint and soft tissue aspirations and injections in patients taking warfarin sodium. Arthritis Rheum. 1998;41:736-9. PMID: 9550485

## Joint Disease Question 25
## Answer: C

**Educational Objective:** *Recognize the musculoskeletal features of patients with hypothyroidism.*

Hypothyroidism is often a cause of stiffness and joint pain. This patient also has symptoms of carpal tunnel syndrome, which hypothyroidism can cause. Carpal tunnel syndrome is usually bilateral when it is caused by systemic disease, and it is the most common cause of a peripheral mononeuropathy. A recent screening in southern Sweden found the prevalence of symptoms to be 14.4%. Clinically certain carpal tunnel syndrome affected 3.8% of subjects; electrophysiology confirmed median nerve damage was found in 4.9% of subjects; and combined clinical and electrically confirmed damage was found in 2.7% of subjects. Of 125 randomly chosen participants without symptoms of carpal tunnel syndrome, 23 subjects had electrophysiologically confirmed median nerve damage. Polymyalgia rheumatica would be one consideration in this elderly patient, but the finding of a viscous, bland synovial fluid is more typical of myxedema. Pseudogout is associated with hypothyroidism, but the decreased leukocyte count in the synovial fluid makes this diagnosis and the diagnosis of gout unlikely.

Polymyositis is associated with proximal muscle weakness, but stiffness, joint effusions, and peripheral neuropathy are not part of this syndrome.

### Bibliography

1. **McLean RM, Podell DN**.Bone and joint manifestations of hypothyroidism. Semin Arthritis Rheum. 1995;24:282-90. PMID: 7740308

2. **Atroshi I, Gummesson C, Johnsson R, Ornstein E, Ranstam J, Rosen I**. Prevalence of carpal tunnel syndrome in a general population. JAMA. 1999;282:153-8. PMID: 10411196

## Joint Disease Question 26
## Answer: C

**Educational Objective:** *Prescribe muscle-strengthening and aerobic exercises to improve pain and disability in osteoarthritis of the knee.*

There have been more than ten controlled trials showing improved outcomes with both aerobic and muscle-building exercise programs for osteoarthritis of the knee. Very few studies have been done for other joints, but limited evidence in hip osteoarthritis suggests that exercise may have similar benefits. Exercise programs must be individualized, taking into account the severity of the arthritis and the patient's comorbidities and level of physical conditioning. The benefits of exercise include improvement in joint pain and mobility, muscle strengthening, and increased bone mineral density.

The alternative recommendations will not contribute to muscle building and its associated benefits. Water exercise programs are preferable for some patients with severe arthritis and deconditioning. There have been only two controlled trials of exercise in osteoarthritis that have been long-term studies; both showed continuing benefit for self-reported pain relief and disability. However, there is very little information on the effect of exercise on disease progression.

### Bibliography

1. **van Baar ME, Assendelft WJ, Dekker J, Oostendorp RA, Bijlsma JW**.Effectiveness of exercise therapy in patients with osteoarthritis of the hip or knee: a systematic review of randomized clinical trials. Arthritis Rheum. 1999;42:1361-9. PMID: 10403263

2. **Ettinger WH Jr, Burns R, Messier SP, Applegate W, Rejeski WJ, Morgan T, et al.** A randomized trial comparing aerobic exercise and resistance exercise with a health education program in older adults with knee osteoarthritis. The Fitness Arthritis and Seniors Trial. JAMA. 1997;277:25-31. PMID: 8980206

3. **Kovar PA, Allegrante JP, MacKenzie CR, Peterson MG, Gutin B, Charlson ME**. Supervised fitness walking in patients with osteoarthritis of the knee. A randomized, controlled trial. Ann Intern Med. 1992;116:529-34. PMID: 1543305

# Fluid, Electrolyte, and Acid-Base Disorders

**Fluid, Electrolyte, and Acid-Base Disorders
Question 1
Answer: A**

**Educational Objective:** *Recognize the mixed acid-base disorder of metabolic (anion gap) acidosis with respiratory alkalosis and volume depletion characteristic of salicylism.*

Early after a salicylate overdose, centrally mediated hyperventilation with respiratory alkalosis occurs. Some renal compensation occurs in response to respiratory alkalosis with retention of hydrogen ions (acids) in exchange for renal wasting of potassium. As salicylate toxicity progresses, metabolic acidosis occurs because of the uncoupling of oxidative phosphorylation and ketosis. Anion gap acidosis with increased lactate and ketones occurs. With progressive acidosis, more salicylate moves into the central nervous system, producing altered mental status and tinnitus. Hyperglycemia may be an acute stress response, but central nervous system hypoglycemia (hypoglycorrhachia) may occur despite a normal to elevated plasma glucose level. This patient with diabetes mellitus who is under stress is most likely to become hyperglycemic. The typical electrolyte picture therefore is option A, with mild hypernatremia (due to renal free water losses), hypokalemia (due to renal losses), and anion gap acidosis (low serum bicarbonate).

## Bibliography

1. **Brenner BE**. Clinical significance of the elevated anion gap. Am J Med. 1985;79:289-96. PMID: 4036980
2. **Gabow PA, Anderson RJ, Potts DE, Schrier RW**. Acid-base disturbances in the salicylate-intoxicated adult. Arch Intern Med. 1978;138:1481-4. PMID: 708168
3. **Hill JB**. Salicylate intoxication. N Engl J Med. 1973;288:1110-3. PMID: 4572648

**Fluid, Electrolyte, and Acid-Base Disorders
Question 2
Answer: C**

**Educational Objective:** *Identify the likely cause of hypercalcemia.*

This patient with a suppressed parathyroid hormone (PTH) level has nonparathyroid hypercalcemia. The only two nonparathyroid causes of hypercalcemia among the choices given are sarcoidosis and malignancy. Of these, sarcoidosis is more compatible with the time course necessary to develop a kidney stone. It would be distinctly unusual for a malignant tumor to present with a kidney stone because of the typically rapid onset of hypercalcemia in such disorders. Hypercalcemia occurs in less than 10% of patients with sarcoidosis, but hypercalciuria is more common. Both disorders result from unregulated synthesis of 1,25-dihydroxyvitamin D, the active metabolite of vitamin D, in macrophages of sarcoid granulomas. As a consequence of excess 1,25-dihydroxyvitamin D, intestinal calcium absorption and bone resorption are increased, and the secretion of PTH is suppressed. Vitamin D intoxication could also cause this complex of symptoms.

Hypercalcemia is not part of the syndrome of idiopathic hypercalciuria, and the PTH level is high or at least normal (and therefore inappropriate) in hypercalcemic patients with hyperparathyroidism and familial benign hypocalciuric hypercalcemia.

## Bibliography

1. **Potts JT Jr**. Hyperparathyroidism and other hypercalcemic disorders. Adv Intern Med. 1996;41:165-212. PMID: 8903589
2. **Rizzato G**. Clinical impact of bone and calcium metabolism changes in sarcoidosis. Thorax. 1998;53:425-9. PMID: 9708239
3. **Sharma OP**. Vitamin D, calcium, and sarcoidosis. Chest. 1996;109:535-9. PMID: 8620732

**Fluid, Electrolyte, and Acid-Base Disorders
Question 3
Answer: A**

**Educational Objective:** *Evaluate hypercalcemia in a patient with breast cancer.*

In an asymptomatic middle-aged woman with hypercalcemia, the most likely diagnosis is primary hyperparathyroidism. With a prevalence of up to 3 per 1000 in middle-aged women, primary hyperparathyroidism can occur coincidentally with breast carcinoma. An elevated parathyroid hormone (PTH) level would be consistent with this diagnosis. A suppressed PTH level in a hypercalcemic patient would indicate that the hypercalcemia is of nonparathyroid origin, and if the patient had a suppressed PTH level in the setting of recent breast carcinoma, a bone scan would be indicated to determine whether osseous metastases from breast cancer were present despite the absence of bone pain or other signs of recurrence.

If the patient had neither hyperparathyroidism nor evidence of recurrent breast carcinoma, other laboratory tests would be indicated to search for rare causes of hypercalcemia, such as vitamin D intoxication, which would be indicated by increased levels of 25-hydroxyvitamin D, the principal circulating form of the vitamin, or sarcoidosis, which results from production of 1,25-dihydroxyvitamin D in sarcoid granulomas.

**Bibliography**

1. **Potts JT Jr**. Hyperparathyroidism and other hypercalcemic disorders. Adv Intern Med. 1996;41:165-212. PMID: 8903589

2. **Silverberg SJ**. Diagnosis, natural history, and treatment of primary hyperparathyroidism. Cancer Treat Res. 1997;89:163-81. PMID: 9204192

## Fluid, Electrolyte, and Acid-Base Disorders
## Question 4
## Answer: D

**Educational Objective:** *Choose the best initial therapy for a patient with malignancy-associated hypercalcemia.*

In this patient, it is important to correct dehydration before instituting therapy with loop diuretics to avoid further impairment of renal function that might result from increased dehydration with vigorous diuresis. Pamidronate will be useful in this patient with severe malignancy-associated hypercalcemia and should be administered early in the hospitalization. However, because pamidronate takes about 3 days to have its full effect, correction of dehydration and institution of a saline diuresis are the first line of therapy. Oral alendronate is ineffective as therapy for severe hypercalcemia. Calcitonin yields only a transient effect for 1 to 2 days and is best used as a supplement to other treatments.

**Bibliography**

1. **Bilezikian JP**. Management of acute hypercalcemia. N Engl J Med. 1992;326:1196-203. PMID: 1532633

## Fluid, Electrolyte, and Acid-Base Disorders
## Question 5
## Answer: D

**Educational Objective:** *Determine the etiology of hypocalcemia.*

This patient has hypocalcemia after correction for mild hypoalbuminemia, suggesting strongly that the ionized calcium level is low. He also has hypophosphatemia and an elevated alkaline phosphatase level. These findings are compatible with osteomalacia from vitamin D deficiency. In osteomalacia, hypocalcemia results from poor intestinal calcium absorption, and hypophosphatemia results primarily from consequent secondary hyperparathyroidism. In this patient with weight loss, vitamin D deficiency osteomalacia is probably caused by malabsorption of vitamin D as part of a generalized malabsorption syndrome. Nutritional vitamin D deficiency would produce a similar syndrome.

The serum phosphorus level would be increased in a patient with hypoparathyroidism, and the serum calcium and phosphorus levels are usually normal in patients with osteoporosis, whether it is caused by hypogonadism or liver disease. Alcoholic liver disease is less likely and most often causes osteoporosis, with normal serum calcium and phosphorus levels, rather than osteomalacia.

**Bibliography**

1. **Bell NH, Key LL Jr**. Acquired osteomalacia. Curr. Ther. Endocrinol. Metab. 1997;6:530-3. PMID: 9174801

## Fluid, Electrolyte, and Acid-Base Disorders
## Question 6
## Answer: B

**Educational Objective:** *Evaluate hypernatremia in an acutely ill patient.*

The most likely cause of hypernatremia in this patient is central diabetes insipidus due to head trauma. This disorder can be diagnosed by finding a high serum osmolality with a high volume of dilute urine. The central (rather than nephrogenic) nature of this disorder will then be confirmed following a diagnostic dose of desmopressin acetate (DDAVP).

However, there are several other possibilities to be considered in this patient. The combination of tube feeding and high-dose dexamethasone may result in glucose intolerance or frank diabetes, which has an osmotic effect. Similarly, his immobilization may result in hypercalcemia, which also has an osmotic diuretic effect. In a patient who was in a coma and unable to drink to thirst, hypernatremia may result. Therefore, measuring plasma glucose and serum calcium is also necessary. Measuring hemoglobin $A_{1c}$ is not useful in this setting, because the patient was healthy before the accident and would be expected to have a normal hemoglobin $A_{1c}$, even if he is now acutely diabetic. Disorders of cortisol, thyroxine, and phosphate do not cause polyuria and hypernatremia.

**Bibliography**

1. **Robertson GL**. Diabetes insipidus. Endocrinol Metab Clin North Am. 1995;24:549-72. PMID: 8575409

## Fluid, Electrolyte, and Acid-Base Disorders
## Question 7
## Answer: A

**Educational Objective:** *Recognize the indications for surgery in a patient with hyperparathyroidism.*

According to the clinical practice guidelines adopted by an NIH Consensus Development Conference, patients with hyperparathyroidism who are younger than 50 years are candidates for surgery because of the long period of risk for development of complications of hypercalcemia if left untreated. Data to support this recommendation are lacking, but it is reasonable and generally accepted. An additional factor in this patient is the presence of nonspecific symptoms. Studies suggest that nonspecific symptoms are more frequently relieved by parathyroidectomy in primary hyperparathyroidism than by thyroidectomy in patients with thyroid disorders, suggesting that the benefit of parathyroidectomy outweighs the placebo effect of having an operation. If this patient's serum calcium concentration were higher than 11.0 to 11.5 mg/dL, that would be an additional indication for surgery. Other studies could be performed as a baseline but would not guide the decision regarding parathyroidectomy. Bisphosphonates do not appear to provide satisfactory medical treatment for hypercalcemia in hyperparathyroidism.

## Bibliography

1. Proceedings of the NIH Consensus Development Conference on diagnosis and management of asymptomatic primary hyperparathyroidism. Bethesda, Maryland, October 29-31, 1990. J Bone Miner Res. 1991;6 Suppl 2:S1-166. PMID: 1763659
2. **Silverberg SJ, Bilezikian JP, Bone HG, Talpos GB, Horwitz MJ, Stewart AF.** Therapeutic controversies in primary hyperparathyroidism. J Clin Endocrinol Metab. 1999;84:2275-85. PMID: 10404790
3. **Chan AK, Duh QY, Katz MH, Siperstein AE, Clark OH.** Clinical manifestations of primary hyperparathyroidism before and after parathyroidectomy. A case-control study. Ann Surg. 1995;222:402-12. PMID: 7677469

## Fluid, Electrolyte, and Acid-Base Disorders
## Question 8
## Answer: C

**Educational Objective:** *Understand the differential diagnosis of hyponatremia and the importance of the urinary sodium concentration, serum uric acid, blood urea nitrogen, and serum creatinine and the assessment of clinical volume status in establishing the diagnosis.*

This patient has the syndrome of inappropriate antidiuretic hormone secretion (SIADH). Patients with lung cancer, especially small cell lung cancer, frequently have SIADH. The syndrome may be clinically quiescent until the patient receives intravenous fluids following admission to the hospital. Although this patient was given normal saline, his serum sodium concentration fell because his kidneys excreted electrolytes at a concentration > 145 meq/L. Therefore, he was retaining electrolyte-free water. Although he has bilateral adrenal masses that are likely due to metastatic disease, he is unlikely to have Addison's disease. Most patients with adrenal metastatic disease do not develop Addison's disease. Furthermore, the low potassium concentration argues against Addison's disease. Extracellular fluid volume depletion is unlikely, given the clinical scenario and the fact that his urinary sodium is 110 meq/L. Although he may have mild heart failure and hepatic disease, the clinical findings, including the high urinary sodium concentration, make cirrhosis and congestive heart failure very unlikely causes of the fall in the serum sodium concentration. A serum uric acid concentration would help to differentiate between these hyponatremic syndromes. Uric

acid concentration is usually elevated when the extracellular fluid volume is contracted or the effective arterial volume is reduced in patients with cirrhosis or congestive heart failure. In contrast, the uric acid concentration is usually reduced when the extracellular fluid volume is expanded, as in patients with SIADH.

## Bibliography

1. **Decaux G, Genette F, Mockel J.** Hypouremia in the syndrome of inappropriate secretion of antidiuretic hormone. Ann Intern Med. 1980;93: 716-7. PMID: 7212483
2. **Schrier RW.** Pathogenesis of sodium and water retention in high-output and low-output cardiac failure, nephrotic syndrome, cirrhosis, and pregnancy (2). N Engl J Med. 1988;319:1127-34. PMID: 3050523
3. **Leier CV, Dei Cas L, Metra M.** Clinical relevance and management of the major electrolyte abnormalities in congestive heart failure: hyponatremia, hypokalemia, and hypomagnesemia. Am Heart J. 1994;128:564-74. PMID: 8074021
4. **Oster JR, Singer I.** Hyponatremia, hyposmolality, and hypotonicity: tables and fables. Arch Intern Med. 1999;159:333-6. PMID: 10030305

## Fluid, Electrolyte, and Acid-Base Disorders
## Question 9
## Answer: C

**Educational Objective:** *Understand how hyperglycemia causes the serum sodium concentration to decrease and how to calculate the expected serum sodium concentration after the hyperglycemia has been corrected.*

The serum sodium concentration is most likely to be 135 to 145 meq/L. Hyperglycemia causes a shift of water from the intracellular space into the extracellular space. This simultaneously dilutes the extracellular sodium salts and increases the intracellular solute concentration. The water shift continues until the extracellular and intracellular osmolalities are similar. It can generally be assumed that in adults each 100 mg/dL increase in plasma glucose will cause a water shift that reduces the serum sodium concentration by approximately 1.6 meq/L. Consequently, if the plasma glucose increases from 100 to 1200 mg/dL, this should reduce the serum sodium concentration by about 18 meq/L. Conversely, if insulin reduces the plasma glucose from 1200 to 100 mg/dL, the serum sodium concentration should increase by about 18 meq/L from 124 to 142 meq/L. Therefore, this patient's hyponatremia can be entirely explained by a shift of water from the intracellular space to the extracellular space, and after correction of hyperglycemia, her serum sodium concentration should be restored to the normal range.

Although one recent study suggests the correction factor may be higher than 1.6 meq/L, and perhaps as high as 2.4 meq/L, this is a single study of acute hyperglycemia in otherwise normal subjects and has not yet been confirmed. The applicability of the new data to diabetic patients with hyperglycemia remains unclear.

## Bibliography

1. **Katz MA**. Hyperglycemia-induced hyponatremia–calculation of expected serum sodium depression. N Engl J Med. 1973;289:843-4. PMID: 4763428

2. **Daugirdas JT, Kronfol NO, Tzamaloukas AH, Ing TS**. Hyperosmolar coma: cellular dehydration and the serum sodium concentration. Ann Intern Med. 1989;110:855-7. PMID: 2655518

3. **Popli S, Leehey DJ, Daugirdas JT, Bansal VK, Ho DS, Hano JE, et al**. Asymptomatic, nonketotic severe hyperglycemia with hyponatremia. Arch Intern Med. 1990;150:1962-4. PMID: 2393329

4. **Hillier TA, Abbott RD, Barrett EJ**. Hyponatremia: evaluating the correction factor for hyperglycemia. Am J Med. 1999;106:399-403. PMID: 10225241

## Fluid, Electrolyte, and Acid-Base Disorders
## Question 10
## Answer: C

**Educational Objective:** *Understand the mechanism of action of calcium salts when used to treat hyperkalemia-induced cardiac toxicity.*

Calcium gluconate is least likely to reduce this patient's serum potassium concentration. The appropriate treatment of hyperkalemia is primarily guided by its cardiac manifestations. If the electrocardiogram shows hyperkalemic cardiac toxicity, intravenous calcium salts are generally indicated. Calcium acts within minutes to reverse the cardiac effects of hyperkalemia. However, this is a direct membrane electrical effect; calcium salts do not reduce the serum potassium concentration. Treatment that shifts potassium from the extracellular fluid into cells should also be started. Such treatment includes glucose and insulin, albuterol, and sodium bicarbonate. If total body potassium stores are increased, potassium must be removed via the kidneys, by dialysis, and/or via the gastrointestinal tract (by administration of sodium polystyrene sulfonate).

## Bibliography

1. **Blumberg A, Weidmann P, Shaw S, Gnadinger M**. Effect of various therapeutic approaches on plasma potassium and major regulating factors in terminal renal failure. Am J Med. 1988;85:507-12. PMID: 3052050

2. **Allon M**. Hyperkalemia in end-stage renal disease: mechanisms and management. J Am Soc Nephrol. 1995;6:1134-42. PMID: 8589279

## Fluid, Electrolyte, and Acid-Base Disorders
## Question 11
## Answer: A

**Educational Objective:** *Recognize the importance of rapid correction of acute severe hyponatremia that is associated with neurotoxicity.*

Patients with schizophrenia often develop symptomatic hyponatremia. This may be due to the effects of psychotropic drugs, increased thirst produced by dry mucous membranes,

and perhaps a direct central nervous system manifestation of schizophrenia itself. These patients sometimes ingest enormous quantities of water over a very short period of time and can develop profound hyponatremia that causes neurologic dysfunction and seizures. If seizures occur, the syndrome of inappropriate antidiuretic hormone secretion (SIADH) may develop because a seizure can cause the release of antidiuretic hormone.

This patient has profound hyponatremia that has probably caused a seizure. We can assume that his hyponatremia is of acute onset. In this setting, the serum sodium concentration should be increased relatively rapidly to approximately 120 to 125 meq/L. This can be accomplished most effectively by infusing hypertonic (3%) saline to increase the sodium concentration by 10 to 15 meq/L over several hours. Although physicians are appropriately concerned about the dangers of increasing sodium concentration too rapidly, this concern should be largely limited to patients with chronic hyponatremia. Under those circumstances, the serum sodium concentration should not be increased by more than 0.5 meq/h or 12 meq/24 h. Parenteral furosemide (to decease maximal renal concentrating mechanisms) with strict water restriction may be useful in some patients with SIADH and chronic hyponatremia. However, a more reasonable level of water restriction is about 500 to 600 mL/24 h. Normal saline is only indicated for the treatment of hyponatremia produced by volume depletion and is contraindicated in this patient.

## Bibliography

1. **Cheng JC, Zikos D, Skopicki HA, Peterson DR, Fisher KA**. Long-term neurologic outcome in psychogenic water drinkers with severe symptomatic hyponatremia: The effect of rapid correction. Am J Med. 1990;88:561-6. PMID: 2189300

2. **Berl T**. Treating hyponatremia: damned if we do and damned if we don't. Kidney Int. 1990;37:1006-18. PMID: 2179612

3. **Karp BI, Laureno R**. Pontine and extrapontine myelinolysis: a neurologic disorder following rapid correction of hyponatremia. Medicine (Baltimore). 1993;72:359-73. PMID: 8231786

4. **Sterns RH**. Severe symptomatic hyponatremia: treatment and outcome. A study of 64 cases. Ann Intern Med. 1987;107:656-64. PMID: 3662278

## Fluid, Electrolyte, and Acid-Base Disorders
## Question 12
## Answer: A

**Educational Objective:** *Recognize the reasons for an elevated blood urea nitrogen:serum creatinine ratio in patients with extracellular fluid volume depletion.*

High fever (increased catabolic state), gastrointestinal bleeding, and treatment with high-dose glucocorticoids may all cause increased production of urea and thus elevate the blood urea nitrogen:serum creatinine ratio. However, the most common reason for an elevated ratio is reduced renal perfusion caused by extracellular fluid volume depletion, as occurred in this patient. Other causes of impaired renal perfusion and an increased blood urea nitrogen:serum creatinine ratio include cardiac failure or cirrhosis in which there is reduced effective circulating volume (arterial under filling). Since urea is a small molecule and freely equilibrates across cell membranes, its elevation could only be due to increased production or diminished excretion, but would not be due to shifts.

### Bibliography

1. **Dossetor JB**. Creatininemia versus uremia: the relative significance of blood urea nitrogen and serum creatinine concentrations in azotemia. Ann Intern Med. 1966;65:1287-99. PMID: 5928490

## Fluid, Electrolyte, and Acid-Base Disorders
## Question 13
## Answer: B

**Educational Objective:** *Know how to treat hypomagnesemia in a patient with heart disease.*

Patients treated with diuretics may develop hypomagnesemia because of increased renal magnesium losses. Magnesium depletion may be worsened because of poor nutrition and a direct renal effect to cause wasting in individuals who consume alcohol. Hypomagnesemia is associated with hypokalemia and hypocalcemia, which may be refractory to electrolyte repletion unless the magnesium deficit is first replaced. There is no indication to stop the diuretic. Calcium repletion is likely to be ineffective if magnesium depletion is causing the hypocalcemia. Magnesium should be replaced to treat the electrolyte disorders and prevent arrhythmias. There is no indication for volume repletion in this patient.

### Bibliography

1. **Elisaf M, Milionis H, Siamopoulos KC**. Hypomagnesemic hypokalemia and hypocalcemia: clinical and laboratory characteristics. Miner Electrolyte Metab. 1997;23:105-12. PMID: 9252977

2. **Agus ZS**. Hypomagnesemia. J Am Soc Nephrol. 1999;10:1616-22. PMID: 10405219

## Fluid, Electrolyte, and Acid-Base Disorders
## Question 14
## Answer: D

**Educational Objective:** *Understand that endocrine paraneoplastic syndromes resolve as the cancer responds to treatment.*

In two thirds of patients with extensive-stage small cell lung cancer who are treated with chemotherapy, their tumor shrinks by more than 50%. The amount of arginine vasopressin produced by small cell lung cancer decreases as the tumor volume shrinks from treatment. Therefore, the serum sodium concentration increases from the presenting level of 122 meq/L and pretreatment level of 129 meq/L to a normal value and is not expected to increase above 148 meq/L (normal, 136 to 145 meq/L).

The common endocrine paraneoplastic syndromes in patients with small cell lung cancer include hyponatremia of malignancy, Cushing's syndrome caused by adrenocorticotrophic hormone, and acromegaly caused by growth hormone-releasing hormone. The severity of the syndrome typically parallels the severity of the cancer. The syndromes resolve when the cancer shrinks after treatment with chemotherapy, radiation therapy, and/or surgical resection. The syndromes are more common in patients with more advanced cancer. Patients with extensive-stage small cell lung cancer are twice as likely to have these syndromes as patients with limited-stage small cell lung cancer.

### Bibliography

1. **Gross AJ, Steinberg SM, Reilly JG, Bliss DP Jr, Brennan J, Le PT, et al**. Atrial natriuretic factor and arginine vasopressin production in tumor cell lines from patients with lung cancer and their relationship to serum sodium. Cancer Res. 1993;53:67-74. PMID: 8380126

2. **Sorensen JB, Andersen MK, Hansen HH**. Syndrome of inappropriate secretion of antidiuretic hormone (SIADH) in malignant disease. J Intern Med. 1995;238:97-110. PMID: 7629492

3. **Johnson BE, Damodaran A, Rushin J, Gross A, Le PT, Chen HC, et al**. Ectopic production and processing of atrial natriuretic peptide in a small cell lung carcinoma cell line and tumor from a patient with hyponatremia. Cancer. 1997;79:35-44. PMID: 8988724

## Fluid, Electrolyte, and Acid-Base Disorders
## Question 15
## Answer: B

**Educational Objective:** *Manage hypercalcemia of malignancy due to a tamoxifen-induced tumor flare.*

This patient developed symptomatic hypercalcemia within 2 weeks of initiating tamoxifen therapy for breast cancer metastatic to bone. Hypercalcemia and increased bone pain are occasionally seen in such patients and constitute the "tumor flare" phenomenon. The flare frequently heralds a subsequent tumor response if tamoxifen therapy is continued. The drug should not be stopped unless the hypercalcemia is life threatening or refractory to treatment; its long half-life of elimination precludes immediate benefit. Vigorous saline hydration, the most important therapeutic intervention, restores plasma volume, renal perfusion, and calcium excretion. Furosemide may be used to control volume overload, but early administration may impede restoration of plasma volume. Inhibition of osteoclast function with bisphosphonates such as pamidronate is effective adjunctive therapy to hydration and has few side effects. Gallium nitrate, which also blocks osteoclastic bone resorption, is another alternative. Calcitonin has a transient effect lasting only one to two days and is used only as a supplement to other therapies.. Phosphate therapy is effective in lowering serum calcium concentration but should not be used when the serum phosphate is normal or elevated to avoid precipitation of ionized calcium in tissues.

Prostaglandin inhibitors such as ibuprofen are occasionally helpful in the chronic management of hypercalcemia, but they have no role in acute management. Mithramycin has significant toxic effects and should be reserved for patients with refractory hypercalcemia.

### Bibliography

1. **Singer FR.** Pathogenesis of hypercalcemia of malignancy. Semin Oncol. 1991;18:4-10. PMID: 1925629
2. **Gucalp R, Ritch P, Wiernik PH, Sarma PR, Keller A, Richman SP, et al.** Comparative study of pamidronate disodium and etidronate disodium in the treatment of cancer-related hypercalcemia. J Clin Oncol. 1992;10:134-42. PMID: 1727915
3. **Warrell RP Jr, Murphy WK, Schulman P, O'Dwyer PJ, Heller G.** A randomized double-blind study of gallium nitrate compared with etidronate for acute control of cancer-related hypercalcemia. J Clin Oncol. 1991;9:1467-75. PMID: 1906532

## Fluid, Electrolyte, and Acid-Base Disorders
### Question 16
### Answer: D

**Educational Objective:** *Understand the acid-base abnormalities that may accompany pulmonary edema and identify their causes.*

This patient is acidemic, and the elevated $P_{CO_2}$ indicates respiratory acidosis. With an elevated $P_{CO_2}$, the serum bicarbonate level would be expected to be above normal indicating metabolic compensation. Because it is less than normal, metabolic acidosis is also present. The patient's blood gas values lie between those of simple respiratory acidosis and metabolic acidosis when plotted on an acid-base map. With severe pulmonary edema, alteration of lung mechanics leads to carbon dioxide retention, and lactic acidosis may also result from poor tissue perfusion and anaerobic metabolism.

### Bibliography

1. **Avery WG, Samet P, Sackner MA.** The acidosis of pulmonary edema. Am J Med. 1970;48:320-4. PMID: 5265250
2. **Sharp JT, Griffith GT, Bunnell IL, et al.** Ventilatory mechanics in pulmonary edema in man. J Clin Invest. 1958;37:111-7.

## Fluid, Electrolyte, and Acid-Base Disorders
### Question 17
### Answer: B

**Educational Objective:** *Understand the relation between airflow obstruction and hypercapnia in chronic obstructive pulmonary disease.*

The arterial blood gas values indicate hypercapnia ($P_{aCO_2}$, 52 mm Hg) and alkalemia (pH, 7.46). The patient has a mixed acid-base disorder with respiratory acidosis (elevated $P_{aCO_2}$) and metabolic alkalosis (an increase in pH greater than expected solely from compensatory metabolic alkalosis with chronic respiratory acidosis). This patient has COPD and this diagnosis is supported by the fact that he is a former cigarette

smoker with airflow obstruction (reduced ratio of forced expiratory volume in 1 sec [$FEV_1$] to forced vital capacity [FVC]) that is minimally reversible with a bronchodilator. However, obesity hypoventilation syndrome, and not COPD, is the most likely primary cause of the hypercapnia.

Carbon dioxide retention in COPD develops as a consequence of severe airflow obstruction. In the absence of medications or other conditions that depress ventilatory drive, hypercapnia usually does not develop in COPD until the $FEV_1$ decreases to less than 1.5 L and less than 50% of the predicted value. Hypercapnia develops in response to the increased work of breathing to maintain a normal minute ventilation in the presence of severe airflow obstruction in COPD. It does not develop in the presence of only mild to moderate degrees of airflow obstruction. Morbid obesity and hypercapnia direct consideration in this case to obesity hypoventilation syndrome (Pickwickian Syndrome).

Respiratory compensation for primary metabolic alkalosis might be expected to cause $P_{aCO_2}$ to increase slightly in response to this degree of alkalemia, but not to 52 mm Hg. Respiratory (diaphragmatic) muscle weakness is a cause of hypercapnia, but the history and examination findings for this patient give no hint of neuromuscular weakness. Congestive heart failure when severe and causing acute pulmonary edema can manifest as hypercapnia. Modest degrees of left ventricular dysfunction, if they influence alveolar ventilation at all, generally cause hyperventilation with hypocapnia.

### Bibliography

1. **Lane DJ, Howell JB, Giblin B.** Relation between airways obstruction and CO2 tension in chronic obstructive airways disease. Br Med J. 1968;3:707-9. PMID: 5673961
2. **Weinberger SE, Schwartzstein RM, Weiss JW.** Hypercapnia. N Engl J Med. 1989;321:1223-31. PMID: 2677729

# Dysuria

## Dysuria Question 1
**Answer: C**

**Educational Objective:** *Manage a urinary track infection in a pregnant woman.*

Amoxicillin is the indicated antibiotic choice for a urinary tract infection in late pregnancy, and 7 days is the appropriate duration of therapy. In the pregnant woman, anatomic changes include dilated ureters and decreased bladder tone. The prevalence of asymptomatic bacteriuria in pregnant women is 7%. Symptomatic infection can occur in 20% to 40% of those patients, and pyelonephritis in 30% of those with symptomatic infection.

Treatment of patients with asymptomatic bacteriuria is generally for 3 days. However, women with symptomatic urinary tract infections in late pregnancy have a 20% to 50% incidence of premature delivery as well as fetal growth retardation and perinatal death. In pregnant patients, treatment should include urinalysis, culture, and 7 days of antibiotic therapy.

Therapy with ciprofloxacin, sulfonamides, and nitrofurantoin should be avoided in the last 6 weeks of pregnancy. Prophylactic therapy in patients with recurrent urinary tract infections during pregnancy is effective.

### Bibliography

1. **Stray-Pederson B, Blakstad M, Bergan.** Bacteriuria in the puerperium. Risk factors, screening procedures, and treatment programs. Am J Obstet Gynecol. 1990;162:792-7. PMID: 2316591

## Dysuria Question 2
**Answer: D**

**Educational Objective:** *Prescribe appropriate oral antimicrobial therapy for chronic bacterial prostatitis.*

This patient most likely has chronic bacterial prostatitis. Although the optimal duration of therapy is uncertain, most authorities recommend at least a 6-week course of an antibiotic known to concentrate well in the prostate and to cover coliform bacteria, the most common cause of bacterial prostatitis. Treatment success rates range from 30% to 40% with trimethoprim-sulfamethoxazole and 60% to 90% with fluoroquinolones. Infections that are not cured are generally managed satisfactorily by continuous, suppressive, low-dose therapy with agents such as trimethoprim-sulfamethoxazole, one single-strength tablet daily, or nitrofurantoin, 100 mg orally once or twice daily.

*Fluoroquir*

### Bibliography

1. **Lipsky BA.** Prostatitis and urinary tract infection in men: what's new; what's true? Am J Med. 1999;106:327-34. PMID: 10190383

## Dysuria Question 3
**Answer: C**

**Educational Objective:** *Push a drug to efficacy, toxicity, target concentration, or dosage before switching to or adding an additional drug to treat the same indication.*

In principle, switching to gentamicin, ampicillin, or gentamicin and ampicillin all would be possible choices for this condition; all are effective. However, the patient is already receiving trimethoprim-sulfamethoxazole, which is a very effective therapy for urinary tract infection and achieves very high concentrations in the urine. Antimicrobial sensitivity testing expresses a relative sensitivity. Most importantly, this patient is responding to therapy with a particular drug. Therefore, there is no reason to change her therapy.

### Bibliography

1. **Hooton TM, Stam WE.** Management of acute uncomplicated urinary tract infection in adults. Med Clin North Am. 1991;75:339-57. PMID: 1996038

## Dysuria Question 4
**Answer: C**

**Educational Objective:** *Differentiate between bacterial colonization and infection of the urinary tract.*

Because long-term indwelling urinary catheters are almost universally associated with bacteriuria, the clinician must differentiate between colonization and infection. In this patient, the lack of fever, tachycardia, and tachypnea argue against infection; the elevated leukocyte count is nonspecific. Appropriate management would include ongoing clinical observation, with antibiotic therapy not being indicated at this time.

### Bibliography

1. **Warren JW.** Catheter-associated urinary tract infections. Infect Dis Clin North Am. 1997;16:609-22. PMID: 9378926

## Dysuria Question 5
## Answer: C

**Educational Objective:** *Choose the preferred management for a young woman with uncomplicated cystitis.*

A 3-day course of trimethoprim-sulfamethoxazole is highly effective for treatment of women with uncomplicated cystitis, which is usually caused by highly susceptible strains of *Escherichia coli* or *Staphylococcus saprophyticus*. Some clinicians would use a more expensive 3-day course of a fluoroquinolone because of increasing resistance of *E. coli* to trimethoprim-sul-famethoxazole, and this would be the appropriate alternative regimen if the patient's symptoms do not improve in 48 hours. Single doses of fluoroquinolones and less than a 7-day course of nitrofurantoin are not as effective, and failures of a single dose of fluoroquinolones are particularly seen in patients with *S. saprophyticus* infections. A urine culture is not necessary in patients of this type because of the generally predictable susceptibility profile of their uropathogens.

### Bibliography
1. **Kunin CM**. Urinary tract infections in females. Clin Infect Dis. 1994;18:1-12. PMID: 8054415
2. **Stamm WE, Hooton TM**. Management of urinary tract infections in adults. N Engl J Med. 1993;329:1328-34. PMID: 8413414

## Dysuria Question 6
## Answer: C

**Educational Objective:** *Determine the best management for a man with sexually transmitted urethritis.*

Urinary tract infections are sufficiently infrequent in previously healthy young adult males that dysuria should always raise primary consideration of urethritis, particularly in the presence of urethral discharge. The urethral discharge should be the primary focus of evaluation, and the presence of polymorphonuclear neutrophils on Gram stain establishes the diagnosis of urethritis. The presence of intracellular gram-negative diplococci in the urethral discharge from a male is highly specific for infection with *Neisseria gonorrhoeae*. Because of the frequency of coinfection with *N. gonorrhoeae* and *Chlamydia trachomatis*, treatment for both is usually indicated with a combination of ceftriaxone and azithromycin given as single doses. Although doxycycline is an acceptable alternative to azithromycin for chlamydial infection, the possibility of noncompliance with a 7-day course of doxycycline makes azithromycin the preferred antichlamydial agent. Ceftriaxone alone or a single dose of ofloxacin is inadequate treatment for chlamydial infection. A 7-day course of ofloxacin is effective in eradicating both gonococcal and chlamydial infections, but the requirement for compliance with a 1-week regimen and the occasional occurrence of ofloxacin-resistant gonococcal infections makes ofloxacin less desirable than the combination of ceftriaxone and azithromycin. A 3-day course of trimetho-

prim–sulfamethoxazole has not been shown to be effective for either gonococcal or chlamydial infections and would also be too brief a course for an older man with a urinary tract infection.

### Bibliography
1. Sexually transmitted diseases treatment guidelines 2002. Centers for Disease Control and Prevention. MMWR Recomm Rep. 2002;51(RR-6):1-78. PMID: 12184549
2. **Burstein GR, Zenilman JM**. Nongonococcal urethritis – a new paradigm. Clin Infect Dis. 1999;28(suppl 1):S66-73. PMID: 10028111

## Dysuria Question 7
## Answer: D

**Educational Objective:** *Recognize the clinical features of struvite stone disease.*

Struvite (infection) stones occur most often in women. *Proteus* species, a urea-splitting organism, is frequently the cause of the chronic urinary tract infection that causes the stones. Patients with medullary sponge kidney and hypercalciuric stone formers have radiopaque stones, but they will not have alkaline urine, pyuria, or bacteriuria unless a superimposed infection is present. Nephrolithiasis associated with renal tubular acidosis will cause an alkaline urine and a low plasma bicarbonate concentration but will not cause pyuria or bacteriuria.

### Bibliography
1. **Schwartz BF, Stoller ML**. Nonsurgical management of infection-related renal calculi. Urol Clin North Am. 1999;26:765-8. PMID: 10584617
2. **Rodman JS**. Struvite stones. Nephron. 1999;81:50-9. PMID: 9873215

## Dysuria Question 8
## Answer: B

**Educational Objective:** *Recognize the urinalysis associated with acute pyelonephritis.*

This patient presents with a typical case of relatively severe acute uncomplicated pyelonephritis. The clinical spectrum attributable to acute uncomplicated pyelonephritis in young women ranges from mild fever and flank pain to severe pyelonephritis associated with gram-negative bacteremia and sepsis. Although a urinalysis demonstrating pyuria and hematuria strongly suggests the diagnosis of acute pyelonephritis, the demonstration of bacteriuria on a Gram stain of unspun urine greatly strengthens the diagnosis. Furthermore, the Gram stain can differentiate the occasional case of gram-positive (staphylococcal, enterococcal, or streptococcal) pyelonephritis from the much more common gram-negative infections due to *Escherichia coli*, *Klebsiella* species, or *Proteus* species. Thus, an initial Gram stain of unspun urine should be done. Option B, with many leukocytes, few or no epithelial cells, and gram-negative bacilli is most consistent with pyelonephritis.

In milder cases, management with oral antimicrobial agents in the outpatient setting can be successful. Oral therapy should be reserved for women with a clear diagnosis of pyelonephritis, no nausea or vomiting, stable vital signs, and no evidence of septicemia clinically. Patients in whom the diagnosis is not certain, in whom nausea or vomiting is present, or in whom severe illness or septicemia may be present should be hospitalized for initial parenteral therapy.

In order to confirm the diagnosis and identify the antimicrobial susceptibility pattern of the infecting strain, urine and blood cultures should be done. The vast majority of women with acute uncomplicated pyelonephritis do not have urologic abnormalities or obstruction, and hence, evaluation of the urinary tract by ultrasonography, intravenous pyelography, or other means is not indicated initially. Such procedures should be considered in patients who fail to improve after 72 hours of antimicrobial therapy.

### Bibliography

1. **Ronald AR, Nicolle LE, Harding GK.** Standards of therapy for urinary tract infections in adults. Infection. 1992;20:S164-70. PMID: 1490743

2. **Stamm WE, McKevitt M, Counts GW.** Acute renal infection in women: treatment with trimethoprim-sulfamethoxazole or ampicillin for 2 or 6 weeks. Ann Intern Med. 1987;106:341-5. PMID: 3492950

3. **Johnson JR, Lions MF II, Pearce W, Gorman P, Roberts PL, White N, et al.** Therapy for women hospitalized with acute pyelonephritis: a randomized trial of ampicillin vs. trimethoprim-sulfamethoxazole for 14 days. J Infect Dis. 1991;163:325-30. PMID: 1988516

# Acute Renal Failure

## Acute Renal Failure Question 1
### Answer: C

**Educational Objective:** *Recognize renal failure in a patient treated with an aminoglycoside antibiotic.*

The time course and urinalysis are consistent with aminoglycoside nephrotoxicity. Prerenal azotemia is unlikely in the absence of signs of volume depletion or volume overload. The specific gravity and high urinary sodium concentration are also inconsistent with prerenal azotemia. Although the patient was treated with ampicillin, which can be associated with acute interstitial nephritis, and the time course is plausible for a diagnosis of acute interstitial nephritis, there is no evidence of rash or eosinophilia to make this diagnosis more likely. In addition, the urinalysis, which does not show pyuria or low-grade proteinuria, would be distinctly unusual in a patient with interstitial nephritis. There is no evidence for rhabdomyolysis in the absence of dipstick-positive heme or for glomerulonephritis in the absence of proteinuria, hematuria, or erythrocyte casts.

### Bibliography
1. **Rybak MJ, Abate BJ, Kang SL, Ruffing MJ, Lerner SA, Drusano GL**. Prospective evaluation of the effect of an aminoglycoside dosing regimen on rates of observed nephrotoxicity and ototoxicity. Antimicrob Agents Chemother. 1999;43:1549-55. PMID: 10390201

## Acute Renal Failure Question 2
### Answer: C

**Educational Objective:** *Treat acute renal failure in a patient treated with an aminoglycoside antibiotic.*

Discontinuation of the aminoglycoside is indicated, and the prognosis for improvement of renal function is good for this patient. Glucocorticoids are not effective for treating aminoglycoside nephrotoxicity and can be deleterious in a patient with infection. The efficacy of dopamine has not been evaluated extensively in patients with aminoglycoside nephrotoxicity, but dopamine has not been shown to be effective in patients with other forms of acute renal failure. There is no evidence that alkalinization of the urine is beneficial in treating aminoglycoside nephrotoxicity.

### Bibliography
1. **Rybak MJ, Abate BJ, Kang SL, Ruffing MJ, Lerner SA, Drusano GL**. Prospective evaluation of the effect of an aminoglycoside dosing regimen on rates of observed nephrotoxicity and ototoxicity. Antimicrob Agents Chemother. 1999;43:1549-55. PMID: 10390201

## Acute Renal Failure Question 3
### Answer: B

**Educational Objective:** *Recognize the characteristics of the urine in patients with acute tubular necrosis and other causes of acute renal failure.*

In contrast-induced acute tubular necrosis (ATN), the urine may be almost normal but often shows muddy brown casts, renal tubular cells, and renal tubular cell casts. There usually is no significant proteinuria. Erythrocyte casts are not seen in patients with ATN and usually imply glomerular injury, as does significant (4+) proteinuria. Leukocytes accompanied by bacteria are typical of urinary tract infection but not of ATN. Urinary eosinophils may be found in patients with acute interstitial nephritis, atheroembolic renal disease, and urinary tract infections. In a study by Corwin et al, 16% of patients whose urine was specifically examined had urinary eosinophils. Of these, 45% had clinical evidence of upper or lower urinary tract infection, and 14% had clinical or biopsy evidence of acute interstitial nephritis. In several small studies, eosinophiluria has been observed in patients with atheroembolic renal disease. Thus, the finding of eosinophiluria in patients with renal disease is nonspecific and must be interpreted based on the clinical context of the particular patient.

### Bibliography
1. **Miller TR, Anderson RJ, Linas SL, Henrich WL, Berns AS, Gabow, PA, Schrier RW**. Urinary diagnostic indices in acute renal failure: a prospective study. Ann Intern Med. 1978;89:47-50. PMID: 666184
2. **Corwin HL, Korbet SM, Schwartz MM**. Clinical correlates of eosinophiluria. Arch Intern Med. 1985;145:1097-9. PMID: 4004436

## Acute Renal Failure Question 4
## Answer: C

**Educational Objective:** *Recognize clinical situations in which the serum creatinine concentration may be elevated without a change in the glomerular filtration rate.*

In patients with extracellular fluid volume contraction, elevations of serum creatinine concentration are due to reductions in the glomerular filtration rate (GFR). In all of the other options listed, the increase in creatinine concentration could be explained by mechanisms other than a reduced GFR. Trimethoprim and cimetidine cause elevations in serum creatinine concentration by inhibition of tubular secretion of creatinine and not by reductions in the GFR. Increased intake of meat or increased muscle mass increase serum creatinine without affecting GFR. Rhabdomyolysis may accompany prolonged seizure activity and causes increased release of creatinine from injured muscle. Severe rhabdomyolysis may also be associated with acute renal failure, which is usually due to accompanying hypotension, drug overdose, or hyperthermia.

### Bibliography

1. **Ducharme MP, Smythe M, Strohs G**. Drug-induced alterations in serum creatinine concentrations. Ann Pharmacother. 1993;27:622-33. PMID: 8347916

## Acute Renal Failure Question 5
## Answer: A

**Educational Objective:** *Recognize the appearance of broad casts and know their diagnostic significance.*

Casts are cylindrical elements comprised of mucoproteins, with or without entrapped intact or decaying cells. Broad casts, which are the largest, are commonly found in acute tubular necrosis. Their size reflects their formation in dilated, injured tubules. They may have a granular appearance or contain damaged tubular cells. If bilirubin, myoglobin, or free hemoglobin is present in the urine, the casts may appear pigmented. The size of these casts and their association with tubular damage allow distinction from smaller red blood cell casts, the hallmark of renal glomerular disease and while blood cell casts, the hallmark of acute interstitial nephritis or infections.

Other types of casts include white blood cell, coarsely granular, finely granular, and hyaline casts. Hyaline casts may be seen when there is no intrinsic renal disease, such as dehydration, and granular casts, when present in large numbers, are nonspecific indicators of kidney disease. Nephrotic syndrome should not cause broad casts, but is associated with casts containing fat globules. Under polarized light, the characteristic "Maltese Crosses" of fat globules can be seen.

### Bibliography

1. **Misdraji J, Nguyen PL**.Urinalysis. When — and when not — to order. Postgrad Med. 1996;100:173-6, 181-2, 185-8. PMID: 8668615

## Acute Renal Failure Question 6
## Answer: B

**Educational Objective:** *Recognize the appearance and implications of red blood cell casts in the urine and know how to distinguish them from other cellular casts.*

The presence of casts in urine is usually indicative of intrinsic renal disease. The geometric shape of the casts reflects their origin in the renal tubules. Some casts are composed of acellular material and are described as hyaline, fatty, waxy, granular, or broad. Hyaline casts may indicate simply dehydration. Granular, waxy, and broad casts represent various stages of degeneration of cells in a protein matrix. Fatty casts (casts with fat globules) are seen in patients with the nephrotic syndrome. Under polarized light, the characteristic "Maltese crosses" of fat globules can be recognized.

Cellular casts provide a clue to the type of the underlying renal disease. Red blood cell casts (whose cells have no nuclei) are seen in glomerular disease and vasculitis. White blood cell casts are found in infections or other tubulointerstitial diseases. Epithelial casts can be seen in various tubular diseases. Rhabdomyolsis results in hemoglobinuria and/or myoglobinuria, but not in red blood cell casts. Pyelonephritis can result in WBC casts, but not isolated RBC casts.

### Bibliography

1. **Misdraji J, Nguyen PL**.Urinalysis. When — and when not — to order. Postgrad Med. 1996;100:173-6, 181-2, 185-8. PMID: 8668615

## Acute Renal Failure Question 7
## Answer: D

**Educational Objective:** *Differentiate between glomerulonephritis and thrombotic microangiopathy.*

This patient's findings of schistocytes on peripheral smear, thrombocytopenia, anemia, elevated liver enzyme levels, and a high lactate dehydrogenase (LDH) concentration point to the hemolytic-uremic syndrome. Patients who have thrombotic microangiopathy, such as hemolytic-uremic syndrome, frequently appear to have glomerulonephritis. The key to the diagnosis of this case rests on finding schistocytes on the peripheral smear associated with thrombocytopenia, which should not occur with nephrotic syndrome, nephritic syndrome, systemic vasculitis, or rhabdomyolysis.

The question is whether or not she has rhabdomyolysis with an elevated creatine phosphokinase. In order for rhabdomyolysis to cause an elevated serum creatinine level of 2.9 mg/dL, her creatine kinase level would have to be in the thousands. Thus, the hemolytic-uremic syndrome is the most likely diagnosis. The creatine kinase may be elevated in some patients with thrombotic microangiopathy for reasons that are not clear.

Hemolytic-uremic syndrome in childhood is among the most common causes of acute renal failure in this age group. Hemolytic-uremic syndrome in this population may be distinguished on the basis of epidemic or sporadic cases. The epidemic disease is accompanied by bacterial infections, such as infectious diarrhea, usually caused by a verotoxin-producing strain of *Escherichia coli*.

Hemolytic-uremic syndrome may also occur in the postpartum period, associated with cancer and chemotherapy, and as a consequence of some drugs, such as penicillin, metronidazole, cyclosporine, and oral contraceptives.

### Bibliography

1. **Remuzzi G**. HUS and TTP: variable expression of a simple entity. Kidney Int 1987; 32:292-308. PMID: 3309432

## Acute Renal Failure Question 8
## Answer: C

**Educational Objective:** *Recognize potential renal complications of nonsteroidal anti-inflammatory drugs in patients with systemic lupus erythematosus.*

Nonsteroidal anti-inflammatory drugs (NSAIDs), including indomethacin, can result in deterioration of renal function. The mechanism appears to be secondary to inhibition of prostaglandin synthesis, with a resulting loss of renal blood flow autoregulation and increasing vasoconstriction. Diseases that result in decreased renal blood flow place the patient at increased risk for this complication. Thus, NSAIDs should be used with caution in patients with hypovolemia, congestive heart failure, cirrhosis, nephrotic syndrome, and preexisting parenchymal renal disease, especially glomerulonephritis. Decreasing renal function secondary to NSAID use is not unusual in the setting of preexisting nephritis. This side effect should not be confused with a much rarer renal complication of these medications, such as interstitial nephritis associated with large amounts of proteinuria. The reversible vasoconstriction observed with NSAIDs is not by itself associated with urinalysis abnormalities, such as an increased level of proteinuria. Early on, there are no abnormalities seen on histologic examination of the kidney. If recognized early and the drug discontinued, this complication of NSAID use is totally reversible. The most prudent course for this patient would be to discontinue the NSAID and see if renal function returns to baseline levels over the next week. Subsequent follow-up and 24-hour urine studies may help determine whether further evaluation or treatment is indicated. Corticosteroids are not indicated in the treatment of this noninflammatory side effect of NSAIDs.

High doses of oral prednisone (1 mg/kg daily) are considered to be a reasonable initial therapy for severe lupus nephritis. In this patient, however, the recent initiation of indomethacin, the absence of severe proteinuria, and the presence of only minimal urinalysis abnormalities suggest that active lupus nephritis is not likely to be the cause of the deterioration in renal function. Therefore, therapy directed at active lupus nephritis, without further investigation or follow up, seems unwarranted. Hospitalization and initiation of pulse methylprednisolone or initiation of prednisone and cyclophosphamide also seem inappropriate in the absence of more evidence that decreasing renal function is secondary to progressive lupus nephritis.

### Bibliography

1. **Clive DM, Stoff JS**. Renal syndromes associated with nonsteroidal anti-inflammatory drugs. N Engl J Med. 1984;310:563-72. PMID: 6363936

2. **Whelton A, Stout RL, Spilman PS, Klassen DK**. Renal effects of ibuprofen, piroxicam, and sulindac in patients with asymptomatic renal failure. A prospective, randomized, crossover comparison. Ann Intern Med. 1990;12:568-76. PMID: 2183665

3. **Balow JE, Austin HA 3d, Tsokos GC, Antonovych TT, Steinberg AD, Klippel JH**. NIH Conference. Lupus nephritis. Ann Intern Med. 1987;106:79-94. PMID: 3789582

## Acute Renal Failure Question 9
## Answer: A

**Educational Objective:** *Recognize that angiotensin-converting enzyme inhibitors can cause acute renal failure.*

Patients with preexisting chronic renal insufficiency should be treated to reduce the progression of renal disease. Control of hypertension by any regimen is effective, but angiotensin-converting enzyme (ACE) inhibitors have been shown to confer enhanced benefits in several studies of patients with and without diabetic renal disease. This patient most likely has chronic renal insufficiency, as evidenced by an increased serum creatinine concentration. The cause is unclear, but hypertensive nephropathy is a possible diagnosis, especially because of the relatively low level of urinary protein excretion. The patient also has a history of hypercholesterolemia and evidence of peripheral vascular disease, raising the possibility of the presence of renal arterial disease. A diagnosis of acute renal failure can be confirmed in this patient, who already has chronic renal failure, because his serum creatinine concentration has increased over a short period. Patients with renal vascular disease or preexisting renal insufficiency, as well as those with decreased renal perfusion because of congestive heart failure, may develop an acute decrease in the glomerular filtration rate when treated with ACE inhibitors (or angiotensin II receptor blockers) because of the hemodynamic effects of these drugs. Physical examination demonstrates that this patient does not have a volume disorder, and his urinalysis does not suggest glomerular, interstitial, or renal tubular disease. Although the diagnosis is likely to be renal vascular disease, the decrement in the glomerular filtration rate associated with blockade of angiotensin synthesis is usually quickly reversed when the ACE inhibitor is discontinued.

Lovastatin has been associated with the development of rhabdomyolysis, but there is no evidence of hemoglobin or myoglobin in this patient's urine or symptoms of muscle pain or weakness. There is also no evidence of volume depletion, and therefore, no indication for administering intravenous fluids. Contrast agents should be used only for the most urgent indications in patients with acute renal failure because of the potential for the development of nephrotoxicity. Finally, there is no evidence that the β-blocker, given in an unchanged dose, has caused this patient's renal function to deteriorate.

## Bibliography

1. **Biesenbach G, Janko O, Stuby U, Zagornik J**. Myoglobinuric renal failure due to long-standing lovastatin therapy in a patient with pre-existing chronic renal insufficiency. Nephrol Dial Transplant. 1996;11:2059-60. PMID: 8918723

2. **Esmail ZN, Loewen PS.**Losartan as an alternative to ACE inhibitors in patients with renal dysfunction. Ann Pharmacother. 1998;32:1096-8. PMID: 9793603

3. **Wynckel A, Ebikili B, Melin JP, Randoux C, Lavaud S, Chanard J**. Long-term follow-up of acute renal failure caused by angiotensin converting enzyme inhibitors. Am J Hypertens. 1998;11:1080-6. PMID: 9752893

4. **van de Ven PJ, Beutler JJ, Kaatee R, Beek FJ, Mali WP, Koomans HA**. Angiotensin converting enzyme inhibitor-induced renal dysfunction in atherosclerotic renovascular disease. Kidney Int. 1998;53:986-93. PMID: 9551408

# Hypertension

## Hypertension Question 1
### Answer: C

**Educational Objective:** *Recognize the benefits of treating hypertension in the old-old.*

Average life expectancy for an 80-year-old woman is almost 9 more years. For patients in there 80s when their hypertension is first treated, the risk of stroke, cardiovascular events, and heart failure decreases. Mortality, however, is not affected.

### Bibliography

1. **Gueyffier F, Bulpitt C, Boissel JP, Schron E, Ekbom T, Fagard R, et al**. Antihypertensive drugs in very old people: a subgroup meta-analysis of randomized controlled trials. INDANA Group. Lancet. 1999;353:793-6. PMID: 10459960

## Hypertension Question 2
### Answer: B

**Educational Objective:** *Recognize the potential interactions between angiotensin-converting enzyme inhibitors and aspirin.*

Angiotensin-converting enzyme (ACE) inhibition reduces the incidence of recurrent myocardial infarction. The mechanisms are unclear, but one possibility is that ACE inhibitors block the breakdown of prostaglandins and kinins, such as bradykinin, a known smooth muscle vasodilator that may act beneficially on the coronary vascular tree. Aspirin counteracts these effects. The evidence regarding the negative interaction between these two agents is circumstantial and retrospective but is a cause for concern. ACE inhibitors are particularly beneficial in patients with diabetes mellitus, and the beneficial effects of aspirin are well recognized. Whether patients receiving an ACE inhibitor should receive a lower dose of aspirin is unknown, but physicians should be cognizant of this potentially important drug interaction.

### Bibliography

1. **Al-Khadra AS, Salem DN, Rand WM, Udelson JE, Smith JJ, Konstam MA**. Antiplatelet agents and survival: a cohort analysis from the Studies of Left Ventricular Dysfunction (SOLVD) trial. J Am Coll Cardiol. 1998;31:419-25. PMID: 9462588
2. **Teerlink JR, Massie BM**. The interaction of ACE inhibitors and aspirin in heart failure: torn between two lovers. Am Heart J. 1999;138:193-7. PMID: 10426826

## Hypertension Question 3
### Answer: B

**Educational Objective:** *Recognize how to identify and treat determinants of myocardial oxygen demand in patients with angina pectoris.*

After inquiring about this patient's compliance with medications, an appropriate strategy is to progressively increase the dose of his antihypertensive medication to achieve a systolic blood pressure of 125 to 130 mm Hg at rest. This patient's blood pressure on exertion will be even higher than the resting value of 170/95 mm Hg recorded on examination at rest. As much as 40 mg of lisinopril can be administered daily, and some patients may even be able to tolerate doses as much as 80 mg daily and/or the addition of another ACE inhibitor. In this patient, one major determinant of myocardial oxygen demand, the heart rate, is well controlled by a β-blocker. He is also taking a lipid-lowering agent, aspirin, and a long-acting nitrate to maintain his ischemic heart disease in a stable state. However, his angina appears to be accelerating. This may be due to the natural progression of his disease, to noncompliance with medication, or to inadequate control of his blood pressure, which is another determinant of myocardial oxygen demand. Prophylactic sublingual nitroglycerin before exertion is also often useful under these circumstances, although the patient's symptoms have worsened despite this maneuver. His other medications (isosorbide mononitrate and atenolol) are already optimal, with good heart rate control. If he continues to have anginal symptoms with progressively milder exertion despite adequate control of heart rate and blood pressure, coronary angiography should be considered.

### Bibliography

1. The sixth report of the Joint National Committee on prevention, detection, evaluation, and treatment of high blood pressure. Arch Intern Med. 1997;157:2413-46. PMID: 9385294
2. **Gibbons RJ, Chatterjee K, Daley J, Douglas JS, Fihn SD, Gardin JM, et al.** ACC/AHA/ACP-ASIM Guidelines for the Management of Patients with Chronic Stable Angina: executive summary and recommendations. A report of the American College of Cardiology/American Heart Association Task Force on Practice Guidelines (Committee on Management of Patients with Chronic Stable Angina). J Am Coll Cardiol. 1999;33:2092-197. PMID: 10362225

## Hypertension Question 4
## Answer: C

**Educational Objective:** *Evaluate a patient with suspected pheochromocytoma.*

This patient has three classic symptoms that suggest pheochromocytoma: headache, sweating, and palpitations, all of an episodic nature. The diagnosis is further suggested by the history of labile blood pressure during a recent surgical procedure. The fact that he is not currently hypertensive does not argue against the diagnosis, because many patients with pheochromocytoma have hypertension only during their episodic paroxysms. Once suspected clinically, the diagnosis is established biochemically with the finding of elevated urinary secretion of catecholamines or their metabolites. Diagnostic yield is highest when the collection is initiated with the onset of an episode. Though rare, pheochromocytoma can be life threatening, and if it is considered in the differential diagnosis of a patient's symptoms, testing should be ordered.

Although some of the patient's symptoms are suggestive of acromegaly or stress, there are no other symptoms, historical features, or physical findings that support these diagnoses. Physical examination does not suggest hypothyroidism, and the normal results of thyroid function tests exclude this diagnosis. A normal plasma glucose concentration during a symptomatic episode excludes insulinoma.

**Bibliography**

1. **Young WF Jr.** Pheochromocytoma and primary aldosteronism: diagnostic approaches. Endocrinol Metab Clin North Am. 1997;26:801-27. PMID: 9429861

## Hypertension Question 5
## Answer: D

**Educational Objective:** *Evaluate a patient with suspected Cushing's syndrome.*

This patient presents with clinical features suggestive of Cushing's syndrome. Urine-free cortisol is the best test to diagnose this disorder. However, because of his recent heavy alcohol use, he may have alcoholic pseudo-Cushing's syndrome. This disorder can mimic endogenous Cushing's syndrome and can only be distinguished from it by having the patient abstain from alcohol for an extended period of time. No evaluation for Cushing's syndrome should be done until after a period of abstinence.

The patient's easy bruising can be explained by excess circulating cortisol. Small vessel vasculitis would produce "palpable purpura" not found in this patient. von Willebrand's disease could produce bruising but not his other symptoms. Platelet dysfunction would produce petechiae, not bruising. Hemochromatosis would be expected to produce liver function abnormalities, heart failure, diabetes, decreased libido, and a bronze discoloration of the skin but not the hyperten-

sion, round face, and abnormal fat deposition of Cushing's syndrome.

**Bibliography**

1. **Meier CA, Biller BM.** Clinical and biochemical evaluation of Cushing's syndrome. Endocrinol Metab Clin North Am. 1997;26:741-62. PMID: 9429858

## Hypertension Question 6
## Answer: A

**Educational Objective:** *Recognize the clinical setting in which primary hyperaldosteronism should be considered and perform appropriate confirmatory testing.*

This patient presents with the typical features of primary hyperaldosteronism (autonomous overproduction of aldosterone). Most patients with this disorder are asymptomatic, and it should be considered in all patients with hypertension and hypokalemia. A paired plasma aldosterone concentration to plasma renin activity ratio of greater than 20 is suggestive of this disorder, and referral to a specialist is advisable because some patients can be cured with unilateral adrenalectomy. Although Cushing's syndrome may cause hypertension and hypokalemia, there are no suggestive clinical features of this disorder on the patient's history and physical examination. Renovascular hypertension and pheochromocytoma are not associated with hypokalemia. Bartter's syndrome is associated with hypokalemia but not hypertension.

**Bibliography**

1. **Young WF Jr.** Pheochromocytoma and primary aldosteronism: diagnostic approaches. Endocrinol Metab Clin North Am. 1997;26:801-27. PMID: 9429861

## Hypertension Question 7
## Answer: C

**Educational Objective:** *Identify autosomal dominant polycystic kidney disease as a secondary form of hypertension.*

This patient with stage 2 hypertension, a normal urinalysis and renal function, and a positive family history for hypertension and renal disease has autosomal dominant polycystic kidney disease (ADPKD). ADPKD may be found in young adults with hypertension, azotemia, or palpable kidneys. In patients with this disorder, hypertension may occur even with a normal urinalysis and serum creatinine level. The positive family history of renal failure is suggestive of an inherited disorder. Establishing the diagnosis of ADPKD may be important for prognosis and for providing family counseling. Renal ultrasonography is indicated, as this study will show multiple cysts in the kidneys. Approximately 50% of patients may also have hepatic cysts. Obtaining a captopril-stimulated renal scan and/or plasma renin activity and aldosterone determinations to search for renal artery stenosis is not warranted. Patients with renal artery stenosis (including fibromuscular hyperplasia in young women) or partial urinary tract obstruction may present with hypertension and a normal urinalysis and kidney function. However, the positive family history of renal failure suggests the correct diagnosis of ADPKD. A 24-hour urine determination for vanillylmandelic acid is also not warranted because the patient does not have signs or symptoms suggestive of pheochromocytoma.

### Bibliography

1. **Gabow PA**. Autosomal dominant polycystic kidney disease. N Engl J Med. 1993;329:332-42. PMID: 8321262

## Hypertension Question 8
## Answer: B

**Educational Objective:** *Recognize the importance of achieving target blood pressure with a minimum number of side effects.*

This patient's blood pressure control while on amlodipine is inadequate (blood pressure has not been reduced to < 140/90 mm Hg), and she has developed pedal edema attributable to the dihydropyridine calcium-channel blocker. Her medication should be changed to another antihypertensive agent that is unlikely to induce edema and will optimize blood pressure control. As reported in the report of the Sixth Joint National Conference on Prevention, Detection, Evaluation, and Treatment of High Blood Pressure (JNC-VI), adequate control of blood pressure to < 140/90 mm Hg is achieved in only 45% of patients treated with medication, which represents only 27% of all patients with hypertension. This has been labeled the "great hypertension disconnect." Almost all physicians know the target blood pressure of < 140/90 mm Hg; however, we are not very successful in achieving this target. When target blood pressure is not attained, the JNC-VI recommends three possible options: 1) increase the dose of the initial agent, 2) add a second agent, or 3) change to another drug or class of agent. This patient requires a change to another antihypertensive agent to achieve a target blood pressure and reduce side effects. Increasing this patient's dihydropyridine calcium-channel blocker is not indicated because this will likely increase her edema. A recent randomized, double-blind, clinical trial demonstrated that thiazide diuretics were superior to calcium channel blockers or angiotensin-converting enzyme inhibitors in lowering systolic blood pressure. The diuretic was superior to calcium channel blockers in preventing heart failure, and superior to angiotensin-converting enzyme inhibitors in reducing combined coronary vascular disease outcomes, stroke, and heart failure. Since diuretics are less expensive and more effective in preventing 1 or more major forms of coronary vascular disease, they should be preferred for first-step anti-hypertensive therapy in most patients. Finally, salt restriction and support hose are unlikely to resolve the medication-induced edema or improve the blood pressure.

### Bibliography

1. The sixth report of the Joint National Committee on Prevention, Detection, Evaluation and treatment of high blood pressure. Arch Intern Med. 1997;157:2413-46. PMID: 9385294

2. **Berlowitz DR, Ash AS, Hickey EC, Friedman RH, Glickman M, Kader B, et al**. Inadequate management of blood pressure in a hypertensive population. N Engl J Med. 1998;339:1957-63. PMID: 9869666

3. Major outcomes in high-risk patients randomized to angiotensin-converting enzyme inhibitor or calcium channel blocker vs diuretic: The Antihypertensive and Lipid-Lowering Treatment to Prevent Heart Attack Trial (ALLHAT). JAMA. 2002;288:3039-42. PMID: 12479763

## Hypertension Question 9
## Answer: D

**Educational Objective:** *Recognize the importance of "white coat" hypertension and its risks for cardiovascular disease.*

Patients with "white coat" hypertension may have subtle functional abnormalities when compared with their normotensive counterparts. Abnormalities include a higher systemic vascular resistance, higher insulin and triglyceride levels, a higher left ventricular mass index, and increased carotid artery intimal medial thickness. These patients are also more likely to develop sustained hypertension. Overall, patients with "white coat" hypertension may have an increased risk for cardiovascular disease, although the risk of cardiovascular complications appears to be relatively low if the ambulatory blood pressure remains normal.

"White coat" hypertension may be defined as the presence of office hypertension when the patient's blood pressure is repeatedly normal when measured by the patient or by others at home, at work, or by 24-hour ambulatory blood pressure monitoring. However, 24-hour ambulatory blood pressure monitoring is not required for the diagnosis. The risk of hypertensive cardiovascular complications (including both the development and regression of left ventricular hypertrophy) correlates more closely with 24-hour or daytime ambulatory blood pressure monitoring than with office pressure readings. "White coat" hypertension may affect up to 20% of patients with mild hypertension. One way to minimize the "white coat" effect is to have blood pressure in the office taken by a nurse rather than by the physician. A study using continuous interarterial monitoring has documented a more pronounced increase in systolic blood pressure (about 22 mm Hg) when blood pressure was measured with a sphygmomanometer by an unfamiliar physician rather than by a nurse.

Bibliography

1. Mancia G, Parati G, Pomidossi G, Grassi G, Casadei R, Zanchetti A. Alerting reaction and rise in blood pressure during measurement by physician and nurse. Hypertension. 1987;9:209-15. PMID: 3818018

2. Palatini P, Mormino P, Santonastaso M, Mos L, Dal Follo M, Zanata G, et al. Target-organ damage in stage I hypertensive subjects with white coat and sustained hypertension: results from the HARVEST study. Hypertension. 1998;31:57-63. PMID: 9449391

3. Julius S, Mejia A, Jones K, Krause L, Schork N, van de Ven C, et al. "White coat" versus "sustained" borderline hypertension in Tecumseh, Michigan. Hypertension. 1990;16:617-23. PMID: 2246029

## Hypertension Question 10
## Answer: C

**Educational Objective:** *Be aware of the clinical presentation of Takayasu's arteritis.*

This patient has typical features of Takayasu's arteritis. More than one half of affected patients have a systemic phase with nonspecific constitutional symptoms. Occlusive disease in the aorta and subclavian and carotid arteries produces bruits and diminished pulses. Hypertension is common and results from aortic constriction or renal artery occlusive disease. Laboratory findings are nonspecific; the erythrocyte sedimentation rate is usually elevated.

Giant cell arteritis may produce features similar to those of Takayasu's arteritis. However, it rarely presents before the fifth decade. Thromboangiitis obliterans primarily affects young male smokers and produces occlusion of medium- and small-caliber vessels in the upper and lower extremities. Aortic arch involvement is rare. Systemic lupus erythematosus may produce this patient's constitutional symptoms and hypertension, but major arterial involvement is rare. Diminished or asymmetric pulses are an important clue to aortic dissection. However, this diagnosis does not explain the constitutional symptoms or elevated sedimentation rate.

Bibliography

1. Shelhamer JH, Volkman DJ, Parrillo JE, Lawley TJ, Johnston MR, Fauci AS. Takayasu's arteritis and its therapy. Ann Intern Med. 1985;103:121-6. PMID: 2860834

## Hypertension Question 11
## Answer: A

**Educational Objective:** *Treat urgent hypertension safely.*

The most common cause of accelerated or urgent hypertension is noncompliance with prescribed therapy, despite frequent patient claims to the contrary. Reasonable blood pressure control at the previous visit suggests that the regimen was effective. The fact that the pulse rate is now 86/min casts some doubt on whether the atenolol has been taken recently. Imme-

diate administration of some or all of the patient's medications will help re-establish that they are effective for this patient.

It is not necessary to lower the blood pressure to normal at this juncture. The use of sublingual nifedipine to lower blood pressure has been condemned by medical experts and the U.S. Food and Drug Administration. The precipitous and uncontrolled decrease in blood pressure frequently produced by sublingual nifedipine presents a risk of myocardial infarction, stroke, or death. Because the patient has no evidence of acute end-organ damage (papilledema, abnormal mental status or neurologic findings), admission to the intensive care unit for treatment of hypertensive crisis is not warranted. Anxiety is not evident, nor is it likely to produce this magnitude of blood pressure elevation; thus, treatment with lorazepam is not indicated. Asking the patient to resume treatment with all medications (option E) is reasonable, but the follow-up period of 2 weeks is unreasonably long. It would be preferable to verify that the patient's regimen is effective before sending him home.

Bibliography

1. Grossman E, Messerli FH, Grodzicki T, Kowey P. Should a moratorium be placed on sublingual nifedipine capsules given for hypertensive emergencies and pseudoemergencies? JAMA. 1996;276:1328-31. PMID: 8861992

2. The sixth report of the Joint National Committee on Prevention, Detection, Evaluation, and Treatment of High Blood Pressure. Arch Intern Med. 1997;157:2413-46. PMID: 9385294

3. Wu SG, Lin SL, Shiao WY, Huang HW, Lin CF, Yang YH. Comparison of sublingual captopril, nifedipine and prazosin in hypertensive emergencies during hemodialysis. Nephron. 1993;65:284-7. PMID: 8247194

## Hypertension Question 12
## Answer: D

**Educational Objective:** *Select the most appropriate initial therapy for treating secondary hypertension in a patient with a pheochromocytoma.*

This woman has a pheochromocytoma, diagnosed by elevated urinary catecholamines and an adrenal mass with the typical clinical history. The mainstay of initial medical treatment is α-blockade, and the drug of choice is phenoxybenzamine. This agent will block both α1 and α2 receptors, which is advantageous, as a small population of α2 receptors may help mediate peripheral vasoconstriction in addition to α1 receptors. Phenoxybenzamine is also an irreversible blocker, causing destruction of the receptor. It is important to remember that patients with pheochromocytoma are volume-depleted and require substantial volume replacement with normal saline solution.

Esmolol (β-blockade without α-blockade) may precipitate a severe hypertensive crisis. Sublingual nifedipine may produce a precipitous fall in blood pressure that will be transient. An angiotensin-converting enzyme (ACE) inhibitor such as captopril is not the drug of choice in this clinical setting because it does not antagonize the α receptors.

**Bibliography**

1. **Werbel SS, Ober KP**. Pheochromocytoma. Update on diagnosis, localization, and management. Med Clin North Am. 1995;79:131-53. PMID: 7808088

## Hypertension Question 13
## Answer: B

**Educational Objective:** *Clinically recognize coarctation of the aorta.*

Coarctation of the aorta is a curable cause of systemic hypertension that is diagnosed clinically by systolic pressure difference between the upper and lower extremities, as in this patient. Normally, the systolic pressure in the lower extremity exceeds the blood pressure in the arms by 5 to 10 mm Hg. In supravalvular aortic stenosis there is commonly a difference in the systolic blood pressures between the right and left arm of several mm Hg but little difference between upper and lower extremities. In this patient, the aortic ejection sound and diastolic murmur suggest a bicuspid valve and the presence of mild aortic regurgitation. The incidence of a bicuspid aortic valve in patients with coarctation varies between 10% and 80%, and these patients should receive endocarditis antibiotic prophylaxis. The diagnosis is confirmed by echocardiography with Doppler flow recordings. The alternative diagnoses may cause systolic and diastolic murmurs but do not produce hypertension.

**Bibliography**

1. **Wren C, Oslizlok P, Bull C**. Natural history of supravalvular aortic stenosis and pulmonary artery stenosis. J Am Coll Cardiol. 1990;15:1625-30. PMID: 2345244

2. **Cohen M, Fuster V, Steele PM, Driscoll D, McGoon DC**. Coarctation of the aorta. Long-term follow-up and prediction of outcome after surgical correction. Circulation. 1989;80:840-5. PMID: 2791247

## Hypertension Question 14
## Answer: D

**Educational Objective:** *Select appropriate therapy for a pregnant woman with chronic hypertension.*

Preexisting hypertension is associated with an increased risk of complications during pregnancy, including fetal growth retardation, premature labor, placental abruption, and acute renal failure. It is defined as blood pressures > 140/90 mm Hg present prior to pregnancy or to the twentieth week of gestation. Drug therapy is recommended for patients with a diastolic blood pressure > 100 mm Hg or > 90 mm Hg in the setting of end-organ involvement.

Methyldopa is the most widely studied antihypertensive agent used in pregnancy, with clear safety and efficacy established. β-Blockers, such as propranolol, appear to be safe as well but may cause fetal growth retardation when used early in gestation. Hydralazine may be used safely as an adjunct to methyldopa and β-blockers and has an established track record in the treatment of preeclampsia. Calcium-channel blockers are probably safe, but insufficient long-term data are available to recommend their use.

Angiotensin-converting enzyme (ACE) inhibitors are contraindicated during pregnancy and have been associated with fetal death in animal models. Selective AT1 subtype angiotensin II receptor antagonists have an effect on the renin-angiotensin system that is similar to that of ACE inhibitors and are therefore contraindicated in pregnancy. Diuretics, such as hydrochlorothiazide, are also generally discouraged, because of potential effects on the fetus and because a fall in central blood volume may interfere with uteroplacental perfusion. In patients with significant volume overload, however, diuretics may be indicated.

**Bibliography**

1. **Lindheimer MD**. Hypertension in pregnancy. Hypertension. 1993;22:127-36. PMID: 8319988

## Hypertension Question 15
## Answer: C

**Educational Objective:** *Manage hypertension in a patient with type 1 diabetes mellitus, and understand the relative benefits and risks of the various classes of antihypertensive agents.*

Several medications are effective in treating hypertension in patients with diabetes. Angiotensin-converting enzyme (ACE) inhibitors, however, have been shown to have selective benefit in this regard: they not only lower blood pressure, but also can retard the rate of progression of any underlying nephropathy. In this patient, the presence of microalbuminuria (albumin level greater than 40 mg/24 h) indicates the presence of early nephropathy. Because ACE inhibitors can retard the progression of nephropathy even in normotensive individuals, these agents should be given even if nonpharmacologic therapy has been successful in lowering the blood pressure to normal levels. However, such use can cause hyperkalemia, and because patients with diabetes are prone to hyporeninemic hypoaldosteronism (type IV renal tubular acidosis), it is important to check potassium levels during therapy.

Other agents lack this selective benefit and are used as second-line treatment or if ACE inhibitors cannot be tolerated.

**Bibliography**

1. **Caldwell BV**. Treating hypertension in the diabetic patient: therapeutic goals and the role of calcium channel blockers. Clin Ther. 1993;15:618-36. PMID: 8221813

2. **Lewis EJ, Unsicker LG, Bain RP, Rohde RD.** The effect of angiotensin-converting-enzyme inhibition on diabetic nephropathy. The Collaborative Study Group. N Engl J Med. 1993;329:1456-62. PMID: 8413456

## Hypertension Question 16
## Answer: A

**Educational Objective:** *Recognize the findings of combined hypertensive retinopathy and retinal arteriolar sclerosis on a funduscopic photograph.*

Characteristic changes are noted in the retinas of patients with longstanding hypertension. Narrowing of the terminal branches of retinal arterioles may be seen, as well as general narrowing of vessels with severe local constriction (as shown in this photograph). As the disease progresses, striate hemorrhages and soft exudates become visible. In a normal eye, retinal arterioles are transparent, so that blood flow is visible during ophthalmoscopy. A light streak from the ophthalmoscope will reflect from the convex wall of the healthy arteriole. In a sclerotic arteriole, thickening and fibrosis of the vessel wall develop as the sclerosis progresses. The central light reflex increases in width, and the walls of the vessel look like burnished copper, producing a "copper-wire" arteriole. With further progression and additional fibrosis, the entire width of the arteriole reflects the white stripe, producing "silver-wire" arteries. This patient's funduscopic photograph shows both the "copper and silver wires" characteristic of arteriolar sclerosis and the characteristic changes of hypertensive retinopathy.

### Bibliography
1. **Dodson PM, Lip GY, Eames SM, Gibson JM, Beevers DG.** Hypertensive retinopathy: a review of existing classification systems and a suggestion for a simplified grading system. J Hum Hypertens. 1996;10:93-8. PMID: 8867562

## Hypertension Question 17
## Answer: D

**Educational Objective:** *Recognize malignant hypertension on a funduscopic photograph.*

The retinal changes associated with malignant hypertension consist of arteriolar narrowing, severe local vasoconstriction, hemorrhages, exudates, and papilledema. The exudates are caused by fibroid necrosis of vessel walls. Papilledema associated with malignant hypertension can be differentiated from papilledema due to other causes by its clinical context. Optic neuritis, generally monocular and another cause of a disk swelling, is not associated with hypertension and will have accompanying afferent pupillary defects and loss of vision. Both papilledema associated with malignant hypertension and optic neuritis can be accompanied by loss of vision. Arteriolar sclerosis is not accompanied by papilledema. Brain tumors can be associated with papilledema but not arteriolar narrowing, vasoconstriction, hemorrhages, or exudates.

### Bibliography
1. **Dodson PM, Lip GY, Eames SM, Gibson JM, Beevers DG.** Hypertensive retinopathy: a review of existing classification systems and a suggestion for a simplified grading system. J Hum Hypertens. 1996;10:93-8. . PMID: 8867562

## Hypertension Question 18
## Answer: A

**Educational Objective:** *Recognize a unilateral adrenal mass and know that, with this patient's presentation, the mass is most likely a primary adrenal tumor causing Cushing's syndrome.*

The differential diagnosis of an adrenal mass includes pheochromocytoma, adrenocortical adenoma, adrenal cancer, malignancy metastatic to the adrenal glands, nonfunctional adrenal tumor, and aldosteronoma. This patient's workup should begin with a hormonal evaluation for Cushing's syndrome before anatomic radiographic imaging is performed. In contrast to Cushing's syndrome, Cushing's disease is a pituitary lesion associated with hypercortisolism due to excess ACTH secretion and is more likely to present as diffuse bilateral enlargement of both adrenal glands than as a focal or unilateral lesion. It is also crucial to rule out a pheochromocytoma by hormonal studies in this patient, however her symptoms are not consistent with pheochromocytoma. Renal call carcinoma and renal artery fibromuscular dysplasia are incorrect answers because the arrows in the CT scan are pointing to the adrenal glands; the tumor is on the left.

### Bibliography
1. **Foo R, O'Shaughnessy KM, Brown MJ.** Hyperaldosteronism: recent concepts, diagnosis, and management. Postgrad Med J. 2001;77:639-44. PMID: 11571370

## Hypertension Question 19
## Answer: A

**Educational Objective:** *Set appropriate treatment goals in a case of a hypertensive emergency.*

This patient reports headache and transient visual loss and is found to be confused. The diagnosis of hypertensive encephalopathy is likely, even in the absence of papilledema. Hypertensive encephalopathy is a diagnosis of exclusion, but there is no a priori evidence of stroke, seizure disorder, or encephalitis. Admission to the intensive care unit and immediate treatment with intravenous nitroprusside are indicated. Mean arterial blood pressure (MAP) should be lowered by no more than approximately 25%. In this case, admission MAP is 207 mm Hg (systolic blood pressure plus twice the diastolic blood pressure, divided by 3) and should be lowered quickly into the range of 150 to 160 mm Hg. A blood pressure of

220/110 mm Hg corresponds to a MAP of 147 mm Hg, which is acceptable. Lowering blood pressure to a level as low as 160/90 mm Hg (MAP, 133 mm Hg) carries the risk of provoking stroke or myocardial infarction. The initial target blood pressure should be maintained for several days, then gradually brought into normotensive range.

Oral or sublingual nifedipine can cause unpredictable falls in blood pressure and should not be used. Labetalol can be useful in cases of hypertensive crisis, but in this case, it would have to be given in the intensive care unit in the form of repeat intravenous boluses for rapid and controlled effect. Oral labetalol followed by continued observation in the emergency department is not adequate therapy in a case of hypertensive encephalopathy.

**Bibliography**

1. **Calhoun DA, Oparil S**. Treatment of hypertensive crisis. N Engl J Med. 1990;323:1177-83. PMID: 2215596
2. **Grossman E, Messerli FH, Grodzicki T, Kowey P**. Should a moratorium be placed on sublingual nifedipine capsules given for hypertensive emergencies and pseudoemergencies? JAMA. 1996;276:1328-31. PMID: 8861992

## Hypertension Question 20
## Answer: A

**Educational Objective:** *Be aware that low-dose estrogen preparations can cause hypertension and that oral contraceptive-induced hypertension resolves within a few months of cessation of the drug.*

Oral contraceptive agents increase the blood pressure slightly in most women, but only about 5% will become hypertensive. With newer low-dose estrogen preparations, the incidence of hypertension may even be lower. However, this patient was on a low-dose estrogen-containing preparation when she developed hypertension, and there is a good possibility that it was the cause of her hypertension. In more than half of all women with oral contraceptive associated hypertension, the blood pressure normalizes within 3 months of cessation of therapy. Therefore, the best strategy is to stop the oral contraceptive and see the patient again in a few weeks to recheck her blood pressure.

It is possible that this patient will turn out to have new-onset essential hypertension. However, 24-hour ambulatory monitoring and echocardiography are not routine screening tests in the work-up of hypertension. The cost of these tests does not justify their use in this situation. Drug therapy would be premature at this time.

In women of childbearing age, angiotensin-converting enzyme inhibitors are a less-than-ideal choice because of their teratogenic potential. In cases in which no other form of contraception is acceptable and the hypertension is not severe, oral contraceptives can be continued together with antihypertensive therapy. In such cases, diuretics would be a good choice.

**Bibliography**

1. The sixth report of the Joint National Committee on Prevention, Detection, Evaluation, and Treatment of High Blood Pressure. Arch Intern Med. 1997;157:2413-46. PMID: 9385294
2. **Dong W, Colhoun HM, Poulter NR.** Blood pressure in women using oral contraceptives: results from the Health Survey for England 1994. J Hypertens. 1997;15:1063-8. PMID: 9350579
3. **Kaplan NM.** The treatment of hypertension in women. Arch Intern Med. 1995;155:563-7. PMID: 7887751
4. **Piper JM, Ray WA, Rosa FW.** Pregnancy outcome following exposure to angiotensin-converting enzyme inhibitors. Obstet Gynecol. 1992;80:429-32. PMID: 1495700

## Hypertension Question 21
## Answer: E

**Educational Objective:** *Diagnose fulminant preeclampsia, and distinguish it from other diseases.*

This woman has fulminant preeclampsia, a multisystem disease caused by widespread endothelial cell dysfunction resulting in fibrin deposits in the small vessels of the kidney, liver, and brain. Microangiopathic hemolytic anemia is present secondary to the widespread fibrin deposits.

Preeclampsia has many similarities to thrombotic thrombocytopenic purpura (TTP), but TTP causes damage to the endothelial cells by an immunologic mechanism. Fever virtually always is present in TTP, and hypertension is rare.

This woman manifests the HELLP syndrome; this acronym indicates hemolysis, elevated liver enzymes, and low platelet count. The HELLP syndrome is always an indication for immediate delivery, which is the definitive treatment for preeclampsia.

Although hypertension occurs in patients with preeclampsia, the pressure does not reach the levels seen in malignant hypertension, in which diastolic pressure is usually above 120 mm Hg and the hypertension itself causes endothelial cell damage. Thus, preeclampsia is not associated with retinal hemorrhages or exudates or papilledema, characteristically seen in malignant hypertension.

The hyperuricemia and proteinuria without microscopic hematuria or casts are typical of preeclampsia; with acute glomerulonephritis, however, microscopic hematuria accompanies proteinuria.

Liver involvement is common in preeclampsia, and fatty deposition in liver cells and fibrin deposits in the sinusoids have been found on percutaneous liver biopsy studies. Thrombocytopenia and elevated fibrin split products are consistent with widespread fibrin deposition, which can lead to a consumptive coagulopathy. Acute pancreatitis cannot explain the hematological, hypertensive, or funduscopic findings of this patient.

**Bibliography**

1. **Martin JN Jr, Blake PG, Perry KG Jr, McCaul JF, Hess LW, Martin RW.** The natural history of HELLP syndrome: patterns of disease progression and regression. Am J Obstet Gynecol. 1991;164:1500-9. PMID: 2048596

2. **Brown MA, Lindheimer MD, de Swiet M, Van Assche A, Moutquin JM**.The classification and diagnosis of the hypertensive disorders of pregnancy: statement from the International Society for the Study of Hypertension in Pregnancy (ISSHP). Hypertens Pregnancy. 2001;20:IX-XIV. PMID: 12044323

## Hypertension Question 22
## Answer: C

**Educational Objective:** *Understand the tests used to evaluate patients for renovascular hypertension.*

The evaluation of patients for suspected renovascular hypertension continues to be controversial, but a consensus is available. Renovascular hypertension is not common; in patients with long-standing hypertension, correction of a renal artery stenotic lesion may not result in significant improvement in blood pressure control. The usual cause of renal artery stenosis in 55-year-old men is atherosclerotic renal artery stenosis. Although blood pressure can often be managed with medication, an additional major reason to be concerned about this type of patient is that renal artery stenosis may result in ischemic nephropathy. Although the ideal test would have a 100% degree of sensitivity and specificity, no such test is available for evaluating patients with suspected renovascular hypertension. Even renal arteriography is not 100% specific because the presence of renal artery stenosis does not guarantee the presence of functional significance of stenotic lesions.

Using standard criteria of delay in uptake of contrast material, hyper concentration, and decreases in kidney size, intravenous pyelography has a 70% degree of sensitivity and a greater than 90% degree of specificity. It is not especially useful for the diagnosis of bilateral renovascular hypertension because most of the criteria depend on comparison between the ipsilateral and contralateral kidneys.

Although the degree of sensitivity of renal scintigraphy is greater than 85%, it is not a particularly specific test because as many as 30% of patients with essential hypertension prove positive.

The addition of converting enzyme inhibitors to renal scintigraphy has greatly enhanced both the sensitivity and specificity of post-converting enzyme inhibitor scintigraphy. In patients with essential hypertension, converting enzyme inhibitors cause small decreases in efferent vascular tone that are offset by decreases in afferent vascular tone, so that renal blood flow remains constant. In contrast, in patients with functionally significant renal artery stenosis, reduction in efferent tone cannot be offset by reductions in afferent tone because of upstream stenosis. This results in decreases in the glomerular filtration rate and the renal blood flow, as well as in a positive test. This test has a degree of sensitivity and specificity greater than 90% and is therefore recommended.

Basal renin values have not been found to be discriminatory. The addition of converting enzyme inhibitors has clearly increased the accuracy of plasma renin activity determinations.

Although the principle is the same as that of post converting enzyme inhibitor scintigraphy (converting enzyme inhibitors cause decreases in efferent tone and, in the presence of fixed upstream stenotic lesions, renal ischemia ensues and results in production of renin), as many as 25% of patients with essential hypertension have a positive post converting enzyme inhibitor renin study.

Although relatively inexpensive and noninvasive, renal ultrasonography is positive only in patients with severe renal artery stenosis resulting in decreases in renal size. Hence, its sensitivity is quite low, especially in diagnosing early renovascular hypertension.

### Bibliography

1. **Svetkey LP, Himmelstein SI, Dunnick NR, Wilkenson RH Jr, Ballinger RR, McCann RL, et al**. Prospective analysis of strategies for diagnosing renovascular hypertension. Hypertension. 1989;14:247-57. PMID: 2670763

2. **Davidson R, Wilcox CS**. Diagnostic usefulness of renal scanning after angiotensin converting enzyme inhibitors. Hypertension. 1991;18:299-303. PMID: 1889844

3. **Mann SJ, Pickering TG**. Detection of renovascular hypertension. State of the art. Ann Intern Med. 1992;117:845-53. PMID: 1416561

# Altered Mental Status

## Altered Mental Status Question 1
## Answer: D

**Educational Objective:** *Differentiate normal from abnormal changes in memory in older adults.*

No further evaluation with MRI or neuropsychologic testing or specific therapy (e.g. antidepressants) is required for this patient at this time. She has no signs of depression or neurophysiologic dysfunction. Normal aging is accompanied by several changes in the ability to learn something new and recall it. Older people need more repetitions to learn something new. With age, "the tip-of-the-tongue phenomenon" becomes more common, manifested as difficulty recalling proper names and specific words. Reaction time slows and there are increased errors on tasks that require dividing or switching attention or that are timed. The ability to store new memories remains intact with normal aging, even if it may take a cue to retrieve the stored memory. When a person with age-associated memory impairment is reminded of what they're forgotten, they generally remember it. A demented person usually has no recollection, even after being reminded.

**Bibliography**
1. **Grady CL, Craik FI**. Changes in memory processing with age. Curr Opin Neurobiol. 2000;10:224-31. PMID: 10753795
2. **Brown AS**. A review of the tip-of-the-tongue experience. Psychol Bull. 1991;109:204-23. PMID: 2034750

## Altered Mental Status Question 2
## Answer: A

**Educational Objective:** *Develop a differential diagnosis for a patient with delirium.*

Hyponatremia is a common and dangerous cause of delirium in hospitalized patients. An undernourished, elderly man would be at particularly high risk. Meningitis may accompany pneumonia; however, because this patient has responded to treatment and has been afebrile for 3 days, meningitis manifesting at this late date is unlikely.

Alcohol abstinence syndrome is always a consideration when delirium develops without a clear explanation in a hospitalized patient. However, most cases become manifest much earlier and are usually accompanied by tachycardia, agitation, tremulousness, and sometimes mild fever.

Pulmonary embolism is always a consideration, when unexplained delirium develops in a hospitalized patient. But, when hypoxemia leads to delirium, the patient is often agitated rather than drowsy. Furthermore, it would be unusual to have normal vital signs with newly worsening hypoxemia. Antibiotic therapy rarely causes delirium.

**Bibliography**
1. **Elie M, Cole MG, Primeau FJ, Bellavance F**. Delirium risk factors in elderly hospitalized patients. J Gen Intern Med. 1998;13:204-12. PMID: 9541379
2. **Inouye SK**. Prevention of delirium in hospitalized older patients: risk factors and targeted intervention strategies. Ann Med. 2000;32:257-63. PMID: 10852142

## Altered Mental Status Question 3
## Answer: C

**Educational Objective:** *Prescribe conservative measures to reduce the risk of delirium.*

In a randomized clinical trial, conservative measures were effective in reducing the risk of delirium in hospitalized patients. Reducing ambient noise, orienting the patient repeatedly, early mobilization, and strategies to improve impaired hearing and vision were important parts of the intervention.

Benzodiazepines and major tranquilizers (such as haloperidol) should never be used to prevent delirium in elderly, demented patients because these agents are reported to cause the syndrome. Physical restraints and urinary catheters may also provoke the syndrome. Limiting fluids has not been shown to help, and dehydration is a risk factor for delirium. Bright illumination all night long would probably interfere with sleep and thus be counterproductive. Sleep-enhancement protocols are part of the effective intervention.

Encouraging family members to stay with the high-risk patient is probably effective, although not rigorously studied.

**Bibliography**
1. **Elie M, Cole MG, Primeau FJ, Bellavance F**. Delirium risk factors in elderly hospitalized patients. J Gen Intern Med. 1998;13:204-12. PMID: 9541379
2. **Inouye SK, Bogardus ST, Charpentier PA, Leo-Summers L, Acampora D, Holford TR, Cooney LM**. A multicomponent intervention to prevent delirium in hospitalized older patients. N Engl J Med. 1999;340:669-76. PMID: 10053175

## Altered Mental Status Question 4
## Answer: E

**Educational Objective:** *Recognize restraints as a danger to many delirious patients.*

Although the use of physical restraints is a very prominent feature in Joint Commission on Accreditation of Healthcare Organizations (JCAHO) inspections and the topic of a JCAHO "Sentinel Event Alert," very few data guide the proper use of restraints in hospitalized patients; most data are generated in long-term care facilities and extrapolated to the acute setting.

In the nursing home, physical restraints do not seem to reduce the risk of injury and have been shown to cause injury and death. Death by fire has been reported in smokers who were restrained and smoked in bed while restrained or used their lighters to attempt to burn off their restraints.

Bedrails present a particular problem. In the nursing home, eliminating bedrails leads to an increase in falls from the bed, but no change or a decrease in injurious falls has been seen. The difference in mechanics between sliding off a mattress and falling from the top of bedrails may explain this difference.

Therapy with benzodiazepines increases the risk of falls. Although direct supervision of this patient is resource-intense, it is probably warranted because this patient is highly vulnerable and at serious risk.

### Bibliography

1. Elie M, Cole MG, Primeau FJ, Bellavance F. Delirium risk factors in elderly hospitalized patients. J Gen Intern Med. 1998;13:204-12. PMID: 9541379
2. Cole MG, Primeau FJ, Bailey RF, Bonnycastle MJ, Masciarelli F, Engelsmann F, et al. Systematic intervention for elderly inpatients with delirium: a randomized trial. CMAJ. 1994;151:965-70. PMID: 7922932

## Altered Mental Status Question 5
## Answer: B

**Educational Objective:** *Recognize the diagnostic features of normal-pressure hydrocephalus.*

The triad of urinary incontinence, gait impairment, and cognitive impairment is typical of normal-pressure hydrocephalus (NPH). In addition, mild, generalized slowness of movement (bradykinesia) and slowness of thought (bradyphrenia) are often present in patients with NPH. The patient's feet often seem to "cling to the floor," as if drawn by a magnet (thus called a "magnetic" or "apractic" gait). The gait in patients with Parkinson's disease is more "shuffling" or "festinating," and asymmetric resting tremor, rigidity, and bradykinesia are more characteristic of Parkinson's disease. A large, bifrontal brain tumor could mimic NPH (which is why CT or MRI scanning is necessary), but a mild headache and papilledema are often present with a tumor. This patient's cognitive impairment cannot be explained by a spinal cord lesion. Multi-infarct dementia is a diagnosis that is often applied incorrectly and is not appropriate in this patient because his course has been gradual and progressive rather than punctuated by discrete events with a "step-wise" progression.

The cause of NPH is not fully understood. Pathophysiology may be due to excessive cerebrospinal fluid (CSF) production, insufficient CSF absorption, or both. The resulting imbalance causes dilatation of the ventricles, which "stretches" the cortical-subcortical neural networks involved in cognition, balance, and continence. By allowing the excessive CSF to flow into the abdomen via a ventriculoperitoneal shunt, the "stretching" effect can be diminished and in some patients completely eliminated, resulting in improvement of some or all symptoms.

When NPH is suspected clinically, the imaging study of choice is an MRI scan of the brain. A neurologic consultation should be sought in most instances. Since degenerative dementia with atrophy and secondary ventricular dilatation as well as NPH tends to occur in patients over the age of 65, neuropsychometric testing is useful in most patients, particularly those with cognitive impairment alone or in combination with only one of the other two diagnostic features. In patients with gait impairment as the major feature, a large-volume lumbar puncture (30 mL), preferably with videotaping of the patient walking before and after CSF is removed, can document any improvement in gait after CSF drainage. Some centers perform serial lumbar punctures or continuous CSF drainage over 2 to 4 days. If unequivocal improvement in gait occurs, the diagnosis of NPH is supported, and the patient is more likely to benefit from ventriculoperitoneal shunting.

NPH can be relatively easy to diagnose, but the determination of "whom to shunt and whom not to shunt" can be challenging. Not all patients with NPH benefit from shunting, and complications such as meningitis, shunt malfunction, and subdural hematoma occur in 30% to 40% of patients. Those who have cognitive impairment for less than 1 year or whose gait impairment precedes cognitive impairment are more likely to respond to shunting. Carbidopa/levodopa may improve symptoms in some patients who do not undergo a shunt procedure.

### Bibliography

1. Graff-Radford NR, Godersky JC, Jones MP. Variables predicting surgical outcome in symptomatic hydrocephalus in the elderly. Neurology. 1989;39:1601-4. PMID: 2586777
2. Vanneste JA. Diagnosis and management of normal-pressure hydrocephalus. J Neurol. 2000;247:5-14. PMID: 10701891

## Altered Mental Status Question 6
## Answer: D

**Educational Objective:** *Distinguish brain abscess from other conditions associated with fever and/or meningeal signs.*

The clinical presentation of brain abscesses is variable and depends on the location of the abscess and the extent of increased intracranial pressure. Although patients may present with fever and meningeal signs, the presence of papilledema is unusual in acute bacterial or aseptic meningitis and mandates that neuroimaging be performed before doing a lumbar puncture. Furthermore, fever and meningismus are not a typical presentation for a cerebral neoplasm. Most brain abscesses are polymicrobial, and anaerobic bacteria are the most common pathogens when the predisposing cause is chronic dental sepsis. Diagnosis of a pyogenic abscess relies on neuroimaging. MRI is superior to CT scans of the brain in characterizing the number and pathologic features of the lesion(s). MRI typically reveals a central zone of hypointensity on T1-weighted images corresponding to purulent material, with a ring of T1-weighted hyperintensity that enhances following gadolinium and delineates the capsule of the abscess. Treatment includes the initiation of broad-spectrum antibiotics, management of increased intracranial pressure, and surgical drainage.

### Bibliography
1. **Mathisen GE, Johnson JP**. Brain abscess. Clin Infect Dis. 1997;25:763-79. PMID: 9356788
2. **Wong J, Quint DJ**. Imaging of central nervous system infections. Semin Roentgenol. 1999;34:123-43. PMID: 10231907

## Altered Mental Status Question 7
## Answer: A

**Educational Objective:** *Recognize the appropriate management strategies for patients with questionable dementia versus pseudodementia.*

This scenario exemplifies a common clinical situation in which the clinician must consider whether pseudodementia or an early degenerative dementing illness best explains a patient's cognitive-behavioral change. Although there are numerous reports in the literature suggesting that certain features are diagnostically helpful for differentiating degenerative dementia from pseudodementia, this distinction is becoming blurred because depression and dementia often coexist, and some evidence suggests that depression is a risk factor for the future development of dementia. In this patient, it is reasonable to initiate an antidepressant agent that has few cognitive side effects. The response to this therapy can then provide diagnostic and therapeutic information. Selective serotonin reuptake inhibitors have less anticholinergic side effects than tricyclic antidepressants and are most appropriate for this patient. Cholinesterase inhibitors are indicated for patients with suspected Alzheimer's disease, but this patient's symptoms and relative preservation of memory on the Mini-Mental State Examination (MMSE) argue against this diagnosis. Although a referral to a psychiatrist is reasonable, proceeding directly to electroconvulsive therapy is inappropriate. Reassurance that nothing is wrong is a common remark in situations such as this. However, although the patient's performance on the MMSE is only borderline abnormal, his marked behavioral changes and loss of employment clearly indicate that an abnormality exists.

### Bibliography
1. **Raskind MA**. The clinical interface of depression and dementia. J Clin Psychiatry. 1998;59:9-12. PMID: 9720476

## Altered Mental Status Question 8
## Answer: C

**Educational Objective:** *Distinguish features of HIV-associated cognitive-motor complex from other causes of cognitive decline in a patient with AIDS.*

The HIV-associated cognitive-motor complex is a syndrome characterized by cognitive, motor, and behavioral dysfunction and is the most common direct central nervous system complication of HIV-1 infection. The syndrome generally occurs during late stages of HIV-1 infection, often at the same time as other AIDS-defining systemic illnesses develop. During early stages, it may be difficult to distinguish the clinical presentation from that of depression or an opportunistic central nervous system infection. These patients may appear depressed because of their lack of interest and initiative but do not fulfill clinical criteria for a depressive disorder.

Imaging studies are essential to rule out mass lesions. Between 20% and 40% of patients demonstrate ill-defined, nonenhancing areas of increased T2 signal in the deep white matter on MRI. In patients with HIV-associated cognitive-motor complex, the neurologic examination demonstrates diffuse central nervous system signs, including slowing of rapid alternating movements of the extremities, a generalized increase in deep tendon reflexes, and the emergence of frontal release signs such as snout, glabellar, and grasp reflexes. This is distinct from the typical focal neurologic findings seen in patients with HIV infection who have a mass lesion caused by cerebral toxoplasmosis. Cerebrospinal fluid abnormalities include an elevated protein concentration in approximately 45% of patients and an increased IgG level in about 80% of patients. The cerebrospinal fluid is usually acellular. Cytomegalovirus (CMV) encephalitis can be confused with the HIV-associated dementia complex. The course of CMV encephalitis is typically rapidly progressive and often occurs in a patient with CMV retinitis or disseminated CMV infection. MRI of the brain demonstrates periventricular white matter lesions with contrast-enhancing lesions in subependymal and cortical regions.

## Bibliography

1. **Adams MA, Ferraro FR**. Acquired immunodeficiency syndrome dementia complex. J Clin Psychol. 1997;53:767-78. PMID: 9356907
2. **Navia BA**. Clinical and biologic features of the AIDS dementia complex. Neuroimaging Clin N Am. 1997;7:581-92. PMID: 9376969

## Altered Mental Status Question 9
## Answer: B

**Educational Objective:** *Recognize the diagnostic utility of currently available ancillary tests for the diagnosis of Alzheimer's disease.*

This patient has features that satisfy all criteria for the diagnosis of Alzheimer's disease, and it is reasonable to make this clinically probable diagnosis. Although an initial report in the literature indicated that a positive pupillary response to tropicamide eyedrop administration confirmed the diagnosis of Alzheimer's disease, these results have been refuted. Unless there are contraindications, vitamin E, 2000 IU daily, and donepezil, 5 mg daily for 1 month followed by 10 mg daily thereafter, would be the most reasonable management. Estrogen failed to improve memory in women with Alzheimer's disease in a clinical trial. Although prior use of nonsteroidal anti-inflammatory drugs has been suggested to decrease the risk of subsequent development of Alzheimer's disease, there are no placebo-controlled trials to date in which any of these drugs has been efficacious once Alzheimer's disease becomes symptomatic. Since *ApoE* is a susceptibility gene and thus affects the *risk* of developing Alzheimer's disease, it has been recommended that *ApoE* genotyping should <u>not</u> be used to diagnose patients with dementia or to assess the risk of developing Alzheimer's disease in asymptomatic individuals. *ApoE4* can also be present in patients with pathologically proven frontotemporal dementia and dementia with Lewy bodies. Recent data have also demonstrated that in patients with dementia, a low cerebrospinal fluid (CSF) amyloid level, a high CSF tau level, and a high CSF or urine neuronal thread level are all suggestive of Alzheimer's disease. However, the sensitivity and specificity of each test are not 100%.

There is no noninvasive or CSF test available to date that will firmly establish or negate the presence of Alzheimer's disease in a patient with dementia. Histologic examination of brain tissue by biopsy or autopsy is required to establish this diagnosis. In choosing whether to perform testing for *ApoE*, amyloid, tau, and neuronal thread levels, one must weigh the slight increase in diagnostic accuracy against the expense and the patient's and family's wishes. (Some children do not want to know their *ApoE* status.)

## Bibliography

1. **Graff-Radford NR, Lin SC, Brazis PW, Bolling JP, Liesegang TJ, Lucas JA, et al**. Tropicamide eyedrops cannot be used for reliable diagnosis of Alzheimer's disease. Mayo Clin Proc. 1997;72:495-504. PMID: 9179132
2. Statement on use of apolipoprotein E testing for Alzheimer disease. American College of Medical Genetics/American Society of Human Genetics Working Group on ApoE and Alzheimer Disease. JAMA. 1995;274:1627-9. PMID: 7474250
3. **Galasko D, Chang L, Motter R, Clark CM, Kaye J, Knopman D, et al**. High cerebrospinal fluid tau and low amyloid beta42 levels in the clinical diagnosis of Alzheimer disease and relation to apolipoprotein E genotype. Arch Neurol. 1998;55:937-45. PMID: 9678311
4. **Mulnard RA, Cotman CW, Kawas C, van Dyck CH, Sano M, Doody R, et al**. Estrogen replacement therapy for treatment of mild Alzheimer disease: a randomized controlled trial. Alzheimer's Disease Cooperative Study. JAMA. 2000;283:1007-15. PMID: 10697060

## Altered Mental Status Question 10
## Answer: D

**Educational Objective:** *Recognize Creutzfeldt-Jakob disease as a cause of rapidly progressive dementia.*

Although there are many potential causes of rapidly progressive dementia with myoclonus, Creutzfeldt-Jakob disease is most likely in this patient. This is a disorder caused by a prion, a small proteinaceous particle that can cause a rapidly progressive dementia many years after exposure. However, in a patient with a dementing illness, other possibilities, including multi-infarct dementia, must be considered. This patient's clinical findings are not compatible with multi-infarct dementia or vitamin $B_{12}$ deficiency. An imaging study that shows increased ventricular size in a patient with dementia may indicate normal-pressure hydrocephalus, which typically presents with the clinical triad of dementia, gait apraxia, and urinary incontinence. The standard cerebrospinal fluid examination parameters are often normal in patients with Creutzfeldt-Jakob disease, but a slightly elevated protein concentration may be present. Neuron-specific-enolase, an enzyme found in neurons and neuroendocrine cells, is typically substantially elevated in the cerebrospinal fluid of patients with Creutzfeldt-Jakob disease but is a nonspecific marker. Finding 14-3-3 brain protein in the cerebrospinal fluid is a more specific marker for this disease. Hypothyroidism, with an increased sensitive thyroid-stimulating hormone level, can cause dementia, but the dementia usually is not rapidly progressive. The electroencephalogram in patients with Creutzfeldt-Jakob disease demonstrates high-amplitude, periodic sharp waves that can progress over several days or weeks. These sharp wave findings are often transient and therefore are not seen in all patients with Creutzfeldt-Jakob disease.

## Bibliography

1. **Prusiner SB**. The prion diseases. Brain Pathol. 1998;8:499-513. PMID: 9669700

2. **Zerr I, Bodemer M, Gefeller O, Otto M, Poser S, Wiltfang J, et al**. Detection of 14-3-3 protein in the cerebrospinal fluid supports the diagnosis of Creutzfeldt-Jakob disease. Ann Neurol. 1998;43:32-40. PMID: 9450766

3. **Zerr I, Bodemer M, Racker S, Grosche S, Poser S, Kretzschmar HA, Weber T**. Cerebrospinal fluid concentration of neuron-specific enolase in diagnosis of Creutzfeldt-Jakob disease. Lancet. 1995;345:1609-10. PMID: 7783539

## Altered Mental Status Question 11
## Answer: A

**Educational Objective:** *Become familiar with the differential diagnosis and evaluation of a patient with metabolic encephalopathy.*

The neurologic findings in this patient are those of a subacute toximetabolic encephalopathy. Encephalopathies are characterized by (1) a decrease in the level of alertness, (2) a global decrease in cognitive functions, (3) fluctuations in alertness and cognitive abilities during the day, and (4), often, asterixis. Focal neurologic signs are usually absent.

In this patient, the most likely diagnosis is hyponatremia related to her water-drinking and renal disease. There is nothing in the account given to suggest that the patient might have hypothyroidism or systemic lupus erythematosus. Although vitamin $B_{12}$ deficiency might explain the absent ankle reflexes and decreased vibration sense in the feet, it would not explain the reduced alertness and encephalopathic findings.

A lumbar puncture would be useful if meningitis, encephalitis, intracranial bleeding, or high cerebrospinal fluid pressure were present. The patient's history and neurologic signs do not suggest any of these conditions.

### Bibliography
1. **Arieff AI, Llach F, Massry SG**. Neurological manifestations and morbidity of hyponatremia: correlation with brain water and electrolytes. Medicine (Baltimore). 1976;55:121-9. PMID: 1256311

## Altered Mental Status Question 12
## Answer: E

**Educational Objective:** *Consider the diagnosis of vitamin $B_{12}$ deficiency in patients with myelopathy, but without anemia or macrocytosis.*

The diagnosis that would explain all of this patient's findings is vitamin $B_{12}$ deficiency, probably secondary to pernicious anemia. Nearly one fourth of patients with vitamin $B_{12}$ deficiency and neurologic disease (combinations of myelopathy, peripheral neuropathy, dementia, psychiatric symptoms, or, infrequently, optic atrophy) have normal hematocrits and hemoglobin levels, and some do not even demonstrate macrocytosis, although high-normal mean corpuscular volumes tend to fall with treatment. A hematologic clue in this patient is the presence of hypersegmented polymorphonuclear leukocytes on blood smear. Serum vitamin $B_{12}$ levels can be falsely nor-

mal in the presence of neurologic or hematologic disease; levels can also be low yet clinically insignificant. In such settings, the diagnosis can be confirmed by obtaining serum concentrations of the metabolites methylmalonic acid and homocysteine, which are nearly always elevated in clinically significant cobalamin deficiency, falling with treatment.

Spastic legs, extensor plantar responses, and a suggestive midthoracic sensory level indicate myelopathy, and an infective or neoplastic cause must be considered. Negative spinal radiographs make such a diagnosis unlikely but do not exclude it. However, the patient also has mild dementia, and her absent lower extremity tendon reflexes in the face of spasticity suggest peripheral neuropathy. Spasticity and extensor plantar responses are not features of tabes dorsalis, and the patient does not report pain. Normal-pressure hydrocephalus causes gait disturbance and dementia (most characteristically abulia rather than memory loss or irritability), but not myelopathy or peripheral neuropathy. Moreover, computed tomography of her head does not support that diagnosis. Alcohol abuse indirectly causes dementia, cerebellar ataxia, and peripheral neuropathy, but not myelopathy.

### Bibliography
1. **Lindenbaum J, Healton EB, Savage DG, Brust JC, Garrett TJ, Podell ER, et al**. Neuropsychiatric disorders caused by cobalamin deficiency in the absence of anemia or macrocytosis. N Engl J Med. 1988;318:1720-8. PMID: 3374544

# Depression

## Depression Question 1
## Answer: B

**Educational Objective:** *Recognize symptoms of grief.*

Hearing the voice of the recently deceased is a common phenomenon of grief. It does not indicate a psychotic disorder unless it is accompanied by other delusions, hallucinations, disorganized speech, or grossly disorganized behavior. Treatment with an antipsychotic agent is not needed.

Depressive symptoms are common in acute grief. Primary depressive disorder should be considered when severe symptoms persist for more than 2 months. Symptoms to consider include persistent thoughts of death, guilt, feelings of worthlessness, psychomotor retardation, marked functional impairment, and hallucinatory experiences other than transiently hearing the voice or seeing the image of the deceased. This patient's grief reaction is not sufficiently severe or prolonged to diagnose major depression. Counseling may be helpful for relief of symptoms such as insomnia.

### Bibliography

1. **Rozenzweig A, Prigerson H, Miller MD, Reynolds CF 3rd.** Bereavement and late-life depression: grief and its complications in the elderly. Ann Rev Med. 1997;48:421-8. PMID: 9046973
2. **Biondi M, Picardi A.** Clinical and biological aspects of bereavement and loss-induced depression: a reappraisal. Psychother Psychosom. 1996;65:229-45. PMID: 8893324
3. **Pasternak RE, Reynolds CF 3rd, Schlernitzauer M, Hoch CC, Buysse DJ, Houck PR, et al.** Acute open-trial nortriptyline therapy of bereavement-related depression in late life. J Clin Psychiatry. 1991;52:307-10. PMID: 2071562

## Depression Question 2
## Answer: E

**Educational Objective:** *Recognize indications for psychotherapy in patients with depression.*

Psychotherapy can improve response to antidepressant medications, decrease the risk of relapse in recurrent depression, and address ongoing interpersonal and intrapsychic conflicts. This patient's psychological suffering and interpersonal difficulties are an indication for psychological therapy in addition to pharmacotherapy. Changing his medication or adjusting the dosage does not address the psychological issues. Increasing the dosage of sertraline should be considered if response to treatment, particularly the somatic symptoms of depression, is inadequate after 6 to 8 weeks. Switching to bupropion, a tricyclic antidepressant, or another agent should also be considered after an adequate trial of the initial agent. This patient has responded well to sertraline previously, a good predictor of subsequent benefit, and most of his depressive symptoms are resolving. Methylphenidate can increase energy and improve mood when a rapid response is needed or to augment treatment with another agent.

### Bibliography

1. **Thase ME, Greenhouse JB, Frank E, Reynolds CF 3rd, Pilkonis PA, Hurley K, et al.** Treatment of major depression with psychotherapy or psychotherapy-pharmacotherapy combinations. Arch Gen Psychiatry. 1997;54:1009-15. PMID: 9366657
2. **Katon W, Robinson P, Von Korff M, Lin E, Bush T, Ludman E, et al.** A multifaceted intervention to improve treatment of depression in primary care. Arch Gen Psychiatry. 1996;53:924-32. PMID: 8857869

## Depression Question 3
## Answer: D

**Educational Objective:** *Understand the indications for maintenance antidepressant therapy.*

After the acute phase of treatment with antidepressant medication (the first 6 to 12 weeks), therapy should be continued for at least 4 to 9 months (continuation phase) to prevent early relapse. Continuation of therapy for at least 1 year reduces the rate of relapse from 50% to 26%. History of previous major depressive episodes increases the risk of relapse, and long-term maintenance therapy should be considered in these patients. Medication should be prescribed at the full dosage during maintenance therapy. Augmentation with methylphenidate or lithium carbonate or switching to another agent should be considered if symptoms are very severe (lack of energy that interferes significantly with professional or personal activities) or if response is not adequate after an adequate trial with the primary antidepressant (8 to 12 weeks at full dosage).

### Bibliography

1. **Reimherr FW, Amsterdam JD, Quitkin FM, Rosenbaum JF, Fava M, Zajecka J, et al.** Optimal length of continuation therapy in depression: a prospective assessment during long-term fluoxetine treatment. Am J Psychiatry. 1998;155:1247-53. PMID: 9734550
2. **Schulberg HC, Katon W, Simon GE, Rush AJ.** Treatment of major depression in primary care practice: an update of the Agency for Health Care Policy and Research Practice Guidelines. Arch Gen Psychiatry. 1998;55:1121-7. PMID: 9862556

## Depression Question 4
## Answer: C

**Educational Objective:** *Distinguish between mental impairment and depression in an elderly patient.*

The Mini-Mental State Examination score ≤ 23 implies cognitive impairment for people with a ninth grade or higher education; however, scores of 18 to 23 may be normal for people with less formal education. In particular, nonworking people may be less aware of the specific date, serial sevens are incorrectly performed by almost 50% of people, and the "s" in "no ifs, ands, or buts" may not be heard by people with presbycusis. This patient, however, has had several losses recently and appears to be less attentive, not paying bills or knowing the location of her current appointment, suggesting that she may be depressed, with concentration impairment and less motivation. There are several screening tools for depression, including the Geriatric Depression Scale. If the results of the screening test for depression are not suggestive of depression, a neuropsychiatric evaluation may be helpful diagnostically.

**Bibliography**

1. **Molloy DW, Standish TIM**. A guide to the standardized Mini-Mental State examination. Int Psychogeriatr. 1997; 9 Suppl 1:87-94. PMID: 9447431

2. **Yesavage JA**. Geriatric Depression Scale. Psychopharmacol Bull. 1988;24:709-11. PMID: 3249773

## Depression Question 5
## Answer: B

**Educational Objective:** *Prescribe urgent psychiatric consultation in elderly patients with severe depression.*

This patient has major depression complicating bereavement. Major depression should be considered when severe symptoms of bereavement persist for more than 2 months after a loss. The risk of depression is 15% to 35% in the first year after death of a spouse. Urgent psychiatric consultation is indicated to ensure this patient's safety and to institute treatment. Hospitalization may be necessary. Reassurance is inappropriate as a single intervention.

Suicide risk increases with age, and 70% of suicides occur in people over age 60 years. Medical illness and social isolation are known risk factors. Direct questioning regarding suicide risk is essential. The potentially suicidal patient should be detained and possibly hospitalized unless the physician is assured that the risk of suicide is low. A plan for intervention and support must be in place. Tricyclic antidepressants should be used with caution in a potentially suicidal patient because these agents are potentially lethal. In this patient, antidepressant medication is indicated, not an anxiolytic. Simply increasing social interactions is not adequate treatment. Close follow-up must be provided. Two weeks is a reasonable interval to assess initial response to antidepressant medication in stable patients, but closer observation is needed in severely depressed patients.

**Bibliography**

1. **Hirschfeld RM, Russell JM**. Assessment and treatment of suicidal patients. N Engl J Med. 1997;337:910-5. PMID: 9302306

2. **Conwell Y**. Management of suicidal behavior in the elderly. Psych Clin North Am. 1997;20:667-83. PMID: 9323319

3. **Muller-Oerlinghausen B, Berghofer A**. Antidepressants and suicidal risk. J Clin Psych. 1999;60(Suppl 2):94-6. PMID: 10073395

## Depression Question 6
## Answer: A

**Educational Objective:** *Determine the most appropriate course of action in evaluating the patient with unintentional weight loss of unknown cause.*

The elderly are susceptible to many physiologic, mental, and social circumstances that cause unintentional weight loss. Important considerations in this age group include cognitive decline, the appearance of important new systemic medical disorders, physiologic changes of aging that affect swallowing or senses of taste or smell, poor dentition, polypharmacy and adverse drug interactions, low income, and new psychiatric disease. This patient has marked signs of depression and social isolation, which can have a serious effect on a previously healthy older person. The appetite-stimulating qualities of tricyclic antidepressants can reestablish healthy eating behaviors relatively quickly. The alteration in taste that occurs with aging is not usually related to zinc deficiency, nor will it improve with a proton-pump inhibitor. Finally, pseudodementia and dementia may initially be confused with depression; it would be reasonable to address cognitive functioning if antidepressant therapy does not succeed.

**Bibliography**

1. **Wallace JI, Schwartz RS**. Involuntary weight loss in elderly outpatients: recognition, etiologies, and treatment. Clin Geriatr Med. 1997;13:717-35. PMID: 9354751

2. **Thompson MP, Morris LK**. Unexplained weight loss in the ambulatory elderly. J Am Geriatr Soc. 1991;39:497-500. PMID: 2022802

## Depression Question 7
## Answer: B

**Educational Objective:** *Recognize adolescent depression.*

Suicide is the third most common cause of death in persons between ages 10 and 24 years, accounting for 13% of all deaths in this age range. Up to 30% of 16-year-old females seriously consider suicide, and 24% make a suicide plan. Adolescents are less likely to show affective change and are more likely to manifest behavioral disturbances as a symptom of depression than adults, making the diagnosis less apparent.

This patient meets the DSM-PC criteria for major depressive episode in adolescents. Her use of alcohol as a soporific is particularly worrisome. Her suicide risk needs to be ascertained urgently. Medical and emotional conditions are not mutually exclusive. She may have additional reasons for fatigue, such as anemia, hepatitis, or lymphoma. The presence of a rash, cold intolerance, or vomiting may help differentiate between the various causes of her weight loss, and may also be clues to an associated eating disorder or the consequences of her drinking. However, none bear the urgency of further assessment of her mental status. Though patients with premenstrual syndrome may experience a premenstrual exacerbation of the affective component of that disorder, it does not preclude the possibility that they also suffer from major depression and are at risk for suicide.

### Bibliography

1. **Perkins K, Ferrari N, Rosas A, Bessette R, Williams A, Omar H**. You won't know unless you ask: the biopsychosocial interview for adolescents. Clin Pediatr (Phila). 1997;36:79-88. PMID: 9118594
2. **Bell CC, Clark DC**. Adolescent suicide. Ped Clin North Am. 1998;45:365-80. PMID: 9568016

## Depression Question 8
**Answer: E**

**Educational Objective:** *Recognize diagnostic features of dysthymia.*

Dysthymia is characterized by chronic (lasting at least 2 years) symptoms of depression that are not severe enough to meet the diagnostic criteria for major depression. Symptoms include alterations of appetite, sleep, energy, self-esteem, concentration, and feelings of hopelessness that are not as severe or disabling as those of a major depressive disorder but that interfere with function and quality of life. Dysthymia often begins in early life, and patients are at increased risk for major depression. Treatment with antidepressant medication, psychotherapy, or both can be effective.

Most patients with major depression have periods of complete remission, but 20% to 30% have chronic depressive symptoms. Patients with atypical depression usually have weight gain, multiple somatic symptoms, sensitivity to interpersonal rejection, and hypersomnia and meet the criteria for major depression. Seasonal affective disorder is cyclical, with predictable improvement in the summer months. In adjustment disorder with depressed mood, there is an identifiable stressor within the preceding 3 months, and symptoms do not persist longer than 6 months.

### Bibliography

1. **Olfson M, Broadhead WE, Weissman MW, Leon AC, Farber L, Hoven C, et al**. Subthreshold psychiatric symptoms in a primary care group practice. Arch Gen Psychiatry. 1996;53:880-6. PMID: 8857864
2. **Thase ME, Fava M, Halbreich U, Kocsis JH, Koran L, Davidson J, et al**. A placebo-controlled randomized clinical trial comparing sertraline and imipramine for the treatment of dysthymia. Arch Gen Psychiatry. 1996;53:777-84. PMID: 8792754

## Depression Question 9
**Answer: B**

**Educational Objective:** *Recognize depression in the Southeast Asian immigrant.*

There is a high prevalence of depression — and a high level of under diagnosis by primary care physicians — among Vietnamese refugees, who may somaticize their dysphoric affect because of their cultural prejudice against mental health problems. Depression can be diagnosed, however, using such instruments as the culturally specific psychologic assessment. Treatment may be difficult if the patient is unwilling to differentiate between psychologic, physiologic, and supernatural causes of illness.

Polymyalgia rheumatica is unlikely with a normal erythrocyte sedimentation rate and no myalgias. The spleen tip is often palpable in persons from areas that are endemic for malaria, such as Vietnam, but malaria would not explain her current symptoms of headache, cough, and difficulty sleeping. In addition, malaria, disseminated tuberculosis, and HIV disease are ruled out by her extensive workup. Hepatitis B related diseases, such as polyarteritis and hepatoma, should also have been ruled out by physical examination or the laboratory studies done to this point.

### Bibliography

1. **Lin EH, Ihle LJ, Tazuma L**. Depression among Vietnamese refugees in a primary care clinic. Am J Med. 1985;78:41-4. PMID: 3966487
2. **Gold SJ**. Mental health and illness in Vietnamese refugees. West J Med. 1992;157:290-4. PMID: 1413772

# Substance Abuse

## Substance Abuse Question 1
## Answer: C

**Educational Objective:** *Determine the most appropriate course of action in the care of at-risk and nondependent drinkers.*

This patient satisfies the definition of an at-risk drinker (>14 drinks per week or four drinks per occasion for a male). Although it is potentially hazardous, his alcohol consumption does not qualify for alcohol abuse or dependence considering the lack of clinically significant impairment or distress, withdrawal, tolerance, or interference with life functioning. The additional information provided by the CAGE questionnaire suggests hazardous drinking in need of intervention. Performing AUDIT or questioning the probably accurate quantity history are unnecessary at this time because a CAGE cut point of 2 is already highly sensitive (>80%) and specific (>90%) in identifying problem drinking in the elderly. Numerous randomized, controlled trials in primary care settings attest to the efficacy of brief counseling interventions and educational pamphlets in changing adverse health behavior. Two 15-minute office visits with follow-up phone calls resulted in approximately a 50% decrease in drinks per week in one study. Referral to Alcoholics Anonymous or other self-help groups may improve abstinence rates, but there is little clinical trial data available to support referral over office-based motivational enhancement programs. Finally, naltrexone, although effective in blunting craving and reducing relapses in alcoholic patients, is effective only when used in inpatient treatment programs.

### Bibliography
1. **O'Connor PG, Schottenfeld RS**. Patients with alcohol problems. N Engl J Med. 1998;338:592-602. PMID: 9475768
2. **Fleming MF, Barry KL, Manwell LB, Johnson K, London R.** Brief physician advice for problem alcohol drinkers. A randomized controlled trial in community-based primary care practices. JAMA. 1997;277:1039-45. PMID: 9091691
3. **Parish DC**. Another indication for screening and early intervention: problem drinking. JAMA. 1997;277:1079-80. PMID: 9091699

## Substance Abuse Question 2
## Answer: E

**Educational Objective:** *Manage cocaine-associated chest pain and arrhythmias.*

Cocaine users commonly present with chest pain and tachycardia. Although myocardial ischemia needs to be ruled out, there are several unique issues in managing the patient who has recently used cocaine. The electrocardiogram may show J-point elevation in the absence of ischemia. Initial treatment with benzodiazepines decreases anxiety and typically decreases heart rate and blood pressure, avoiding the need for specific antihypertensive medications. Although aspirin and blood pressure control are not contraindicated, the routine use of β-blockers may be detrimental. Propranolol may block the tachycardia but unmask α-adrenergic stimulatory effects of cocaine and worsen hypertension. Diltiazem is useful for atrial fibrillation, and adenosine may be used for supraventricular tachycardia, but neither helps cocaine-induced sinus tachycardia. Nifedipine, either sublingually or orally, may risk precipitating severe hypotension with subsequent ischemia-induced, end-organ damage.

### Bibliography
1. **Hollander JE**. The management of cocaine-associated myocardial ischemia. N Engl J Med. 1995;333:1267-72. PMID: 7566005
2. **Grossman E, Messerli FH, Grodzicki T, Kowey P**. Should a moratorium be placed on sublingual nifedipine capsules given for hypertensive emergencies and pseudoemergencies? JAMA. 1996;276:1328-31. PMID: 8861992

## Substance Abuse Question 3
## Answer: C

**Educational Objective:** *Diagnose and manage alcohol withdrawal as a cause of delirium in the hospital.*

This patient has become delirious with confusion and abnormalities of alertness and attentiveness. Alcohol withdrawal, without a confirmatory history, remains a diagnosis of exclusion, but the syndrome is common and sometimes overlooked.

Venous thromboembolism is less likely because the injury and surgical repair are so recent, the blood gases are normal, and the delirium is so prominent. Fat embolism is a consideration but is less likely than alcohol withdrawal.

Because the patient was fully alert and able to leave the recovery room so promptly after surgery, an anesthetic complication is unlikely. Transfusion reactions are very rarely responsible for delirium. Late hemolytic reactions, due to an anamnestic response that develops against the transfused blood, are usually not apparent for at least 5 days. Acute hemolytic reactions generally present with fever, hemolysis, and renal injury; delirium is rare in this situation.

## Bibliography

1. **Elie M, Cole MG, Primeau FJ, Bellavance F**. Delirium risk factors in elderly hospitalized patients. J Gen Intern Med. 1998;13:204-12. PMID: 9541379

2. **Kraemer KL, Conigliaro J, Saitz R**. Managing alcohol withdrawal in the elderly. Drugs Aging. 1999;14:409-25. PMID: 10408740

## Substance Abuse Question 4
## Answer: E

**Educational Objective:** *Recognize the syndrome of acute Wernicke's disease in the absence of a history of alcohol abuse.*

This patient has the classic clinical triad of acute thiamine deficiency — altered mentation, ophthalmoparesis, and truncal ataxia. His mental abnormalities include more than impaired memory: he has decreased alertness, and he is inattentive and abulic. Wernicke's disease can progress to the point at which altered sensorium and attentiveness make it difficult to assess memory or other cognitive abilities.) The more purely amnesic Korsakoff's syndrome is a chronic manifestation of thiamine deficiency, often affecting patients who have been treated one or more times for acute Wernicke's disease. The eye movement abnormalities here are also characteristic: restricted horizontal movements (abducens or lateral gaze paresis) nearly always precede vertical gaze abnormalities. The ataxic gait is likely secondary to both cerebellar and vestibular dysfunction; it often occurs in the absence of limb ataxia. Although hardly pathognomonic, the enlarged liver and the likely sensory polyneuropathy in this patient offer clues to an alcoholic past.

Vitamin $B_{12}$ deficiency can cause altered mentation, peripheral neuropathy, and ataxia, but symptoms would not progress to this degree over 3 days, and ophthalmoplegia is not part of the clinical picture. Wilson's disease causes hepatic damage, and its major neurologic symptoms are mental, but its clinical manifestations are of insidious onset and progression, with extrapyramidal and cerebellar signs (tremor, rigidity, dystonia, dysarthria). Although hepatic encephalopathy secondary to alcoholic liver damage could cause the patient's altered mentation, it would not account for his eye movement abnormalities or ataxic gait, and there was no asterixis. Similarly, alcohol withdrawal, although possibly contributing to his altered mentation, would not explain his other signs, and there is no tremor.

## Bibliography

1. **Lieber CS**. Medical disorders of alcoholism. N Engl J Med.1995;333:1058-65. PMID: 7675050

2. **Thomson AD**. Mechanisms of vitamin deficiency in chronic alcoholic misusers and the development of the Wernicke-Korsakoff Syndrome. Alcohol Alcohol 2000; 35: 1-27. PMID: 11304071

## Substance Abuse Question 5
## Answer: C

**Educational Objective:** *Identify the clinical features of recreational drug toxicity and withdrawal.*

This patient is suffering from cocaine toxicity. She was treated first for opiate overdose, which had caused the familiar triad of coma, respiratory depression, and pinpoint pupils. Naloxone administration produced overshoot into a withdrawal state, which was treated with methadone. Neither opiate overdose nor opiate withdrawal would be the likely cause of her seizure, however. Although in some animal models opiates lower seizure threshold, seizures are sufficiently unusual in clinical overdose that an additional cause must always be sought. Except possibly in newborns, seizures are not a feature of opiate withdrawal. Unlike sedative or ethanol withdrawal, which can cause seizures, hallucinations, and fatal delirium tremens, opiate withdrawal symptoms resemble a severe case of the flu and are hardly ever life-threatening.

Perhaps related to its local anesthetic properties, cocaine is the most epileptogenic of recreationally used psychostimulants. Seizures can occur many hours after acute psychic effects have worn off, perhaps reflecting the epileptogenicity of less psychotomimetic metabolites. Seizures are not a feature of cocaine withdrawal, which produces only subjective symptoms of hunger, depression, and craving.

## Bibliography

1. **Spivey WH, Eurele B**. Nerologic complications of cocaine abuse. Ann Emerg Med. 1990;19:1422-8. PMID: 2240756

## Substance Abuse Question 6
## Answer: B

**Educational Objective:** *Recognize and initiate proper therapy for alcoholic ketoacidosis.*

This patient presents with abdominal pain, nausea, and vomiting. Physical examination and laboratory testing suggest alcoholic hepatitis. Alcoholic ketoacidosis is usually seen in the setting of binge drinking with cessation of food intake for an extended period and vomiting. It appears to be more common in women than in men. Hyperglycemia is inconsistent and may be present in diabetics or mildly present in nondiabetics. This patient's slightly elevated glucose level makes diabetic ketoacidosis unlikely, and insulin therapy is not appropriate.

In a patient such as this, ingestion of other alcohols (ethylene glycol and methanol) should be considered, and it would be worthwhile to test for these alcohols.

Treatment of alcoholic ketoacidosis consists of rehydration with normal saline and intravenous administration of glucose after the administration of thiamine. The ketosis will clear rapidly with therapy, and sodium bicarbonate usually is not indicated unless the acidosis is very severe. β-Blockers have no place in this situation. Corticosteroids seem to benefit patients with severe alcoholic hepatitis but will not treat the acidosis.

### Bibliography

1. **Fulop M**. Alcoholic ketoacidosis. Endocrinol Metab Clin North Am. 1993;22:209-19. PMID: 8325283
2. **Hooper RJ**. Alcoholic ketoacidosis: the late presentation of acidosis in an alcoholic. Ann Clin Biochem. 1994;31:579-82. PMID: 7880081

## Substance Abuse Question 7
## Answer: C

**Educational Objective:** *Identify possible drug or alcohol abuse in an older person with cognitive impairment.*

Alcohol or drug use should be considered in any older person who presents with a history of fairly acute onset of irritability, distractability, and memory problems. Toxicity from multiple medications often produces the same symptoms. In this 89-year-old woman, the findings of an elevated serum alanine aminotransferase concentration and mean corpuscular volume, although not specific, suggest alcohol abuse.

Chronic dementia, such as Alzheimer's disease and multi-infarct dementia, does not present with an acute onset. Subdural hematoma can present in this way but usually includes focal neurologic findings. Although other acute disorders such as stroke or delirium from an underlying medical disorder should also be considered, alcohol abuse is a prime diagnosis in this patient and the most likely of the options presented.

### Bibliography

1. **Widner S, Zeichner A**. Alcohol abuse in the elderly: review of epidemiology, research and treatment. Clin Gerontol. 1991;11:3-18. PMID: 2650501
2. **Willenbring ML**. Organic mental disorders associated with heavy drinking and alcohol dependence. Clin Geriatr Med. 1988;4:869-87. PMID: 3066465

## Substance Abuse Question 8
## Answer: E

**Educational Objective:** *Recognize and understand how to manage heroin-induced pulmonary edema.*

This patient presents with hypotension, hypoxia, and pulmonary infiltrates in the setting of injection drug use. This clinical picture is most consistent with heroin-induced pulmonary edema. Patients with heroin-induced pulmonary edema do not have increased central venous pressures. The onset of pulmonary edema can be up to 6 to 10 hours after the heroin is injected. Patients can have a rapid improvement following administration of naloxone (a narcotic antagonist) and oxygen. These patients have a low intravascular volume and hypovolemia, so diuretics are not beneficial and can lead

to vascular collapse. A minority of patients do not improve with supportive therapy and die.

Dopamine might be useful in supporting the blood pressure but would not be the first treatment of heroin-induced pulmonary edema. Treatment of the underlying hypotension (i.e., drug overdosage) would be more appropriate.

Digitalis administration would be appropriate for treatment of cardiogenic pulmonary edema; however, there is no evidence of cardiac failure, as demonstrated by the lack of a gallop and a normal cardiac silhouette.

Flumazenil is used to reverse the respiratory suppression caused by benzodiazepines but would have no effect on heroin overdosage.

### Bibliography

1. **Cherubin CE, Sapira JD.** The medical complications of drug addiction and the medical assessment of the intravenous drug user: 25 years later. Ann Intern Med. 1993;119:1017-28. PMID: 8214979
2. **Stein MD.** Medical complications of intravenous drug use. J Gen Intern Med. 1990;5:249-57. PMID: 2187962

## Substance Abuse Question 9
## Answer: D

**Educational Objective:** *Manage drug (alcohol) withdrawal.*

This patient is exhibiting signs of alcohol withdrawal. The increased heart rate and blood pressure, tremors, and hallucinations are most likely secondary to withdrawal and not due to other primary disorders requiring treatment. A benzodiazepine such as lorazepam is the safest therapy to mitigate withdrawal symptoms and facilitate detoxification. Chlorpromazine is used in the treatment of psychoses but is not indicated in the treatment of alcohol withdrawal syndrome. It also could lower seizure threshold and would therefore be contraindicated in this patient. The fact that the patient previously experienced a seizure while withdrawing from ethanol does not in itself warrant prophylactic phenytoin. Naltrexone may help reduce alcohol craving and prevent relapse drinking in alcoholics, but it has no useful role in treatment of alcohol withdrawal. Captopril is used to treat hypertension but would not treat his alcohol withdrawal syndrome (which is the likely cause of his elevated blood pressure).

### Bibliography

1. **Litten RZ, Allen J, Fertig J.** Pharmacotherapies for alcohol problems: a review of research with focus on developments since 1991. Alcohol Clin Exp Res. 1996;20:859-76. PMID: 8865961
2. **Miller NS.** Pharmacotherapy in alcoholism. J Addict Dis. 1995;14:23-46. PMID: 7632745
3. **Brewer C.** Second-line and 'alternative' treatments for alcohol withdrawal: alpha-agonists, beta-blockers, anticonvulsants, acupuncture and neuro-electric therapy. Alcohol Alcohol. 1995;30:799-803. PMID: 8679022

# Smoking

## Smoking Question 1
## Answer: A

**Educational Objective:** *Select the most appropriate approach to smoking cessation during pregnancy.*

This patient has moved from precontemplation and contemplation to determination to change her smoking behavior; therefore, assessing her smoking behavior and advising her to change her habits are unnecessary. The issue now is to facilitate a safe, successful quitting strategy and set achievable goals. In pregnant patients, the primary approach should be intensive smoking-cessation counseling, with nicotine replacement therapy used only in the heaviest smoker if the increased likelihood of smoking cessation with its potential benefits outweighs the risks of nicotine replacement and potential concomitant smoking. In a nonpregnant patient, nicotine replacement therapy or bupropion as an initial strategy should be routinely offered in addition to counseling. Although referral to a smoking-cessation program might be useful, such programs have success rates similar to physician minimal-contact strategies. The longer the physician counsels the patient, the greater the potential for success.

### Bibliography

1. The Agency for Health Care Policy and Research Smoking Cessation Clinical Practice Guideline. JAMA. 1996;275:1270-80. PMID: 8601960
2. **Hughes JR, Goldstein MG, Hurt RD, Shiffman S**. Recent advances in the pharmacotherapy of smoking. JAMA. 1999;281:72-6. PMID: 9892454
3. **Law M, Tang JL**. An analysis of the effectiveness of interventions intended to help people stop smoking. Arch Intern Med. 1995;155:1933-41. PMID: 7575046
4. **Kendrick JS, Merritt RK**. Women and smoking: an update for the 1990s. Am J Obstet Gynecol. 1996;175:528-35. PMID: 8828410

## Smoking Question 2
## Answer: D

**Educational Objective:** *Assist a smoker to quit smoking who has been unsuccessful with the use of over-the-counter treatment.*

Patients who fail to quit smoking after using an over-the-counter preparation now constitute a large percentage of patients seen in physicians' offices requesting other modalities of therapy. In such patients, it is necessary to explore compliance issues as well as assess the patient for psychiatric illnesses, such as depression, that may direct further therapy. There is strong evidence for bupropion alone or in combination with concurrent nicotine replacement therapy as an effective means of doubling quit rates. Tapering cigarette use is not associated with improved opportunities for success as compared with abrupt cessation and initiation of nicotine replacement therapy. Smoking-cessation programs do not improve quit rates over physician counseling. Alternative therapies without evidence for improved efficacy over bupropion or nicotine replacement therapy in the general population include minor tranquilizers, clonidine, tricyclic antidepressant agents, and hypnotism.

### Bibliography

1. **Jorenby DE, Leischow SJ, Nides MA, Rennard SI, Johnston JA, Hughes AR, et al**. A controlled trial of sustained-release bupropion, a nicotine patch, or both for smoking cessation. N Engl J Med. 1999;340:685-91. PMID: 10053177
2. **Hurt RD, Sachs DP, Glover ED, Offord KP, Johnston JA, Dale LC, et al**. A comparison of sustained-release bupropion and placebo for smoking cessation. N Engl J Med. 1997;337:1195-202. PMID: 9337378
3. **Cinciripini PM, McClure JB**. Smoking cessation: recent developments in behavioral and pharmacologic interventions. Oncology (Huntingt). 1998;12:249-56, 259. PMID: 9507525
4. **Kattapong VJ, Locher TL, Secker-Walker RH, Bell TA**. American College of Preventive Medicine practice policy. Tobacco-cessation patient counseling. Am J Prev Med. 1998;15:160-2. PMID: 9713673

## Smoking Question 3
## Answer: D

**Educational Objective:** *Know the management having the highest priority for a patient with intermittent claudication who smokes cigarettes.*

Treatment goals in patients with peripheral arterial disease include prevention of atherosclerosis (especially in the coronary and cerebrovascular beds), reduction of morbidity and morality from coronary and other cardiovascular diseases, limb preservation in *severely* symptomatic patients, and functional improvement in patients with moderate limitation or symptoms.

To prevent disease progression and reduce the risk of major atherosclerotic events, medical management should include intensive risk factor reduction regardless of symptom severity (even in an asymptomatic patient with an ankle-brachial index of < 0.90). Smoking cessation, blood pressure and serum lipid control, and management of diabetes mellitus are strongly indicated. Thus, this patient should first be reassessed for his willingness to stop smoking.

ANSWERS and CRITIQUES • *Smoking*

Pentoxifylline is thought to improve symptoms of peripheral arterial disease by increasing erythrocyte flexibility and improving capillary blood flow, but clinical results are not striking. Although administration of pentoxifylline may be indicated, it is not as high a priority as smoking cessation. Anticoagulants such as warfarin have not been shown to alter the natural history of peripheral arterial disease and are not recommended because of their potential complications. Cilostazol is a relatively new drug for treatment of claudication. It is a phosphodiesterase inhibitor that inhibits platelet aggregation, increases vasodilatation, and inhibits smooth muscle proliferation. It also has beneficial effects on high-density lipoprotein cholesterol and triglyceride levels. The drug appears superior to pentoxifylline in improving walking distance and treadmill time. It is possibly indicated in this patient, but as stated above, smoking cessation is a higher priority.

In *severely* compromised patients, revascularization of the lower limbs can be accomplished surgically or by percutaneous transluminal angioplasty. However, this patient has relatively mild symptoms and is not receiving adequate medical therapy. Revascularization therefore is currently inappropriate.

**Bibliography**

1. **Hiatt WR, Hirsch AT, Regensteiner JG, Bress EP**. Clinical trials for claudication. Assessment of exercise performance, functional status and clinical endpoints. Vascular Clinical Trialists. Circulation. 1995;92:614-21. PMID: 7634476

## Smoking Question 4
## Answer: D

**Educational Objective:** *Recognize risk factors for pancreatic cancer.*

Cigarette smoking is a strong risk factor for pancreatic cancer that can be eliminated. Other identified risk factors for pancreatic cancer are advanced age, male gender, black ethnicity, type 1 diabetes mellitus, chronic pancreatitis, hereditary/familial pancreatitis, pancreatic cancer in close relatives, and industrial exposures to petroleum compounds and leather tanneries. A high-red meat, high-fat diet and heavy alcohol consumption may also be weakly associated with increased risk of pancreatic cancer. Coffee consumption is not a risk factor. Obesity is associated with an increased risk of death from cancer in general. However, the relationship of obesity and pancreatic cancer risk is not well defined. The benefits of weight loss are less significant than those of quitting smoking.

**Bibliography**

1. **Silverman DT, Schiffman M, Everhart J, Goldstein A, Lillemoe KD, Swanson GM, et al.** Diabetes mellitus, other medical conditions and familial history of cancer as risk factors for pancreatic cancer. Br J Cancer. 1999;80:1830-7. PMID: 10468306

2. **Calle EE, Thun MJ, Petrelli JM, et al.** Body-mass index and mortality in a prospective cohort of U.S. adults. N Engl J Med. 1999;341:1097-105. PMID: 10511607

## Smoking Question 5
## Answer: E

**Educational Objective:** *Recognize the most effective intervention known to decrease the risk of lung cancer.*

Transdermal nicotine replacement therapy has been shown in randomized trials to increase the quit rate of cigarette smoking, especially when combined with counseling programs on tobacco cessation. Since most lung cancers are caused by cigarette smoking and the risk of lung cancer decreases over the decade following cigarette smoking cessation, nicotine replacement therapy is the most effective known strategy to decrease the risk of lung cancer. Tobacco cessation is a form of primary prevention. Tobacco cessation also decreases the risk of dying of a number of tobacco-related diseases.

Randomized, prospective trials have shown that despite the fact that chest radiograph and sputum cytology can pick up a substantial number of asymptomatic lung cancers, using these screening tests does not decrease lung cancer death rates. At best, screening for lung cancer only decreases the risk of death from a single disease. 13-*cis*-Retinoic acid has been shown in randomized trials to decrease the risk of getting upper aerodigestive cancers, including lung cancer, after the treatment of head and neck cancer. It has also been shown to increase the regression rate of the premalignant lesion, oral leukoplakia. However, it does not decrease mortality from lung cancer. Finally, lung cancer incidence and mortality are actually increased by β-carotene administration, as shown in two randomized, placebo-controlled trials in men at high risk of lung cancer due to smoking or asbestos exposure. Therefore, β-carotene is contraindicated in a cigarette smoker.

**Bibliography**

1. **Wolpaw DR.** Early detection in lung cancer. Case finding and screening. Med Clin North Am. 1996;80:63-82. PMID: 8569301

2. The effect of vitamin E and beta carotene on the incidence of lung cancer and other cancers in male smokers. The Alpha-Tocopherol, Beta Carotene Cancer Prevention Study Group. N Engl J Med. 1994;330:1029-35. PMID: 8127329

3. **Omenn GS, Goodman GE, Thornquist MD, Balmes J, Cullen MR, Glass A, et al.** Effects of a combination of beta carotene and vitamin A on lung cancer and cardiovascular disease. N Engl J Med. 1996;334:1150-5. PMID: 8602180

4. **Benner SE, Pajak TF, Lippman SM, Earley C, Hong WK.** Prevention of second primary tumors with isotretinoin in patients with squamous cell carcinoma of the head and neck: long term follow-up. J Natl Cancer Inst. 1994;86:140-1. PMID: 8271298

## Smoking Question 6
**Answer: A**

**Educational Objective:** *Recognize the percentage of persons who stop smoking in the United States each year.*

The prevalence of cigarette smoking in the United States is different in men and women. In 1997, 26% of adult men and 21% of women were cigarette smokers. Approximately 2% of current cigarette smokers stop each year.

Smoking-cessation interventions have a 1-year post intervention success rate of 5% to 15%. These interventions include smoking-cessation classes, nicotine replacement, and antidepressant therapy. This is compared to a smoking cessation rate of only 2% for cigarette smokers who try to quit on their own. Most cigarette smokers need multiple attempts to stop smoking and should be encouraged to quit even if they are unsuccessful in their initial attempts.

Current mortality differs between men and women in the United States. The risk of men dying from lung cancer began falling in the 1980s and is now declining by approximately 2% per year. In contrast, the risk of women dying from lung cancer has increased by 1% per year. The risk for women of dying from lung cancer has exceeded the risk of dying from breast cancer for approximately 5 years.

### Bibliography

1. **Landis SH, Murray T, Bolden S, Wingo PA**. Cancer statistics, 1999. CA Cancer J Clin. 1999;49:8-31,1. PMID: 10200775

2. **Wingo PA, Ries LA, Giovino GA, Miller DS, Rosenberg HM, Shopland DR, et al**. Annual report to the nation on the status of cancer, 1973-1996, with a special section on lung cancer and tobacco smoking. J Natl Cancer Inst. 1999;91:675-90. PMID: 10218505

# The Healthy Patient

## The Healthy Patient Question 1
### Answer: C

**Educational Objective:** *Recognize the infection and malignancy health risks in the lesbian population.*

It is important to screen lesbian women with Pap smears, especially if there has been past evidence of heterosexual coitus. Lesbian women undergo Pap tests at longer intervals than do heterosexual women and often conceal their sexual orientation from their physicians. If the woman does not engage in sex with men, the risk of human papillomavirus infection and, hence, cervical carcinoma is lowered. On the other hand, breast and ovarian cancer rates may be higher (because of nulliparity), but population-based evidence does not support this hypothesis yet.

With regard to infections, women who have sex only with women are at less risk for contracting syphilis and chlamydia. HIV transmission, while believed to be rare, can occur through exposure to cervical and vaginal secretions of an HIV-infected woman. Bacterial vaginosis is often diagnosed in the female partners of lesbians with this condition, suggesting that sexual transmission may occur. Finally, although gay men are at markedly increased risk for hepatitis B infection (whether they inject drugs or not), such risk does not apply to lesbians who are not bisexual.

### Bibliography

1. Health care needs of gay men and lesbians in the United States. Council on Scientific Affairs, American Medical Association. JAMA. 1996;275:1354-9. PMID: 8614123

2. **Berger BJ, Kolton S, Zenilman JM, Cummings MC, Feldman J, McCormack WM.** Bacterial vaginosis in lesbians: a sexually transmitted disease. Clin Infect Dis. 1995;21:1402-5. PMID: 8749623

## The Healthy Patient Question 2
### Answer: B

**Educational Objective:** *Recognize the leading cause of death in adolescents and young adults.*

One in two hundred 19-year-old young adults will die in the next 5 years. The leading causes of death from ages 10 to 24 years are motor vehicle accidents (30%), other unintentional injuries (10%), homicide (20%), and suicide (13%). AIDS joins these in the ensuing years as the fifth leading cause of death between the ages of 25 and 44 years, frequently reflecting HIV infection acquired during adolescence. Alcohol, drug abuse, social circumstance, and personal lifestyle are confounding variables that contribute to each of these causes of death and modify individual patients' probabilities of dying. Significant segments of this population, however, do not fit these categories. Homicide has been the leading cause of death among blacks aged 15 to 24 years for over a decade. Gay, lesbian, and bisexual adolescents manifest a higher prevalence of all risk-taking behaviors, are victims of violence at levels that are still being quantified, and are two to three times more likely to attempt suicide than their heterosexual peers. Suicide and death from motor vehicle accidents trail the incidence of AIDS in gay or bisexual men, whose lifetime risk of AIDS, though diminished in recent years, is estimated to be 20% to 30%.

It is generally wise to work on whichever risk behavior the patient is most prepared to address, but when equally contemplative/precontemplative for all, decreasing motor vehicle accidents holds the greatest potential for reducing deaths in young adults, particularly in the patient described with alcohol use problems.

### Bibliography

1. **Hoyert DL, Kochanek KD, Murphy SL.** Deaths: final data for 1997. Natl Vital Stat Rep. 1999;47:1-104. PMID: 10410536

2. **Dahlberg LL.** Youth violence in the United States. Major trends, risk factors, and prevention approaches. Am J Prev Med. 1998;14:259-72. PMID: 9635070

3. **Garofalo R, Wolf RC, Kessel S, Palfrey SJ, DuRant RH.** The association between health risk behaviors and sexual orientation among a school-based sample of adolescents. Pediatrics. 1998;101:895-902. PMID: 9565422

4. **Holmberg SD.** The estimated prevalence and incidence of HIV in 96 large US metropolitan areas. Am J Public Health. 1996;86:642-54. PMID: 8629714

## The Healthy Patient Question 3
### Answer: D

**Educational Objective:** *Recognize the leading cause of premature death in adolescents and young adults over a lifetime.*

One half of cigarette smokers die from a disease causally related to smoking, making it the number-one preventable cause of premature death in the United States and the most lethal of this patient's habits. Death from tobacco use has a long latency and is infrequent in young adults, although it could occur in the next 5 years of this patient's life as the result of oropharyngeal carcinoma, peptic ulcer disease, thromboembolic disease, or cardiovascular disease. All the other risk behaviors the patient manifests pale in comparison. In 1997 in the United States, chronic liver disease and cirrhosis accounted for 1.1% of all deaths; accidents including motor vehicle accidents, 4.1%; HIV infection, 0.7%; homicide, 07.9%; and suicide, 1.3%.

The risks of marijuana and cocaine use are best quantified in long-term narcotic addicts who use cocaine concurrently with other drugs. Most addicts initiated use before 20 years of age. In this group, the mortality rate over 24 years of follow-up is approximately 25%. Of these, 29% of the deaths are the result of homicide, suicide, or accidents; 32% are from drug overdose or toxicity; and 39% are related to smoking, alcohol use, or other causes. The risks to occasional users include HIV infection and serious cardiac, cerebrovascular, pulmonary, hepatic, and gastrointestinal disorders, which have been difficult to quantify.

The lifetime risk of acquiring hepatitis A in the United States is 45%. It has a mortality rate of less than 0.2% secondary to fulminant hepatitis. This patient is at average risk of hepatitis A, with a less than 5% risk of acquiring it and less than 0.01% risk of dying from it in the next 5 years. The lifetime risk of acquiring hepatitis B varies greatly. Middle class whites have a 5% prevalence; middle class blacks, 12%; and homosexual men, 48%. Chronic liver disease leading to cirrhosis or hepatocellular carcinoma develops in 5% to 10% of infected adults, leading to an overall mortality rate of 0.3% to 1.5%. Neither of those end points would be expected to be reached in the next 5 years. Vaccination for hepatitis B is warranted but will not reduce this patient's short-term risk of death.

The only common fatal sexually transmitted diseases are AIDS and hepatitis B. The risk of AIDS acquisition by heterosexuals has been hard to quantify and varies extensively by geographic region, largely paralleling the distribution of patients with AIDS who use intravenous drugs. The highest risk group is women with five or more sex partners per year. HIV seroprevalence ranges from 0.7% to 6.4% among heterosexual persons at high risk. Even if HIV infection were acquired immediately, death from it would not be expected in an adult over a 5-year time span.

Modifying the behavior of adolescents requires recognition of their motivation for the behavior. They must be ready to change and to develop self-efficacy. Strategies that enhance their sense of empowerment and commitment, identify triggering behaviors, reinforce partial successes, and facilitate change prove the greatest success. Adolescents try to stop risk-taking behaviors impulsively and without adequate preparation, making it necessary for the physician to be adaptable to their efforts.

### Bibliography

1. **Hoyert DL, Kochanek KD, Murphy SL.** Deaths: final data for 1997. Natl Vital Stat Rep. 1999;47:1-104. PMID: 10410536
2. **Dahlberg LL.** Youth violence in the United States. Major trends, risk factors, and prevention approaches. Am J Prev Med. 1998;14:259-72. PMID: 9635070
3. **Garofalo R, Wolf RC, Kessel S, Palfrey SJ, DuRant RH.** The association between health risk behaviors and sexual orientation among a school-based sample of adolescents. Pediatrics. 1998;101:895-902. PMID: 9565422
4. **Holmberg SD.** The estimated prevalence and incidence of HIV in 96 large US metropolitan areas. Am J Public Health. 1996;86:642-54. PMID: 8629714

## The Healthy Patient Question 4
## Answer: D

**Educational Objective:** *Perform an appropriate preparticipation assessment in a middle-aged, sedentary man with cardiovascular risk factors.*

This middle-aged man, although apparently healthy, has risk factors for the development of coronary artery disease, namely, his sex and history of hypertension. Unless previous laboratory testing has indicated otherwise, the presence or absence of hypercholesterolemia and diabetes mellitus are also unknown. The basic assessment should focus on detecting and managing these additional risk factors. A resting electrocardiogram should be done to assess for left ventricular hypertrophy, given the history of hypertension, and evidence of ischemia, before performing a graded exercise test. However, the electrocardiogram lacks sufficient sensitivity for silent coronary artery disease to be used alone in this situation. There are no randomized controlled clinical trials addressing the specific question of preparticipation electrocardiograms and graded exercise tests in asymptomatic persons, and the recommendations for their use is a consensus opinion, based on the underlying risk of undetected coronary artery disease and engaging in vigorous physical activity.

If this patient had no other cardiovascular risk factors and he were to embark on a more modest exercise program such as walking, a graded exercise test would be optional, unless his evaluation suggested underlying coronary artery disease. There is no clear role for exercise testing in young, healthy asymptomatic men.

### Bibliography

1. **King CN, Senn MD.** Exercise testing and prescription: practical recommendations for the sedentary. Sports Med. 1996;21:326-36. PMID: 8724201
2. **Katzel LI, Sorkin JD, Goldberg AP.** Exercise-induced silent myocardial ischemia and future cardiac events in healthy, sedentary, middle-aged and older men. J Am Geriatr Soc. 1999;47:923-9. PMID: 10443851
3. **Pilote L, Pashkow F, Thomas JD, Snader CE, Harvey SA, Marwick TH, et al.** Clinical yield and cost of exercise treadmill testing to screen for coronary artery disease in asymptomatic adults. Am J Cardiol. 1998;81:219-24. PMID: 9591907
4. **Livschitz S, Sharabi Y, Yushink J, Bar-On Z, Chouraqui, P, et al.** Limited clinical value of exercise stress test for the screening of coronary artery disease in young, asymptomatic adult men. Am J Card 2000;86:462-4. PMID: 10946046

## The Healthy Patient Question 5
## Answer: C

**Educational Objective:** *Recognize which vaccines are indicated for late adolescence.*

The Advisory Committee on Immunization Practices (ACIP) of the Centers for Disease Control and Prevention (CDC) sets the standards for vaccination in the United States. After years of unsuccessful attempts to diminish the incidence of hepatitis B by targeting vaccination to high-risk groups, universal hepatitis B vaccination was recommended by the ACIP in 1991. Hepatitis B vaccine is now routinely given during infancy and is universally recommended for all adolescents aged 12 years and older who have not been previously vaccinated. Vaccination requires three doses; the second and third given 1 and 6 months after the first.

In 1999, the ACIP, citing the results of two CDC studies done in 1998 that identified a slightly higher risk among college freshman dormitory residents, recommended that physicians give information to students and their parents about meningococcal disease and the benefits of vaccination. Colleges have also been directed to inform parents of the dangers of meningococcal meningitis. A single dose of quadrivalent vaccine is 85% effective in preventing disease, with immunity diminishing rapidly over approximately 3 years. The ACIP stopped short of recommending universal vaccination of college freshman due to the low prevalence of disease and the fact that vaccination is not likely to be cost effective. College students comprise 3% of the 2400 to 3000 patients who develop meningococcal disease annually. The overall risk among undergraduates is actually lower than the rate among noncollege students aged 18 to 23 years (0.7/100,000 vs. 1.1/100,000) but significantly higher among freshman living in dormitories (5.4/100,000). The CDC estimates that it would cost $474,000 to $1.6 million per case prevented if all freshmen living in dormitories were vaccinated and $1.4 to $2.9 million per case prevented if all college freshmen were immunized. This patient living off-campus is at no higher risk for meningococcal disease than the general population. Vaccination should be discussed with her.

Having completed an initial series of diphtheria-pertussis-tetanus vaccine, a tetanus booster is recommended at age 12 years and at 10-year intervals thereafter, although recent tests have focused on the effectiveness of a strategy of giving a booster once during the early adult years and once during midlife. The recommendation for the first tetanus booster has been shifted from age 14 to 12 years because of concerns over waning immunity. A second dose of varicella vaccine is recommended for susceptible persons who receive their initial dose of varicella vaccine at age 13 years or older.

Hepatitis A vaccine is now recommended not only for persons at high risk but universally for children ages 2 to 15 residing in states or regions where the incidence of hepatitis A is greater than or equal to 20 per 100,000. Rarely has this rate been exceeded east of the Mississippi and most consistently on the west coast and southwestern United States. Persons at high risk include gay and bisexual men, patients with chronic liver disease, and travelers to areas with a high prevalence of hepatitis A, including Mexico, South and Central America, and much of Africa and Asia. Europe has a low prevalence of hepatitis A. Hepatitis A vaccine is given in a two-dose schedule with protective antibody levels developing in 94% to 100% of adults 1 month after the first dose.

**Bibliography**

1. American Academy of Pediatrics. Committee on Infectious Diseases. Recommended childhood immunization schedule, United States, January-December 2000. Pediatrics. 2000;105(1 Pt 1):148-51. PMID: 10617721

2. Prevention of hepatitis A through active or passive immunization: Recommendations of the Advisory Committee on Immunization Practices (ACIP). MMWR Morb Mortal Wkly Rep.1999;48(RR-12):1-37. PMID: 10543657

3. Hepatitis B virus: a comprehensive strategy for eliminating transmission in the United States through universal childhood vaccination. Recommendations of the Immunization Practices Advisory Committee (ACIP). MMWR Morb Mortal Wkly Rep. 1991;40(RR-13):1-25. PMID: 1835756

## The Healthy Patient Question 6
## Answer: B

**Educational Objective:** *Recognize which preventive services are indicated for young adults.*

The use of questionnaires offers the opportunity to acquire a knowledge base of a multitude of patient behaviors, risk factors, and concerns. In the absence of such supplemental information in a busy practice, physicians must make choices about how they spend their time when performing periodic health appraisals. Recommendations of what should be included in interview-based screening and counseling of young adults are based almost exclusively on burden of illness, because few outcome data support specific recommendations. There is some consensus about what physicians should include in historical assessment.

All major North American prevention guideline-writing organizations recommend universal interview-based screening and counseling for alcohol use, contraception, sexually transmitted disease prevention, exercise, injury prevention, and substance abuse. Although most groups recommend nutrition and obesity counseling, the Canadian Task Force on the Periodic Health Examination, the U.S. Preventive Services Task Force, and the American Academy of Family Practice do not recommend screening for an eating disorder. Breast and testicular self-examination similarly remains controversial in this age group in the absence of outcome data to support it. No group yet routinely recommends screening for gambling problems, although it has been suggested as a nonthreatening introduction to risk behavior assessment and implicit gambling. The Canadian Task Force on the Periodic

Health Examination and the U.S. Preventive Services Task Force recommend that physicians be alert to possible physical or sexual abuse but do not recommend universal interview-based screening for it.

## Bibliography

1.  **Shafer MA.**Annual pelvic examination in the sexually active adolescent female: what are we doing and why are we doing it? J Adolesc Health. 1998;23:68-73. PMID: 9714168
2.  **Cleeman JI, Grundy SM.**National Cholesterol Education Program recommendations for cholesterol testing in young adults. A science-based approach. Circulation. 1997;95:1646-50. PMID: 9118536

## The Healthy Patient Question 7
## Answer: C

**Educational Objective:** *Recognize which preventive services are indicated for young adults.*

Recommendations for what should be included in routine physical examinations and laboratory assessments of adolescents and young adults are also based on burden of illness and limited outcomes data. All major North American groups who write preventive care guidelines for these groups recommend routine blood pressure measurement, height and weight assessment, and universal assessment for chlamydia infection and gonorrhea in sexually active patients. Urine leukocyte esterase measurement is a sufficient initial screening for chlamydia and gonorrhea in men but lacks sufficient specificity in women. Most recommend assay of cervical swabs for gonorrhea and chlamydia in sexually active women using cultures or gene amplification techniques such as polymerase chain reaction or ligase chain reaction. The latter, when performed on the first sample of voided urine, offers nearly as sensitive a screening for patients unwilling to undergo a pelvic examination. Routine urinalysis is not routinely recommended for young adults. Hearing and vision screening is generally recommended for those at high risk based on occupation or personal or family history.

The timing of initiation of universal cholesterol screening is the subject of controversy. The American Medical Association's Guide to Adolescent Preventive Services (GAPS) recommends universal screening of adolescents at age 19 years. The National Cholesterol Education Program (NCEP) recommends that all adults age 20 years or older have their plasma cholesterol checked. The American College of Physicians and U.S. Preventive Services Task Force have recommended deferring universal screening until age 35 years in men and 45 years in women.

## Bibliography

1.  **Shafer MA.**Annual pelvic examination in the sexually active adolescent female: what are we doing and why are we doing it? J Adolesc Health. 1998;23:68-73. PMID: 9714168

2.  **Cleeman JI, Grundy SM.**National Cholesterol Education Program recommendations for cholesterol testing in young adults. A science-based approach. Circulation. 1997;95:1646-50. PMID: 9118536
3.  The American Medical Association Guidelines for Adolescent Preventative Services. Arch Pediatr Adolesc Med. 1997;151:958-9. PMID: 9308880

## The Healthy Patient Question 8
## Answer: D

**Educational Objective:** *Understand the approach to cervical cancer screening in patients who have had hysterectomy for benign disease.*

At one time, it was mistakenly believed that vaginal hysterectomy for benign disease was associated with an increased incidence of vaginal malignancy. The observational study designs did not control for detection bias, recall bias, or history of dysplasia. The prevalence of abnormal findings on cytopathologic examination of vaginal Pap smears in this setting is extremely low. Not only is the burden of suffering from vaginal cancer low, there is no evidence that early detection is effective. In fact, the positive predictive value of an abnormal vaginal smear for vaginal cancer approaches zero. Therefore, screening for vaginal cancer in women who have undergone hysterectomy for benign disease is not recommended.

Although such patients remain at risk for ovarian cancer, there is currently no evidence that an annual pelvic examination has adequate sensitivity or specificity to warrant its performance, and the sensitivity of the Pap smear for detecting malignant ovarian cells is extremely poor. The U.S. Preventive Services Task Force and the American College of Physicians argue against routine pelvic examination.

## Bibliography

1.  **Pearce KF, Haefner HK, Sariwar SF, Nolan TE.** Cytopathological findings on vaginal Papanicolaou smears after hysterectomy for benign gynecologic disease. N Engl J Med. 1996;335:1559-62. PMID: 8900088
2.  **Fetters MD, Fischer G, Reed BD.** Effectiveness of vaginal Papanicolaou smear screening after total hysterectomy for benign disease. JAMA. 1996;275:940-7. PMID: 8598623
3.  U.S. Preventive Services Task Force. Report of the U.S. Preventive Services Task Force, Guide to Clinical Prevention Services, Second Edition. Screening for Ovarian Cancer. Alexandria, VA: International Medical Publishing, Inc;1996. p. 159-167.

## The Healthy Patient Question 9
## Answer: B

**Educational Objective:** *Initiate a sound immunization course in an adult patient.*

The age of 50 years is ideal for reviewing a patient's immunization status. At this age, the adequacy of immunization may be reviewed, and risk factors that might indicate a need for certain vaccines such as pneumococcus and influenza may be determined. If a patient has completed the pediatric primary immunization series with tetanus diphtheria, a single booster may be provided to renew immunity. This patient should certainly have such a booster, which is recommended every 10 years in adults.

The patient is younger than 65 years and has no specific chronic diseases or immune system compromise to warrant immunization with a pneumococcal vaccine. Other risk factors favoring pneumococcal vaccination include alcoholism, organ transplant, and functional or anatomic asplenia.

Because the patient cannot recall whether he had chicken pox, a reasonable office strategy would be to offer the vaccine if serology reveals he has not been infected previously, because illness in the adult can produce increased morbidity. Antibody assays are accurate and relatively inexpensive and identify as immune adults who do not have a reliable history of varicella, preventing unnecessary vaccination.

Because this patient is traveling to a third world country, hepatitis A and B vaccinations are a safe and highly effective immunization.

### Bibliography

1.  Guide for adult immunization. American College of Physicians Task Force on Adult Immunization and Infectious Diseases Society of America. Philadelphia, PA. American College of Physicians. 1994.
2.  **Gardiner P, Eickhoff T, Colon GA, et al**. Adult immunizations. Ann Intern Med. 1996;124:35-40. PMID: 7503476

## The Healthy Patient Question 10
## Answer: B

**Educational Objective:** *Understand the role of prostate-specific antigen screening in the early detection of prostate cancer.*

There is no definitive proof that screening for prostate cancer by measuring serum prostate-specific antigen (PSA) decreases the mortality rate from prostate cancer. It is possible that morbidity may increase from treating PSA-detected cancers. The American College of Physicians guidelines emphasize increased patient participation in the decision regarding prostate cancer screening. For men aged 50 to 69 years, the physician should be particularly guided by the patient's preference and the physician's and patient's interpretation of the risk/benefit equation, a policy of shared decision making, personalized treatment, and counseling.

Although the American Cancer Society and the American Urologic Association recommend average-risk men begin screening at age 50 years, these groups balance this recommendation by stating it should be limited to men with a life expectancy greater than 10 years. Because of this patient's age and the severity of the chronic obstructive pulmonary disease, he may have a life expectancy of less than 10 years and, therefore, a suboptimal candidate for screening.

Although black men and men with a family history of prostate cancer have a higher lifetime risk, available evidence does not suggest that they should be cared for differently from men at average risk. Men who have lower urinary tract symptoms consistent with benign prostatic hyperplasia are not more likely to have prostate cancer; the absence of lower urinary tract symptoms does not predict cancer occurrence, although the specificity of PSA measurements in these men may be higher.

If a combined strategy of digital rectal examinations and PSA screening is adopted, approximately 25% of screened men older than 50 years may be subject to the cost and risk associated with transrectal needle biopsy (with the percentage increasing by age). Most proponents of screening favor a program of office-based early detection with digital rectal examination and PSA measurements, followed by transrectal ultrasonography to direct needle biopsy if either test result is abnormal.

### Bibliography

1.  **Catalona WJ, Richie JP, Ahmann FR, Hudson MA, Scardino PT, Flanigan RC, et al**. Comparison of digital rectal examination and serum prostate specific antigen in the early detection of prostate cancer: results of a multicenter clinical trial of 6,630 men. J Urol. 1994;151:1283-90. PMID: 7512659
2.  **Harris R, Lohr KN**. Screening for prostate cancer: an update of the evidence for the U.S. Preventive Services Task Force. Ann Intern Med. 2002;137:917-29. PMID: 12458993

## The Healthy Patient Question 11
## Answer: D

**Educational Objective:** *Determine optimal screening for a patient at average risk for ovarian cancer.*

The U.S. Preventive Services Task Force and the American College of Physicians, in opposition to the American Cancer Society, recommend against routine pelvic examination, Pap smear, CA-125 testing, or ultrasound for early diagnosis of ovarian cancer in asymptomatic patients. Women with familial cancer syndromes and other strong risk factors should be counseled about the benefits and risks of ovarian cancer screening and referral to specialty care may be appropriate. The sensitivity and specificity of bimanual pelvic examination are believed to be poor but are not well characterized in the literature. Under unusual circumstances, a Pap smear with very low sensitivity, may incidentally detect malignant ovarian cells. CA-125 testing is far less effective in women with localized disease than in those with advanced disease, and in asymptomatic postmenopausal women, the positive predictive value is below 3%. Abdominal ultrasound has a sensitivity of 62% to 100%, depending upon the study, however it is not very specific. Transvaginal ultrasound has a sensitivity of nearly 100% with a specificity of 97%. Because of the very low prevalence of disease, the positive predictive value remains low at 22% for transvaginal ultrasound and 2.6% for transabdominal ultrasound in studies of asymptomatic women. In such persons, the proportion of women who would then require surgical exploration would be unacceptably high.

### Bibliography

1. U.S. Preventive Services Task Force. Report of the U.S. Preventive Services Task Force, Guide to Clinical Prevention Services, Second Edition. Screening for Ovarian Cancer. Alexandria, VA: International Medical Publishing, Inc;1996. p. 159-167.

2. Ferrini R. Screening asymptomatic women for ovarian cancer: American College of Preventive Medicine practice policy. Am J Prev Med. 1997;13:444-6. PMID: 9415790

3. Guerra CE. Ovarian cancer. In: Diagnostic strategies for common medical problems. 2nd ed. Black ER, Bordley DR, Tape TG, Panzer RJ, editors. American College of Physicians: Philadelphia; 1999. p. 563-574.

## The Healthy Patient Question 12
## Answer: C

**Educational Objective:** *Recognize which older women need Pap smears.*

Although there is insufficient evidence to recommend for or against an upper age limit for Pap testing, the U. S. Preventive Services Task Force, American College of Preventive Medicine, and the American College of Physicians (ACP) recommend discontinuing it after age 65 years in women who have had regular previous screening in which the smears have been consistently normal. Some experts suggest that screening resume if new sexual relationships are started. More than 25% of invasive cervical cancers occur in women older than age 65, and 40% to 50% of all women who die of cervical cancer are older than age 65. Most of these women did not have regular Pap screening. Older women who have not been regularly screened should have two Pap smears a year apart. Further screening depends on the patient's risk factors and the results of these tests. The ACP recommends screening women 66 to 75 years old every 3 years if they have not been screened in the 10 years before age 66 years.

### Bibliography

1. U.S. Preventive Services Task Force. Report of the U.S. Preventive Services Task Force, Guide to Clinical Prevention Services, Second Edition. Screening for Cervical Cancer. Alexandria, VA: International Medical Publishing, Inc;1996. p. 105-119.

## The Healthy Patient Question 13
## Answer: C

**Educational Objective:** *Learn the components of a comprehensive "sun-protection" program.*

This professional golfer will be unable to totally avoid sun exposure. However, he can modify his behavior to limit his exposure. Scheduling tee times during tournaments is out of his control, but he can arrange practice rounds early or late in the day, when the sun is not overhead. Avoiding outdoor activ-

ities during the times of most intense ultraviolet radiation exposure, between 10:00 AM and 4:00 PM (depending on the time of year and latitude), reduces the total lifetime exposure significantly. High-risk behaviors such as sun tanning or going to a tanning salon should be avoided. A "sun-savvy" attitude is also helpful, for example, walking on the shady side of the street, using a sun umbrella at the beach or when spending time at outdoor sporting events, and purchasing tickets on the shady side of the field for outdoor sporting events. This patient can stand in the shade of tree or under an umbrella when his partners are on the putting green.

Protective clothing is probably the soundest strategy and best line of defense for this patient when sun avoidance is a problem. Articles of clothing should be worn that limit exposure to high-risk portions of the exposed skin that are prone to photoaging and skin cancers. These include the scalp, ears, neck, forearms, and the V of the neck. In general, regular use of wide-brimmed hats and long-sleeved shirts and blouses help accomplish this goal. These articles of clothing and hats with wide brims or neck-protective extensions are readily available and fashionable enough for any outdoor activity.

Sunscreen use can be added as the final strategy in a comprehensive, sun-smart approach to life. Regular and proper application of high-potency and wide-spectrum sunscreens supplements the effects of sun avoidance and protective clothing. High-risk areas such as the nose, ears, scalp, and neck can be covered quickly and easily. The three strategies of sun avoidance, protective clothing, and sunscreens are important. Tailoring their proportional use to a specific lifestyle is critical. This patient must rely on protective clothing as a primary strategy, with sunscreen an important adjunct. Over a lifetime, paying attention to sun avoidance maneuvers saves hours of cumulative ultraviolet radiation exposure. Tanning salons play no role in a sun-smart program. This patient cannot select where and when he wants to play.

### Bibliography

1. Guercio-Hauer C, Macfarlane DF, Deleo VA.Photodamage, photoaging and photoprotection of the skin. Am Fam Physician. 1994;50:327-32, 334. PMID: 8042567

## The Healthy Patient Question 14
## Answer: A

**Educational Objective:** *Recognize the difference between perimenopausal mood disturbances and major depression.*

Epidemiologic studies have confirmed that there is not a significant increase in the incidence of major depression associated with the perimenopause. However, there may be an increase in dysphoric mood, thought to be related to sleep deprivation. The best therapy is not medication for sleep, but estrogen replacement for the underlying disorder. Studies have suggested that estrogen replacement is effective in perimenopausal mood disorders, when major depressive symptoms have been ruled out.

In this patient, estrogen replacement is being used short-term, both as a diagnostic test (to determine whether the patient responds) and to relieve acute symptoms. Short-term estrogen replacement therapy is not associated with the same risk profile as is long-term use. Thus, patients can be counseled that short-term use is likely to be safe, and that a discussion of long-term risks and benefits can begin after short-term relief is achieved.

### Bibliography

1. **Burt VK, Altshuler LL, Rasgon N**. Depressive symptoms in the perimenopause: prevalence, assessment, and guidelines for treatment. Harv Rev Psychiatry. 1998;6:121-32. PMID: 10372280

2. **Avis NE, Brambilla D, McKinlay SM, Vass K.** A longitudinal analysis of the association between menopause and depression. Results from the Massachusetts Women's Health Study. Ann Epidemiol. 1994;4:214-20. PMID: 8055122

## The Healthy Patient Question 15
## Answer: E

**Educational Objective:** *Recommend a course of action for a menopausal woman concerned about the risk of osteoporosis.*

Although studies of cost-effectiveness suggest that in women without additional risk factors for osteoporosis, it is most cost effective to defer screening bone densitometry and treatment until age 65 years, a bone density study is reasonable in younger women if they desire it, and a determination of bone mineral density by dual-energy x-ray absorptiometry (DXA) or other methods may be helpful in their decision-making process.

Testing to screen for secondary causes of osteoporosis is unnecessary in the absence of evidence of osteoporosis.

### Bibliography

1. **Miller PD, Zapalowski C, Kulak CA, Bilezikian JP**. Bone densitometry: the best way to detect osteoporosis and to monitor therapy. J Clin Endocrinol Metab. 1999;84:1867-71. PMID: 10372677

## The Healthy Patient Question 16
## Answer: B

**Educational Objective:** *Know how primary prevention can be achieved in the office setting.*

Accumulated evidence that most colorectal cancers arise from adenomatous polyps shows that detection and removal of polyps is an effective primary prevention strategy. Colorectal polyps can be detected by fecal occult blood testing or endoscopy in the office setting. Several randomized trials have shown that fecal occult blood testing performed either annually or every 2 years can decrease colorectal cancer mortality.

Mortality is decreased by early detection of cancers, but large polyps can bleed and offer an opportunity for primary prevention. Case control studies show that sigmoidoscopy is associated with decreased colorectal cancer mortality. The reduced risk persists for a decade or more after the last sigmoidoscopy; therefore, many organizations recommend sigmoidoscopy every 5 years. Other forms of colorectal screening, such as colonoscopy and air-contrast barium enema, are not practical for the average practitioner's office setting, although colonoscopy is rapidly becoming the preferred screening modality. Although smoking-cessation programs can decrease the incidence of pancreatic, bladder, and gastric cancers, smokers represent a high-risk, not an average risk population for these diseases. Routine work-up and antibiotic treatment for the many adults who have been infected with *Helicobacter pylori* could theoretically decrease the incidence of gastric cancer, but the risks and benefits of such a strategy have not been tested. Hepatitis vaccination could logically decrease the risk of liver cancer, but this is more likely in high-risk persons than in those at average risk.

### Bibliography

1. **Pignone M, Rich M, Teutsch SM, Berg AO, Lohr KN.** Screening for colorectal cancer in adults at average risk: a summary of the evidence for the U.S. Preventive Services Task Force. Ann Intern Med. 2002;137:132-41. PMID: 12118972

## The Healthy Patient Question 17
## Answer: E

**Educational Objective:** *Understand the inherent weakness in even the strongest study design and know the difference between efficacy and effectiveness.*

Randomized studies are the best way to avoid lead time bias, length bias, overdiagnosis, and selection bias. Because all events are measured from the time of randomization in both the screened and control study groups, the potential to introduce artifactual lead time due to earlier diagnosis in the screened arm is eliminated. Length bias is avoided because the specific mortality end points are corrected for the different spectrum of disease that may be detected by screening compared to the diagnosis of more aggressive symptomatic disease detected in the control population. Overdiagnosis is an extreme form of length bias (the detection of disease that would not affect life expectancy even if never detected), and therefore, it would also be eliminated. Selection bias is eliminated provided that the randomization procedure does not allow systematic, unbalanced allocation of study subjects with predictive factors for cancer mortality into one of the study groups. In large, randomized screening studies, which typically must include thousands of participants, randomization is the most efficient way to ensure equal balance of both known and unknown risk factors in each study arm. To eliminate this bias, analysis of the results must be by "intent to treat" rather than according to whether screening was actually received or not.

Comparison of results between those actually screened and those not screened does not correct for selection biases, because such an analysis is not protected by randomization.

However, randomization of volunteers in a screening study does not necessarily eliminate generalizability problems. Often people who volunteer for clinical studies have a lower than expected cancer mortality than that of the general population. This is known as the healthy volunteer effect. One study design that can help correct for this is the use of population-based, rather than volunteer, study populations. In this case, potential study subjects are randomly assigned to the study groups from population-based registries, and study end points are analyzed by the "intent to treat" method. However, this study design is rarely practical in the United States. Because of the generalizability issue, trials performed using volunteers are called efficacy studies, whereas trials using population-based subjects are called effectiveness studies.

**Bibliography**

1. **MacLean CD**. Principles of cancer screening. Med Clin North Am. 1996;80:1-14. PMID: 8569290
2. **Kramer BS, Brawley OW**. Cancer screening. Hematol Oncol Clin North Am. 2000;14:831-48. PMID: 10949776

**The Healthy Patient Question 18**
**Answer: A**

**Educational Objective:** *Recognize the relative importance of the most commonly reported end points in cancer screening studies.*

Although overall mortality is the best indicator of improvement in life expectancy, screening for any particular cancer is unlikely to improve mortality in any cancer screening study. This is because competing causes of death are likely to dilute the effect of screening for a single cancer, which would account for only a small proportion of overall deaths. Therefore, cause-specific mortality would be the best end point to measure the effect of the screening tool. The case fatality ratio (the number of deaths from a specific cancer divided by the number of patients with that cancer) is subject to the serious artifacts from length bias, which is the preferential detection of asymptomatic, more indolent cancers by any screening test. Likewise, patient survival after cancer diagnosis is artificially prolonged by screening due to length bias and lead time bias—an advance in the date of cancer diagnosis without necessarily changing the patient's outcome. For this same reason, the relative shift in the proportion of patients diagnosed at early stages is not a good assessment of screening test efficacy. Absolute decrease in the incidence of late-stage (metastatic) cancer is an early indicator that a test may be effective because metastatic cancer frequently leads to death. However, using the absolute incidence of late-stage disease may still be confounded by lead time bias and the result-

ing stage shift. Cause-specific mortality is least subject to the above potentially confounding effects.

**Bibliography**

1. **MacLean CD**.Principles of cancer screening. Med Clin North Am. 1996;80:1-14. PMID: 8569290
2. **Kramer BS, Brawley OW**. Cancer Screening. Hematol Oncol Clin North Am. 2000;14:831-48. PMID: 10949776

**The Healthy Patient Question 19**
**Answer: C**

**Educational Objective:** *Recognize which of the commonly employed early detection tools are most likely to benefit patients who come to an internist for routine medical care.*

Annual and biannual screening with tests for fecal occult blood have been shown in randomized trials to decrease colorectal cancer mortality. Routine screening with this test in patients at average risk is therefore well supported. Testicular clinical examination has never been rigorously studied in the screening setting. However, since testicular germ cell cancer is extremely rare and usually curable even when diagnosed at advanced stages, screening is very unlikely to make an impact on mortality. Breast self-examination is intuitively appealing, but randomized trials have had disappointing results on breast cancer mortality. A randomized study performed in China in which female factory workers were taught how to perform a careful breast self-examination regularly showed no decrease in mortality after 5 years of follow-up. Although twice as many biopsies were performed, the number of cancers diagnosed was similar (the excess numbers of biopsies revealed benign conditions), and there was very little shift to earlier stages of disease at diagnosis. Regular screening of the oral cavity for cancer has not been studied for its ability to decrease head and neck cancer mortality. In randomized trials, chest radiography has been shown to shift lung cancer diagnosis to earlier, more operable stages. Five-year lung cancer survival rates were also increased from 13% to 30%. However, lung cancer mortality rates were the same in screened patients as in control patients. Improved survival and stage shift may have been due to lead and length biases, which can occur in any screening test.

**Bibliography**

1. **Towler B, Irwig L, Glasziou P, Kenwenter J, Weller D, Silagy C**. A systematic review of the effects of screening for colorectal cancer using the faecal occult blood test, hemoccult. BMJ. 1998;317:559-65. PMID: 9721111

# Diabetes Mellitus

## Diabetes Mellitus Question 1
**Answer: C**

**Educational Objective:** *Understand the revised criteria for diagnosing diabetes mellitus.*

The revised criteria for the diagnosis of diabetes mellitus include 1) a fasting plasma glucose concentration of 126 mg/dL or greater, 2) symptoms of diabetes mellitus and a random plasma glucose concentration of 200 mg/dL or greater, and 3) a 2-hour plasma glucose concentration greater than 200 mg/dL during an oral glucose tolerance test. Although the hemoglobin $A_{1C}$ level is statistically related to the plasma glucose level as a predictor of risk, it is not currently recommended as a screening tool because of difficulties in measurement standardization.

The risk of vascular complications increases dramatically at a fasting plasma glucose level greater than or equal to 126 mg/dL. A significant proportion of patients are asymptomatic but remain at high risk, and 50% of patients with type 2 diabetes mellitus remain undiagnosed and may present with diabetic tissue damage at the time of diagnosis.

Patients older than 45 years who have a body mass index greater than 27, who have first-degree relatives with diabetes mellitus, who are members of high-risk ethnic populations, or who have other cardiovascular risk factors are all considered to be at high risk. How often this group should be screened has not been definitively determined. The U.S. Preventive Services Task Force and the ACP believe that screening adults with these risk factors is reasonable, although they do not recommend universal screening for type 2 diabetes mellitus in asymptomatic, nonpregnant adults. The American Diabetes Association suggests screening all adults age 45 years and older for diabetes every 3 years.

### Bibliography

1. Report of the expert committee on the diagnosis and classification of diabetes mellitus. Diabetes Care. 2003;26 Suppl 1:S5-20. PMID: 12502614

## Diabetes Mellitus Question 2
**Answer: C**

**Educational Objective:** *Understand the indications for initiation of combination therapy in a patient with type 2 diabetes.*

Type 2 diabetes mellitus is a progressive disorder, and studies have documented that response to monotherapy is lim-

ited. The rate of failure to respond to sulfonylureas is 5% to 10% per year so that "secondary failure" to sulfonylureas in this case is expected. Four options are available to obese patients who have become unresponsive to sulfonylureas: 1) add metformin, 2) add a thiazolidinedione, 3) add an α-glucosidase inhibitor, and 4) add insulin. Arguably the best treatment could be to initiate insulin at bedtime and continue the sulfonylurea. However, when presented with the benefits and potential adverse effects (weight gain and hypoglycemia), the patient selected a combination of oral therapies rather than insulin and an oral agent.

There is no consensus about which option is most effective. Adding metformin to the regimen provides an effective agent that complements the action of sulfonylurea. Several studies document that fasting plasma glucose and hemoglobin $A_{1C}$ values decline with this combination of sulfonylurea and metformin in patients with body mass indexes in the range of 27 to 30 kg/m$^2$. Maximum dosages (2000 mg) of metformin should be administered in divided doses. A trial of this combination for 6 to 8 weeks should determine its effectiveness. If hemoglobin $A_{1C}$ values do not fall to the 7.0% to 7.5% range, the patient should be encouraged to start insulin therapy.

A thiazolidinedione and acarbose (an α-glucosidase inhibitor) are less powerful as hypoglycemic agents than sulfonylureas and metformin, and probably would be less effective in this patient than combination therapy. The patient's obesity indicates that insulin resistance is a likely factor in the progressive hyperglycemia, and a thiazolidinedione warrants consideration; however, if it is used, greater laboratory monitoring is required.

### Bibliography

1. **DeFronzo RA**. Pharmacologic therapy for type 2 diabetes mellitus. Ann Intern Med. 1999;131:281-303. PMID: 10454950
2. **Hermann LS, Schersten B, Bitsen PO, Kjellstrom T, Lindgarde F, Melander A**. Therapeutic comparisons of metformin and sulfonylurea, alone and in various combinations. A double blind controlled study. Diabetes Care. 1994;17:1100-9. PMID: 7821128

## Diabetes Mellitus Question 3
**Answer: A**

**Educational Objective:** *Understand the criteria for the diagnosis of diabetes and the appropriate tests to determine that diagnosis.*

An expert committee of the American Diabetes Association has recommended the fasting plasma glucose as the primary diagnostic test for diabetes mellitus in asymptomatic persons. Fasting values were considered to be a simpler, economically more feasible measure than an oral glucose tolerance test and to yield an earlier diagnosis. Values of 126 mg/dL or higher were suggested as diagnostic because that fasting value predicts a 2-hour postmeal value of 200 mg/dL, a glucose level that correlates with diabetic vascular complications. The suggested fasting value of 126 mg/dL (7.0 mmol/L) replaced the older standard of 140 mg/dL (7.6 mmol/L) and is intended to diagnose diabetes at an earlier stage and afford opportunity for intervention. Controversy about this diagnostic approach centers on those patients whose 2-hour values exceeds 200 mg/dL but whose fasting values are below 126 mg/dL. The expert committee also introduced the concept of impaired fasting glucose – values from 110 to 126 mg/dL – to replace the older concept of impaired glucose tolerance. Patients with impaired fasting glucose are at risk for diabetes and its vascular complications.

Oral glucose tolerance tests are often inconvenient and costly and require a defined protocol so that their use in office practice is not feasible. The rare patient who on repeated fasting or casual testing has values in the uncertain range may warrant such a test. Although glycohemoglobin measurements have been advocated by some as a criterion for the diagnosis of diabetes, the concept has not received widespread acceptance. Measuring a single fasting plasma glucose and corresponding insulin values provides no more information than the glucose measurement alone.

**Bibliography**

1. Report of the expert committee on the diagnosis and classification of diabetes mellitus. Diabetes Care. 2003;26 Suppl 1:S5-20. PMID: 12502614

## Diabetes Mellitus Question 4
## Answer: D

**Educational Objective:** *Adjust insulin schedule to avoid nocturnal hypoglycemia in type 1 diabetes.*

Nocturnal hypoglycemia is a common complication of an insulin treatment schedule that combines an intermediate- and rapid-acting insulin before supper. The actions of the two insulins may overlap and cause hypoglycemia in the early hours of the morning. This patient's experience emphasizes the reasons for the use of intermediate-acting insulin and the importance of the timing of doses. Hypoglycemia can be prevented if insulins mimic the normal physiology of insulin secretion. NPH or lente insulins are intended to simulate the basal insulin secretion of nondiabetic persons. Basal insulin secretion modulates hepatic gluconeogenesis, a major determinant of fasting glucose concentration. During the early hours of the morning, hepatic gluconeogenesis peaks under the influence

of cortisol; insulin blunts or buffers that process. To determine the timing of the evening dose of intermediate-acting insulin, it is important that the peak action of that insulin coincide with the early morning surge in hepatic gluconeogenesis (the so-called dawn phenomenon) and that it not augment the action of presupper regular insulin. Most patients achieve that balance when intermediate-acting insulin is administered at bedtime. Because there is individual variation in the time of the peak action of the intermediate-acting insulins, patients often determine the most suitable hour. When an intermediate-acting insulin is administered early in the evening or before supper, a bedtime snack is advisable.

**Bibliography**

1. **Bolli GB**. How to ameliorate the problem of hypoglycemia in intensive as well as non-intensive treatment of type 1 diabetes. Diabetes Care. 1999;22(Suppl 2):B43-52. PMID: 10097899

## Diabetes Mellitus Question 5
## Answer: D

**Educational Objective:** *Recognize a preventable cause of blindness in patients with diabetes mellitus.*

In patients with diabetes mellitus, blindness occurs not only as a consequence of proliferative retinopathy, but also macular edema, cataracts, and glaucoma.

After 20 years of diabetes mellitus in patients with the onset before age 30 years, retinopathy is present in almost all, and proliferative retinopathy in 50%. Proliferative retinopathy is characterized by the formation of new blood vessels on the surface of the retina or optic disk. These vessels usually are in the posterior portion of the retina and are associated with retinal ischemia. Loss of vision from proliferative retinopathy relates usually to the traction caused by the new vessels rather than the new vessels themselves. Traction leads to retinal detachment or vitreous hemorrhages. Control of hyperglycemia, hypertension, and dyslipidemia reduces the likelihood of proliferative retinopathy. Argon laser is the preferred treatment for high-risk patients with neovascularization accompanied by vitreous hemorrhage or new vessels on or near the optic disk. Tighter glycemic control does not improve glaucoma, retinal edema, or cataracts.

**Bibliography**

1. **Ferris FL 3rd, Davis MD, Aiello LM**. Treatment of diabetic retinopathy. N Engl J Med. 1999;341:667-78. PMID: 10460819

## Diabetes Mellitus Question 6
## Answer: A

**Educational Objective:** *Manage a patient with diabetic ketoacidosis.*

The most common cause of increase in the plasma glucose concentration in a hospitalized patient with diabetic ketoacidosis is the failure to administer subcutaneous insulin at the time the infusion of insulin was discontinued. Under normal conditions insulin has a very short half-life (3 to 5 minutes) in the circulation, so that even in sick patients without a capacity for endogenous insulin production, discontinuing an infusion causes circulating levels to fall precipitously. Consequently, gluconeogenesis and ketogenesis resurge, glucose levels rise (see flow chart), and ketones reappear in the plasma. An insulin infusion should never be discontinued under these circumstances without a simultaneous injection of subcutaneous insulin. In a young woman with recurrent ketoacidosis, the presence of an occult infection, hyperthyroidism, and pregnancy all warrant consideration. The initial good response to the insulin infusion makes each of these causes of insulin resistance unlikely in this instance. Adequate potassium replacement is a prerequisite in the management of diabetic ketoacidosis; the serum potassium concentration should be maintained between 4 and 5 meq/L.

### Bibliography

1. **Lebovitz HE**. Diabetic ketoacidosis. Lancet. 1995;345:767-72. PMID: 7891491

## Diabetes Mellitus Question 7
## Answer: C

**Educational Objective:** *Treat a symptomatic patient with newly diagnosed type 2 diabetes mellitus.*

The therapeutic goals in this patient are to alleviate symptoms and control hyperglycemia. When a newly diagnosed patient has symptoms, evidence of a urinary tract infection and markedly elevated plasma glucose concentration, treatment with insulin is the best assurance that symptoms will resolve and that the infection will respond readily to appropriate therapy. Hospitalization is usually not warranted unless ketoacidosis or severe dehydration and hypotension are present. Some patients will respond to oral agents, such as metformin, but that response may be slow and insufficient to alleviate symptoms. After prolonged periods of markedly elevated glucose, the response to sulfonylureas is blunted as the beta cells of the pancreas produce little or no insulin because of the glucose toxicity. After 6 to 8 weeks of good glycemic control effected by insulin, therapy may be switched to an oral agent if the patient prefers. A benefit of tight glycemic control with intensive insulin therapy in such patients is the reversal of glucose toxicity, with the improvement of both insulin sensitivity and insulin secretion. α-Glucosidase inhibitors like acarbose, reduce postprandial hyperglycemia by delaying glucose absorption, but do no affect glucose utilization or insulin secretion. They are less potent agents and therefore would not be the correct agents to use to control her hyperglycemia.

Every patient with newly diagnosed diabetes mellitus should be offered an educational program that emphasizes the importance of diet and exercise. In symptomatic patients

with this severe a degree of hyperglycemia, diet and exercise are inadequate to achieve the desired goals.

### Bibliography

1. **Ilkova H, Glaser B, Tunckale A, Gabriacik N, Cirasi E**. Induction of long-term glycemic control in newly diagnosed type 2 diabetic patients by transient intensive insulin treatment. Diabetes Care. 1997;20:1353-6. PMID: 9283777

## Diabetes Mellitus Question 8
## Answer: B

**Educational Objective:** *Manage foot pain in a patient with diabetes mellitus.*

This patient has evidence of peripheral neuropathy. In the western world, diabetes is the most common cause of peripheral neuropathy. It is characterized by symmetrical "pins and needles" sensation of the distal extremities, often worse at night and the cause of sleeplessness with consequential fatigue. On examination there is always evidence of additional sensory disturbances including loss of vibration or position sensation, or loss of the ankle stretch reflexes.

Cauda equina syndrome will produce bilateral pain, loss of stretch reflexes, and loss of sensation in the perineum. Sphincter tone may be lax. An L3-L4 herniated disk will result in weakness in extension of the great toe and, usually, loss of the patellar stretch reflex. Spinal cord infarction is associated with the sudden onset of back pain, deep aching pain in the legs, paresthesias, and weakness of the legs soon resulting in the inability to walk.

### Bibliography

1. **Baconja M, Beydoun A, Edwards KR, Schwartz SL, Fonseca V, Hes M, et al**. Gabapentin for the symptomatic treatment of painful neuropathy in patients with diabetes mellitus: a randomized controlled trial. JAMA. 1998;280:1831-6. PMID: 9846777

## Diabetes Mellitus Question 9
## Answer: B

**Educational Objective:** *Recognize the place of sliding scale insulin for inpatients with concurrent illness.*

Sliding scale regimens are prescribed for most patients with diabetes in many hospitals, but there is no evidence that this approach provides benefit when used without a standing dose of intermediate-acting insulin. Sliding scales are associated with fluctuations in plasma glucose and often shifts in potassium. An intermediate-acting dose of insulin adjusted to the intensity of the patient's illness should always be administered and supplemented by a schedule of rapid-acting insulin based upon the method and quantity of the caloric intake. The intermediate-acting insulin is intended to emulate the normal basal secretion of insulin, whereas the supplemental injections are intended to simulate the spurts in insulin secretion that follow meals.

The patient's prehospital insulin schedule may not be adequate for this postoperative patient. An insulin infusion will not be necessary to control the patient's glucose. Metformin is not indicated in patients with type 1 diabetes mellitus.

Coronary artery bypass grafting is associated with severe insulin resistance. When glucose-insulin infusions are given intra- and postoperatively, larger quantities of insulin are required than when diabetic patients undergo routine elective surgery. In patients who receive glucose-insulin-potassium infusions during surgery, plasma glucose should be measured every 2 hours and serum potassium every 4 to 6 hours. Postoperatively, efforts should be made to stabilize the plasma glucose concentration below 200 mg/dL to reduce the risk of infection and to stimulate protein synthesis and healing.

Insulin treatment during major surgery is now standard in patients with type 1 diabetes mellitus. Insulin may be administered subcutaneously with an infusion of glucose to cover the insulin or with a combined infusion of glucose. In patients with type 2 disease who do not take insulin, the determinants of therapy are the nature of the surgery and the preoperative metabolic state of the patient. Patients with type 2 disease who do take insulin should be treated as type 1 patients. Patients on diet alone or diet plus an oral agent do not require any specific therapy for minor surgery; however, the poorly controlled patient ideally should be regulated before surgery with short-acting insulin.

### Bibliography

1. **Queale WS, Seidler AJ, Brancati FL.** Glycemic control and sliding scale insulin use in medical inpatients with diabetes mellitus. Arch Intern Med. 1997;157:545-52. PMID: 9066459

2. **Hirsch IB, Paauw DS, Brunzell J.** Inpatient management of adults with diabetes. Diabetes Care. 1995;18:870-8. PMID: 7555517

## Diabetes Mellitus Question 10
## Answer: D

**Educational Objective:** *Determine the best regimen of insulin in a patient with type 2 diabetes mellitus taking combination oral medications.*

Type 2 diabetes mellitus is a progressive disorder, the course of which is not halted by sulfonylurea or metformin therapy. The United Kingdom Prospective Diabetes Study demonstrated that the deterioration in glycemic control is the result of progressive failure of the pancreatic beta cells. When fasting hyperglycemia develops, the decline in glucose regulation is relentless. Multiple factors such as the duration and severity of the hyperglycemia, the degree of adiposity, and lifestyle of the patient account for the variability in the rate of decline of beta-cell function. The presence of symptoms and/or progressive rise in hemoglobin $A_{1C}$ levels are indicators for the initiation of insulin therapy.

Bedtime intermediate-acting insulin is selected to effect a dampening of usual early morning increments in glucose (the so-called dawn phenomenon). The objective of bedtime insulin is to reduce fasting glycemia within the physiologic range without inducing nocturnal hypoglycemia. Increasing the bedtime insulin steadily every 5 to 7 days by 3 to 5 units to achieve this goal has been recommended.

When clinical symptoms and corresponding laboratory data confirm the likelihood of beta-cell failure, sulfonylurea therapy probably has little place. Sulfonylureas are insulin secretogogues that bind to sulfonylurea receptors on beta cells and depolarize the membranes of these cells to induce the secretion of insulin through exocytosis. If the beta cells have been dysfunctional, as in this patient, sulfonylureas are ineffective and should be discontinued. On the other hand in some patients, responsiveness to sulfonylureas is restored when glycemic control is achieved. In patients taking a sulfonylurea and metformin in whom therapeutic goals are not achieved, the options include adding a third agent (for example, a thiazolidinedione), or starting either bedtime insulin or multiple doses of insulin. If the beta cells are failing and insulin deficiency is progressive, the effectiveness of a third agent is questionable. A study from Finland showed glycemic control in such patients is substantially improved with the bedtime insulin-metformin regimen, in contrast to metformin and multiple doses of insulin. The latter regimen causes significant weight gain, whereas the bedtime insulin and metformin regimen did not.

### Bibliography

1. **Baldeweg SE, Yudkin JS.** Implications of the United Kingdom prospective diabetes study. Prim Care. 1999;26:809-27. PMID: 10523461

2. **King P, Peacock I, Donnelly R.** The UK prospective diabetes study (UKPDS): clinical and therapeutic implications for type 2 diabetes. Br J Clin Pharmacol. 1999;48:643-8. PMID: 10594464

3. **DeFronzo RA.** Pharmacologic therapy for type 2 diabetes mellitus. Ann Intern Med. 1999;131:281-303. PMID: 10454950

4. **Yki-Jarvinen H, Ryysy L, Nikkila K, Tulokas T, Vanamo R, Heikkila M.** Comparison of bedtime insulin regimens in patients with type 2 diabetes mellitus. A randomized, controlled trial. Ann Intern Med. 1999;130:389-96. PMID: 10068412

## Diabetes Mellitus Question 11
## Answer: A

**Educational Objective:** *Initiate pharmacotherapy in a patient with type 2 diabetes mellitus who has failed to respond to a trial of diet and exercise therapy.*

Monotherapy with an oral hypoglycemic agent is indicated after 6 to 8 weeks of a trial educational nutritional-exercise program if that regimen fails. Most studies suggest metformin as the initial monotherapy in obese patients because it reduces body weight as well as serum triglyceride and LDL cholesterol levels. Metformin therapy decreases the fasting plasma glucose by 60 to 70 mg/dl and the hemoglobin $A_{1C}$ by 1.5% to 2.0%.

Sulfonylurea therapy equally reduces fasting plasma glucose levels and hemoglobin $A_{1C}$, but it induces weight gain and has no effect on serum triglycerides or cholesterol. Metformin is the monotherapy of choice in obese patients, sulfonylureas in normal-weight or slightly overweight patients. Metformin at standard dosage is twice as costly as generic sulfonylureas.

An α-glucosidase inhibitor like acarbose delay glucose absorption but do not affect glucose utilization or insulin secretion. They are less potent than other single agents and are unlikely to control her blood glucose or symptoms.

Thiazolidinedione therapy improves insulin sensitivity in the liver, muscle, and adipose tissue, but is less effective as monotherapy in reducing fasting plasma glucose concentration than sulfonylurea or metformin.

Insulin therapy lowers plasma glucose concentration and may be the choice of some patients, although the great majority elect an oral agent. Insulin causes weight gain when glycemic control is achieved, although it may reduce levels of serum triglycerides and LDL cholesterol.

**Bibliography**

1. **DeFronzo RA**. Pharmacologic therapy for type 2 diabetes mellitus. Ann Intern Med. 1999;131:281-303. PMID: 10454950

2. Effect of intensive blood glucose control with metformin in complications in overweight patients with type 2 diabetes (UKPDS 34). UK Prospective Diabetes Study (UKPDS) Group. Lancet. 1998;352:854-65. PMID: 9742977

## Diabetes Mellitus Question 12
## Answer: D

**Educational Objective:** *Manage metformin therapy in the diabetic patient undergoing radiocontrast studies.*

Radiocontrast dyes may cause acute renal failure in diabetic patients, especially those with decreased glomerular filtration rates, albuminuria, and elevated blood urea nitrogen. If renal failure is unrecognized after a radiocontrast dye study and metformin is being used, the plasma levels of metformin increase progressively, and in some cases lactic acidosis develops. In diabetic patients with normal renal function who, in the setting of an acute illness, require a study that uses radiocontrast dye, metformin should be withheld on the day of the procedure and then on the following day (24 hours), serum creatinine should be measured and if normal, metformin treatment should be reinstated. Usually no hypoglycemic agent is required while the metformin is withheld.

Metformin as monotherapy is particularly effective in patients with type 2 diabetes mellitus. The drug inhibits hepatic gluconeogenesis and glycogenolysis, and enhances the sensitivity to insulin in both hepatic and muscle tissue. Fasting plasma glucose falls by 60 to 70 mg/dL and hemoglobin $A_{1C}$ by 1.5% to 2.0% in poorly controlled patients when the drug is given as monotherapy. The drug should not be started or continued if the serum creatinine level is 1.5 mg/dL or

higher. About one third of the patients who start the drug have gastrointestinal side effects which are usually mild and transient.

**Bibliography**

1. **DeFronzo RA**. Pharmacologic therapy for type 2 diabetes mellitus. Ann Intern Med. 1999;131:281-303. PMID: 10454950

2. **Bailey CJ, Turner RC**. Metformin. N Engl J Med. 1996;334:574-9. PMID: 8569826

## Diabetes Mellitus Question 13
## Answer: C

**Educational Objective:** *Recognize the cause of postprandial hypoglycemia in type 1 diabetes mellitus.*

Early satiety and vomiting are prominent indicators that gastroparesis has developed in this patient. Gastroparesis causes poor metabolic control, especially hypoglycemia, because of dyssynchrony between gastric emptying and the absorption of rapid-acting insulin. Gastroparesis is a complication of autonomic neuropathy and is often accompanied by other manifestations of that neuropathy, including orthostatic hypotension or a neurogenic bladder. Dopamine antagonists such as metoclopramide and domperidone may be helpful. There is no evidence that this young patient who has had diabetes mellitus for 12 years has developed diabetic nephropathy or retinopathy. While she may have peripheral neuropathy it does not account for her hypoglycemic reactions.

**Bibliography**

1. **Enck P, Frieling T**. Pathophysiology of diabetic gastroparesis. Diabetes. 1997;46(Suppl 2):S77-81. PMID: 9285504

2. **Cucchiara S, Franzese A, Salvia G, Alfonsi L, Iula VD, Montisci A, et al.** Gastric emptying delay and gastric electrical derangement in IDDM. Diabetes Care. 1998;21:438-43. PMID: 9540029

## Diabetes Mellitus Question 14
## Answer: D

**Educational Objective:** *Understand the mechanisms of action of the thiazolidinedione group of hypoglycemic agents.*

Resistance to the action of insulin is a prime cause of the hyperglycemia in most patients with type 2 diabetes. The thiazolidinediones are a group of drugs that improve sensitivity to insulin in several tissues by binding to PPAR-γ receptors, leading to increased expression of glucose transporters. The agent causes weight gain when used as monotherapy and in combination with insulin. Serum triglyceride values fall, whereas both LDL and HDL cholesterol values increase; the rise in LDL cholesterol in several studies is about 10% to 15%. The currently available thiazolidinediones, rosiglitazone and proglitazone, are equally effective in lowering glucose in patients with type 2 diabetes mellitus. Hemoglobin $A_{1C}$ levels fall about 1.5% in studies of these agents. Several cases of severe liver toxicity have been reported after troglitazone therapy, so it was removed from the market in March of 2000. The U.S. Food and Drug Administration recommends baseline and every 2 month monitoring of liver function tests during the first year of therapy if this class of drugs is used. The incidence of elevated liver enzyme levels in patients treated with proglitazone and rosiglitazone are 0.25% and 0.2% respectively, values similar to those in patients receiving placebos.

### Bibliography

1. **Saltiel AR, Olefsky JM**. Thiazolidinediones in the treatment of insulin resistance and type II diabetes. Diabetes. 1996;45:1661-9. PMID: 8922349

2. **DeFronzo RA**. Pharmacologic therapy for type 2 diabetes mellitus. Ann Intern Med. 1999;131:281-303. PMID: 10454950

## Diabetes Mellitus Question 15
## Answer: C

**Educational Objective:** *Understand the pathogenesis of hypoglycemia unawareness.*

Intensive treatment of diabetes mellitus with episodes of hypoglycemia leads to the loss of the release of epinephrine, which is the essential neurogenic warning signal in type 1 disease. Repeated occurrences of low plasma glucose result in diminished autonomic responses to hypoglycemia. The mechanism for this shift is not known. Normal persons demonstrate a rise in glucagon and epinephrine when plasma glucose falls below 65 to 70 mg/dL. In patients with type 1 diabetes, the glucagon response to hypoglycemia is markedly impaired or is absent after the first several years of the disease, so that epinephrine becomes the sole warning signal when hypoglycemia develops. But recurrent hypoglycemia impairs the release of epinephrine at the usual levels of glycemia — in essence, hypoglycemia begets hypoglycemia as the threshold for the release of epinephrine becomes a lower level of glucose. The treatment of hypoglycemia unawareness is to ease the intensive control of glucose and attempt to maintain meticulous control yet avoid hypoglycemia. Improvement may occur in several days but usually requires weeks of avoidance of low plasma glucose.

The frequency of severe hypoglycemia during intensive insulin therapy may be as much as 25 times that of conventional treatment. Hypoglycemia unawareness frequently occurs at night during sleep; another complication of hypoglycemia unawareness is the prevalence of motor vehicle accidents among intensively treated patients. In normal persons, early cognitive dysfunction begins when plasma glucose declines to 50 to 55 mg/dL; that does not change in diabetic individuals, but when warning signals are absent and glucose falls to 20 to 30 mg/dL, cognitive dysfunction is profoundly impaired. Efforts to avoid hypoglycemia reverse hypoglycemia unawareness despite only marginal improvement in epinephrine responses.

### Bibliography

1. **Gerich JE, Mokan M. Veneman T, Korytkowski M, Mitrakou A.** Hypoglycemia unawareness. Endocr Rev. 1991;12:356-71. PMID: 1760993

2. **Taverna MJ, M'Bemba J, Sola A, Chevalier A, Slama G, Selam JL.** Insufficient adaptation of hypoglycaemic threshold for cognitive impairment in tightly controlled type 1 diabetes. Diabetes Metab. 2000;26:58-64. PMID: 10705105

## Diabetes Mellitus Question 16
## Answer: B

**Educational Objective:** *Prevent progression of diabetic nephropathy in a patient with type 2 diabetes mellitus who takes insulin.*

This patient has already started on the path to progressive diabetic nephropathy. Although all of the preventive measures still warrant attention, blood pressure control at this stage is most important. From the onset, good glycemic control (hemoglobin $A_{1C}$ 7% to 7.5%), a protein-regulated diet to reduce intraglomerular pressure as well as antihypertensive therapy with an angiotensin-converting enzyme (ACE) inhibitor should be considered.

Antihypertensive therapy attenuates the decline in renal function in patients with all forms of diabetes. The United Kingdom Prospective Diabetes Study (UKPDS) suggests that tight control ($\leq 144/82$ mm/Hg) of blood pressure decreases the chances of macrovascular and microvascular consequences. While intensive glycemic control delays or prevents the development of nephropathy, it is not certain that such control blunts the disintegration of renal function as nephropathy progresses.

In patients with type 1 diabetes mellitus, a large study revealed that after 4 years of treatment with an ACE inhibitor (captopril), patients had a slower rate of rise in serum creatinine and a lower likelihood of progressing to end-stage renal disease than the placebo group. In patients with creatinine concentrations of 1.5 mg/dL or greater, the rate of rise was reduced by 50%. The UKPDS found that in patients with type 2 disease there was no difference in the outcome between captopril and atenolol, a β-blocker. Two small studies showed that restriction of dietary protein slows the long-term decline in glomerular filtration rate by 60% to 75%, from approximately 12 mL/min/year to 3 mL/min/year. However, there are potential complications with a protein-restricted diet (0.6 g/kg per day) because compliance also results in a reduction in fat and possibly an essential deficiency in the amino acid L-arginine, which is the precursor of the vasodilator nitric oxide. Aspirin and lipid-lowering drugs are effective in diabetics as well as in nondiabetics, but have little or no role in the progression of diabetic nephropathy.

## Bibliography

1. **Cooper ME**. Pathogenesis, prevention, and treatment of diabetic nephropathy. Lancet. 1998;352:213-9. PMID: 9683226
2. **DeFronzo RA**.Pharmacologic therapy for type 2 diabetes mellitus. Ann Intern Med. 1999;131:281-303. PMID: 10454950

## Diabetes Mellitus Question 17
## Answer: C

**Educational Objective:** *Prescribe an optimal oral hypoglycemic agent for a patient with newly diagnosed type 2 diabetes.*

Persistent hyperglycemia and hypertriglyceridemia in an obese patient make metformin an ideal agent. The drug will facilitate weight loss and have beneficial effects on the hypertriglyceridemia. The United Kingdom Prospective Diabetes Study indicated that insulin and sulfonylureas equally lower plasma glucose but do not help weight loss or prevent weight gain. The thiazinolinediones as monotherapy also increase weight as well as possibly adversely affecting serum cholesterol levels. Although metformin as well as insulin and sulfonylureas reduce hyperglycemia and consequently lower the risk for the several microvascular complications, these agents do not significantly alter the risk for myocardial infarction.

Insulin is most effective as the first choice in symptomatic patients, especially those who are normal weight or only slightly overweight. In the setting of infection, a vascular accident, or other medical problem, the patient with recent-onset type 2 disease benefits from insulin as first treatment.

Sulfonylureas would also probably lower plasma glucose in this patient, but weight gain or inability to lower weight are possible complications. In 10% to 15% of recently diagnosed patients, sulfonylureas are ineffective as hypoglycemic agents. The exact cause of this primary failure is unclear, although beta cells exposed to hyperglycemia for prolonged periods will not respond to sulfonylureas.

Acarbose is reserved for patients with type 2 diabetes mellitus in whom postprandial hyperglycemia is the major problem. In patients with elevated fasting glucose levels, acarbose will have limited effect.

The thiazolidinediones effectively reduce fasting plasma glucose concentration. These agents increase serum LDL-and HDL cholesterol slightly and lower triglycerides by about 10-15%.

## Bibliography

1. **Bailey CJ, Turner RC**. Metformin. N Engl J Med. 1996;334:574-9. PMID: 8569826
2. **DeFronzo RA**. Pharmacologic therapy for type 2 diabetes mellitus. Ann Intern Med. 1999;131:281-303. PMID: 10454950

## Diabetes Mellitus Question 18
## Answer: A

**Educational Objective:** *Know the clinical implications of microalbuminuria and subsequent risk of renal and cardiovascular disease.*

Increased urinary protein excretion is the earliest marker of diabetic nephropathy. However, the urine dipstick measurement is a relatively insensitive marker because it does not become positive until protein excretion exceeds 300 mg/d. A specific assay for albumin is more sensitive because the normal rate of albumin excretion is less than 20 mg/d. Persistent values between 30 and 300 mg/d in a patient with diabetes mellitus is termed "microalbuminuria" and is usually indicative of early diabetic nephropathy. Patients with values above 300 mg/d are considered to have overt macroscopic proteinuria.

A 24-hour urine collection is the gold standard for the detection of microalbuminuria. However, screening can be done simply by using a timed urine collection or an early morning specimen to minimize changes in urine volume. Use of the albumin:creatinine ratio has recently been recommended as the preferred screening strategy for all patients with diabetes mellitus. An albumin: creatinine ratio above 30 mg/g represents an albumin excretion of more than 30 mg/d and is diagnostic of microalbuminuria.

Not all patients with diabetes mellitus and microalbuminuria develop overt nephropathy over the next decade. Less than 50% of patients with type 1 diabetes mellitus and microalbuminuria are at risk for progression. Progression to overt nephropathy occurs in 20% to 40% of white patients with type 2 diabetes mellitus. Risk factors contributing to progression include hyperglycemia, hypertension, and tobacco use.

The presence of microalbuminuria is an important risk factor for the development of cardiovascular disease and early cardiovascular mortality in patients with both type 2 diabetes mellitus and essential hypertension. For example, patients with type 2 diabetes mellitus and microalbuminuria who were followed for 3.4 years had a mortality rate of 28%, compared with a mortality rate of 4% for patients with type 2 diabetes mellitus without microalbuminuria. The increased risk appeared to be independent of other cardiovascular risk factors.

Optimal therapy for hypertensive patients with type 2 diabetes mellitus and microalbuminuria is an angiotensin-converting enzyme (ACE) inhibitor. Patients treated with an ACE inhibitor had a slower progression to overt proteinuria and a slower increase in serum creatinine levels over a 3-year period.

## Bibliography

1. **Keane WF, Eknoyan G**. Proteinuria, albuminuria, risk, assessment, detection, elimination (PARADE): a position paper of the National Kidney Foundation. Am J Kidney Dis. 1999;33:1004-10. PMID: 10213663

2. **Mogensen CE, Vestbo E, Poulsen PL, Christiansen C, Damsgaard EM, Eiskjaer H, et al**. Microalbuminuria and potential confounders. A review and some observations on variability of urinary albumin excretion. Diabetes Care. 1995;18:572-81. PMID: 7497874

3. **Mogensen CE**. Microalbuminuria predicts clinical proteinuria and early mortality in maturity-onset diabetes. N Engl J Med. 1984;310:356-60. PMID: 6690964

4. **Lebovitz HE, Wiegmann TB, Cnaan A, Shahinfar S, Sica DA, Broadstone V, et al**. Renal protective effects of enalapril in hypertensive NIDDM: role of baseline albuminuria. Kidney Int Suppl. 1994;45:S150-5. PMID: 8158885

## Diabetes Mellitus Question 19
## Answer: C

**Educational Objective:** *Understand the variety of lipid disorders in a patient with type 2 diabetes mellitus.*

This patient has type 2 diabetes mellitus complicated by significantly elevated total cholesterol levels, and he has a strongly positive family history of coronary artery disease. He had rather remarkable success with his initial attempts at weight loss and exercise, and these efforts should be strongly encouraged. In fact, the success was so good that there is no need to start an oral hypoglycemic agent or restrict alcohol for his diabetes.

Alcohol restriction may help reduce triglyceride levels, but he has already done so simply by losing weight and improving his glucose control, so further restriction would not be necessary. Restricting alcohol intake would not be expected to substantially affect his still-elevated cholesterol levels, nor would further weight loss or further improvement in diabetic control.

The initially fairly high level and relatively small decline in his cholesterol with weight loss and improvement in diabetic control suggest that his hypercholesterolemia is a coexisting primary disorder, rather than one solely secondary to diabetes. The strong family history also supports this possibility. Therefore, measurements of high-density lipoprotein (HDL) and low-density lipoprotein (LDL) cholesterol fractions should be performed. If, indeed, his LDL cholesterol levels are elevated, this condition should be treated very aggressively. He has four risk factors for cardiovascular disease: male gender, family history of early coronary artery disease, diabetes, and the elevated LDL cholesterol levels. It is common to ascribe all lipid abnormalities in diabetic patients to their diabetes, and it is important to recognize when there are independent lipid disorders coexisting with the diabetes that may need additional treatment. Measuring his fasting C-peptide level will not contribute to the understanding or control of his lipid disorder.

### Bibliography

1. Role of cardiovascular risk factors in prevention and treatment of macrovascular disease in diabetes. American Diabetes Association. Diabetes Care. 1989;12:573-9. PMID: 2673697

2. **Dunn FL**. Hyperlipidemia in diabetes mellitus. Diabetes Metab Rev. 1990;6:47-61. PMID: 2192855

3. **Garber AJ, Vinik AI, Crespin SR**. Detection and management of lipid disorders in diabetic patients. A commentary for clinicians. Diabetes Care. 1992;15:1068-74. PMID: 1303635

## Diabetes Mellitus Question 20
## Answer: D

**Educational Objective:** *Know the criteria for initiating insulin therapy.*

A physician can manage a new patient with type 1 diabetes initially without knowing more than the history, physical examination, and plasma glucose level.

Although serologic evidence of autoimmunity in a newly diagnosed diabetic patient is interesting, at present it is not pertinent to the management of the decompensated glycemic state. Measurement of the circulating antibodies to islet cell proteins may be pertinent clinically at some future time in order to use immunomodulating drugs to control further β-cell destruction; however, use of such drugs now is inappropriate apart from a controlled clinical trial.

Often in the decompensated diabetic patient, C-peptide will be measurably absent. Even if it is present, the need for insulin and its appropriate use will relate to the degree of hyperglycemia and to the clinical state.

### Bibliography

1. **Zinman B**.Insulin regimens and strategies for IDDM. Diabetes Care. 1993;16:24-8. PMID: 8299474

2. **Santiago JV**. A pediatric perspective. Insulin therapy in the last decade. Diabetes Care. 1993;16:143-54. PMID: 8299471

## Diabetes Mellitus Question 21
## Answer: B

**Educational Objective:** *Recognize fat droplets in the urine, and differentiate them from other elements in the urine.*

The typical "Maltese cross" appearance of a fat droplet under polarized light microscopy is shown. Fat droplets are composed primarily of cholesterol esters and cholesterol and are commonly found in patients with the nephrotic syndrome or with diabetic nephropathy. They are not found in pyelonephritis, cancer, interstitial nephritis, or hypertensive renal disease. Under routine light microscopy, fat droplets appear as rounded structures and can easily be confused with red blood cells. However, fat droplets have greater variability in size and a darker outline than do red blood cells. Under polarized light microscopy, fat droplets are doubly refractile and have a characteristic "Maltese cross" appearance that clearly differentiates them from red blood cells.

### Bibliography

1. **Hudson JB, Dennis AJ Jr, Gerhardt RE**. Urinary lipid and the Maltese cross. N Engl J Med. 1978;299:586. PMID: 683225

## Diabetes Mellitus Question 22
## Answer: B

**Educational Objective:** *Recognize proliferative diabetic retinopathy on a fundoscopic photograph and distinguish it from the nonproliferative form.*

Proliferative diabetic retinopathy is characterized by the ischemia-induced development of a network of new vessels (neovascularization) protruding from the optic disk. These vessels can rupture and lead to preretinal or vitreous hemorrhage, resulting in severe compromise of vision. In addition, the fibrous tissue that accompanies the new vessels can contract and cause a traction retinal detachment.

Proliferative diabetic retinopathy typically develops after the onset and progression of mild, moderate, or severe forms of nonproliferative diabetic retinopathy. The second funduscopic photograph (right image) shows the mild stage of nonproliferative diabetic retinopathy. The multiple red dots are microaneurysms or microhemorrhages. Flame hemorrhages (intraretinal hemorrhages) and hard exudates (yellowish in appearance) are also present. In moderate nonproliferative diabetic retinopathy, these findings will appear together with cotton-wool spots caused by microinfarction of the nerve fiber layer. In severe nonproliferative diabetic retinopathy, these findings will be present in addition to increased vascular tortuosity, hemorrhages, venous beading, and widespread intraretinal microvascular abnormalities. In mild cases of papilledema, the optic disc appears elevated and its margins are blurred. In more advanced cases, hemorrhages and focal infarcts are present. There is often striking hyperemia of the optic disc from dilation of blood vessels. A macular star may develop from leakage of exudate. It is helpful to search for spontaneous pulsation of the retinal veins as they emerge from the center of the optic disc signifying normal intracranial pressure and thereby helps to exclude the diagnosis of papilledema. In chronic papilledema, optic disc swelling may subside and be replaced by optic atrophy. Hemorrhages are resorbed and the optic disc assumes a pale, gliotic appearance. Small, glittering, drusen-like bodies form on the surface of the optic disc. The retinal vessels become narrowed and sheathed.

Macular degeneration occurs most commonly as a nonexudative and rarely as an exudative form. The nonexudative process begins with the accumulation of extracellular deposits, called drusen, underneath the retinal pigment epithelium. On ophthalmoscopy, they are pleomorphic but generally appear as small discrete yellow lesions clustered in the macula. With time they become larger, more numerous, and confluent. The retinal pigment epithelium becomes focally detached and atrophic.

Exudative macular degeneration, which develops in only a minority of patients, occurs when neovascular vessels from the choroid grow through defects in Bruch's membrane into the potential space beneath the retinal pigment epithelium. Leakage from these vessels produces elevation of the retina and pigment epithelium.

**Bibliography**

1. Ferris FL 3rd, Davis MD, Aiello LM. Treatment of diabetic retinopathy. N Engl J Med. 1999;341:667-78. PMID: 10460819

## Diabetes Mellitus Question 23
## Answer: D

**Educational Objective:** *Become familiar with the differential diagnosis of neuropathy in diabetics.*

This woman has chronic inflammatory demyelinating polyneuropathy predominantly affecting motor fibers, causing significant limb paralysis. The combination of greater distal than proximal muscle weakness, areflexia, and distal loss of vibration sense is characteristic of a peripheral polyneuropathy that affects mostly myelinated fibers. A muscle disease such as polymyositis would cause greater proximal than distal weakness. A spinal cord lesion would not be symmetric, and sensory loss would not be limited to vibration. A hemispheric stroke would produce unilateral signs and symptoms. The differential diagnosis is between a demyelinating polyneuropathy and a diabetic peripheral polyneuropathy.

Diabetic peripheral polyneuropathy is most often a rather mild disorder that causes some decreased sensation in the toes and feet and a loss of ankle reflexes. More severe polyneuropathies do occur, especially in long-standing diabetes, especially if diabetic control is poor. This woman had very mild diabetes that is well controlled. A rapidly progressive, severe, paralyzing polyneuropathy explained by diabetes would be extremely rare in her circumstances. Chronic inflammatory demyelinating polyneuropathy is a relatively common polyneuropathy presumed to be of an autoimmune basis in which proximal and distal weakness and areflexia are common. Usually sensory loss is limited to vibration and position sense, sensory functions mediated by large myelinated fibers within peripheral nerves. Some have thought of this disorder as a kind of chronic Guillain-Barré syndrome. The history and physical examination presented are typical of chronic inflammatory demyelinating polyneuropathy. Electrophysiologic studies will document widespread decrease in motor and sensory nerve conduction velocities indicative of a demyelinating polyneuropathy.

**Bibliography**

1. Dyck PJ, Dyck PJ, Grant IA, Fealey RD. Ten steps in characterizing and diagnosing patients with peripheral neuropathy. Neurology. 1996;47:10-7. PMID: 8710060

2. Gorson KC, Allam G, Ropper AH. Chronic inflammatory demyelinating polyneuropathy: clinical features and response to treatment in 67 consecutive patients with and without monoclonal gammopathy. Neurology. 1997;48:321-8. PMID: 9040714

3. Barohn RJ, Kissel JT, Warmolts JR, Mendell JR. Chronic inflammatory demyelinating polyradiculoneuropathy. Clinical characteristics, course, and recommendations for diagnostic criteria. Arch Neurol. 1989;46:878-84. PMID: 2757528

# HIV Disease

## HIV Disease Question 1
### Answer: C

**Educational Objective:** *Understand that the level of immunosuppression correlates with HIV-associated skin disease and that highly active antiretroviral therapy (HAART) may reverse these manifestations.*

Skin lesions in patients with HIV infection correlate with the level of immunosuppression, and effective therapy can result in a "spontaneous" healing of the lesions. In this case, the patient presented with seborrheic dermatitis that was associated with a high level of immunosuppression. Fortunately, with the newer forms of therapy, viral loads and the level of immune dysfunction may be reversed, and uncontrollable cutaneous disorders, including viral infections, may resolve or be controlled more easily. Seborrheic dermatitis has no potential for malignant transformation.

### Bibliography
1. **Goldstein B, Berman B, Sukenik E, Frankel SJ.** Correlation of skin disorders with CD4 lymphocyte counts in patients with HIV/AIDS. J Am Acad Dermatol. 1997;36:262-4. PMID: 9039183
2. **Hicks CB, Myers SA, Giner J.** Resolution of intractable molluscum contagiosum in a human immunodeficiency virus-infected patient after institution of antiretroviral therapy with ritonavir. Clin Infect Dis. 1997;24:1023-5. PMID: 9142826

## HIV Disease Question 2
### Answer: D

**Educational Objective:** *Recognize the relationship between CD4 cell count and the risk of opportunistic infection.*

This presentation is most consistent with focal lymphadenitis caused by *Mycobacterium tuberculosis* in a patient who is experiencing a good clinical response to therapy. The diagnosis would be determined by a lymph node aspirate, which should be stained and cultured for both acid-fast bacilli and bacteria. The most important clues to the diagnosis in this case are the CD4 cell count, both the pretreatment and the current value, and the clinical features of the lymphadenitis.

The risk for developing non-Hodgkin's lymphoma is increased in patients with HIV infection. In fact, systemic, high-grade, B-cell non-Hodgkin's lymphoma was included in the 1985 Centers for Disease Control and Prevention (CDC) AIDS definition. Non-Hodgkin's lymphoma had been reported to occur in 5% of patients with HIV infection before the development of more potent antiretroviral therapy. Almost all patients with HIV-related non-Hodgkin's lymphoma present with widespread disease, and the majority have constitutional symptoms at diagnosis. Lymphoma can present as an enlarging lymph node; however, the lymph node is not likely to be tender or indurated. Therefore, lymphoma is not the most likely diagnosis. Histoplasmosis is a disseminated infection, and lymphadenitis is not an expected finding. In addition, histoplasmosis occurs at lower CD4 cell counts (generally < 100/µL). Toxoplasmosis can occasionally present as disease outside the central nervous system (CNS). The most common extra-CNS presentation is pulmonary toxoplasmosis. In normal hosts, toxoplasmosis can present as enlargement of a single lymph node; however, the node is not indurated or tender. In patients with HIV infection, toxoplasmosis is generally a reactivation of latent infection that occurs when the CD4 cell count drops below 100/µL.

Prior to the advent of potent antiretroviral therapy, *Mycobacterium avium* complex usually presented clinically as a disseminated infection, with fever, diarrhea, night sweats, and anemia being the most common symptoms. Recently, there have been reports of patients with a history of low CD4 cell counts who developed localized disease caused by *Mycobacterium avium* complex upon initiating potent antiretroviral therapy. The most common presentation has been a focal inflammatory lymphadenitis. For this patient, the lowest known CD4 cell count prior to beginning therapy was 240/µL, which is well above the level at which *Mycobacterium avium* complex is likely to be seen. Therefore, *Mycobacterium avium* complex infection is not a likely diagnosis. If this patient had previously had a CD4 cell count of < 50/µL, *Mycobacterium avium* complex would be in the differential diagnosis and could not be distinguished clinically from *M. tuberculosis*.

### Bibliography
1. **Race EM, Adelson-Mitty J, Kriegel GR, Barlam TF, Reimann KA, Letvin NL, et al.** Focal mycobacterial lymphadenitis following initiation of protease-inhibitor therapy in patients with advanced HIV-1 disease. Lancet. 1998;351:252-5. PMID: 9457095
2. **Jacobson MA, French M.** Altered natural history of AIDS-related opportunistic infections in the era of potent combination antiretroviral therapy. AIDS. 1998;12:S157-63. PMID: 9632998

## HIV Disease Question 3
## Answer: A

**Educational Objective:** *Understand the utility of laboratory tests for diagnosing acute HIV infection.*

The correct answer is the p24 antigen test since the presence of this antigen is diagnostic for HIV infection, although the presence of p24 antigen does not necessarily indicate acute infection. A plasma HIV viral load can also be useful, but neither the polymerase chain reaction (PCR) nor the branched-chain DNA (bDNA) assay is meant to be a diagnostic test. Low titers of virus found in this setting may represent false-positive results. Repeating the ELISA or Western blot 3 days after nondiagnostic results is unlikely to be useful.

Symptoms due to acute HIV infection characteristically occur within 2 to 6 weeks of exposure. This patient's incubation period is within this window, and he could have acute HIV infection despite the initial negative ELISA. Within 2 to 4 weeks of infection, high levels of circulating virus can be detected, with the peak occurring at the time of clinical manifestations. Therefore, a positive repeat ELISA is incorrect. Antibody to p24 and gp160 usually appears within 10 to 21 days, but a definitive ELISA or Western blot may not manifest for many weeks; most patients are seropositive by these techniques by 12 weeks, a few require 24 weeks, and patients very rarely seroconvert at a later date. CD4 counts may be depressed in illnesses other than HIV and are not indicated in making an initial diagnosis HIV.

### Bibliography

1. **Schacker TW, Hughes JP, Shea T, Coombs RW, Corey L.** Biologic and virologic characteristics of primary HIV infection. Ann Intern Med. 1998;128:613-20. PMID: 9537934

## HIV Disease Question 4
## Answer: A

**Educational Objective:** *Distinguish true-positive serologic tests for HIV from nonspecific or indeterminate results.*

Multiparous women occasionally have false-positive ELISA tests for HIV. Their Western blots characteristically show a band against either p24 or gp41. Therefore, this patient almost certainly does not have HIV, since her Western blot has not changed over 6 weeks. Telling the patient that she almost certainly does not have HIV is correct. Obtaining a p24 antigen or plasma HIV viral load is very unlikely to be helpful. This pattern on Western blot is not typical for HIV-2, with one stable band against gp41 for 6 weeks. In addition, HIV-2 is typically found in Africa; it is extremely rare in the Americas. Initiating anti-retroviral therapy would not be indicated in a patient with a false-positive HIV test.

### Bibliography

1. **Brown AE, Jackson B, Fuller SA, Sheffield J, Cannon MA, Lane JR.** Viral RNA in the resolution of human immunodeficiency virus type 1 diagnostic serology. Transfusion. 1997;37:926-9. PMID: 9308639

2. **Davey RT Jr, Deyton LR, Metcalf JA, Easter M, Kovacs JA, Vasudevachari M, Psallidopoulos M, et al.** Indeterminate western blot patterns in a cohort of individuals at high risk for human immunodeficiency virus (HIV-1) exposure. J Clin Immunol. 1992;12:185-92. PMID: 1400898

3. **Gurtler L.** Difficulties and strategies of HIV diagnosis. Lancet. 1996;348:176-9. PMID: 8684160

## HIV Disease Question 5
## Answer: B

**Educational Objective:** *Identify options for managing occupational exposure to HIV infection.*

The prompt initiation of antiretroviral therapy is recommended in the event of a deep injury with a hollow-bore needle from a known HIV-infected source patient with an elevated plasma HIV viral load. Several factors may affect the risk for HIV transmission after an occupational exposure. It has been estimated that the risk for HIV transmission from exposures that involve a larger volume of blood, particularly when the source patient's viral load is high, exceeds the average risk of 0.3%. To maximize efficacy, therapy needs to be started as soon as possible after the injury (ideally within 4 hours). The choice of regimen when the source patient is known to be on therapy should be based on the known treatment history. In this case, the source patient may harbor virus that is resistant to his current drugs; therefore, the choice of zidovudine, lamivudine, and nelfinavir would be appropriate for the resident. Because of the possibility of nucleoside cross-resistance and the inferior potency of monotherapy, the choice of zidovudine monotherapy would not be ideal. Similarly, while baseline HIV testing should be performed on the resident, the decision to start postexposure prophylaxis should not be delayed while awaiting these results.

### Bibliography

1. Updated U.S. Public Health Service Guidelines for the Management of Occupational Exposures to HBV, HCV, and HIV and Recommendations for Postexposure Prophylaxis. MMWR Recomm Rep. 2001;50(RR-11):1-52. PMID: 11442229

2. **Cardo DM, Culver DH, Ciesielski CA, Srivastava PU, Marcus R, Abiteboul D, et al.** A case-control study of HIV seroconversion in health care workers after percutaneous exposure. Centers for Disease Control and Prevention Needlestick Surveillance Group. N Engl J Med. 1997;337:1485-90. PMID: 9366579

## HIV Disease Question 6
### Answer: D

**Educational Objective:** *Identify appropriate testing for HIV exposures that occur in the health-care setting.*

The evaluation of health-care workers at the time of exposure to blood should include an HIV antibody test (ELISA) and testing for protection against hepatitis B. It is important to document the patient's HIV antibody status at the time of injury. The routine use of direct virus assays (for example, HIV p24 antigen assay or polymerase chain reaction [PCR] for HIV RNA) to detect infection in exposed health-care workers is generally not recommended. Although direct virus assays could potentially detect HIV infection earlier than an antibody test, the infrequency of seroconversion in health-care workers and increased costs of these tests do not warrant their routine use in this setting. HIV RNA PCR is only approved for use in monitoring established HIV infection, and false-positive low-level results in this setting can have devastating consequences.

**Bibliography**
1. Busch MP, Satten GA. Time course of viremia and antibody seroconversion following human immunodeficiency virus exposure. Am J Med. 1997;102:117-24. PMID: 9845513
2. Updated U.S. Public Health Service Guidelines for the Management of Occupational Exposures to HBV, HCV, and HIV and Recommendations for Postexposure Prophylaxis. MMWR Recomm Rep. 2001;50(RR-11):1-52. PMID: 11442229

## HIV Disease Question 7
### Answer: D

**Educational Objective:** *Identify the appropriate timing and choice of initial antiretroviral therapy in an asymptomatic patient with HIV infection.*

This asymptomatic patient has probably acquired HIV infection within the past 2 years. She has no signs or symptoms of primary HIV infection, and since her antibody test is positive, it is not likely that her infection is of recent onset. Her current CD4 cell count and plasma HIV viral load suggest that her prognosis over the next 5 years is very good. The best strategy would be to observe the patient with repeat plasma HIV viral load and CD4 cell count in 3 to 6 months. Although this is not a contraindication, her extensive travel schedule may preclude adherence to a complex treatment regimen. The treatment regimens of zidovudine, lamivudine, and either abacavir or nevirapine would be reasonable initial treatment regimens in a patient with early-stage HIV infection. A two-drug regimen of zidovudine and lamivudine is not currently considered a standard of care because of the inferior potency and limited subsequent treatment options following this combination in which one of the drugs, lamivudine, is prone to the development of resistance with a single mutation at codon 184. This is less of a problem when the drug is used as a part

of a completely suppressive regimen (for example, in a three-drug combination).

**Bibliography**
1. **Mellors JW, Munoz A, Giorgi JV, Margolick JB, Tassoni CJ, Gupta P, et al**. Plasma viral load and CD4+ lymphocytes as prognostic markers of HIV-1 infection. Ann Intern Med. 1997;126:946-54. PMID: 9182471
2. **Yeni PG, Hammer SM, Carpenter CC, Cooper DA, Fischl MA, Gatell JM, et al**. Antiretroviral treatment for adult HIV infection in 2002: updated recommendations of the International AIDS Society-USA Panel. JAMA. 2002;288:222-35. PMID: 12095387

## HIV Disease Question 8
### Answer: C

**Educational Objective:** *Understanding when to initiate antiretroviral therapy.*

The current U.S. Public Health Service, Department of Health and Human Services guidelines on antiretroviral therapy suggest that aggressive antiretroviral therapy initiated as soon as possible after the diagnosis is established may be beneficial. However, the decision to start therapy in this setting must be made in conjunction with the patient. The benefits of therapy at this early stage include the potential to preserve critical CD4-specific immune responses that may improve the natural history of infection. There are currently no randomized controlled trials that confirm this benefit. Given the complexity of therapy and the need for strict adherence, it is important that the patient is ready and willing to start therapy. Strong evidence to begin antiretroviral therapy exists for patient with CD4 counts below 200. At counts > 200 and < 500 data is controversial. Initiation of drug therapy for these patients should weigh the risks, benefits, and patients preferences. Development of oral thrush is not an indicator for initiation of antiretroviral therapy.

**Bibliography**
1. **Yeni PG, Hammer SM, Carpenter CC, Cooper DA, Fischl MA, Gatell JM, et al**. Antiretroviral treatment for adult HIV infection in 2002: updated recommendations of the International AIDS Society-USA Panel. JAMA. 2002;288:222-35. PMID: 12095387

## HIV Disease Question 9
### Answer: D

**Educational Objective:** *Recognize the appropriate interventions for a patient with pneumonia and HIV infection.*

The patient is at high risk for *Pneumocystis carinii* pneumonia (PCP) because of her previously low CD4 cell count, lack of prophylaxis, and presenting symptoms. It is essential to determine the degree of hypoxemia when initiating therapy for PCP, since the use of adjunctive glucocorticoids has been shown to reduce mortality during acute PCP. Adjunctive therapy with prednisone is indicated when the arterial blood $P_{O_2}$ is less than 70 mm Hg or the arterial alveolar gradient (a-A gradient) is greater than 35 mm Hg. The lactate dehydrogenase level is a marker of severity during PCP; however, only the a-A gradient has been used to determine the need for adjunctive glucocorticoids. The treatment of choice for PCP is trimethoprim-sulfamethoxazole. T-cell subsets would confirm that the CD4 cell count is within the range where PCP occurs; however, the history of a CD4 cell count less than 200/μL and no intervening therapy are strong evidence that this patient is at risk for developing PCP. A complete blood count should be obtained; however, in the absence of recent chemotherapy the finding of a low absolute neutrophil count would not alter the initial choice of therapy.

### Bibliography

1. **Bozzette SA, Sattler FR, Chiu J, Wu AW, Gluckstein D, Kemper C, et al.** A controlled trial of early adjunctive treatment with corticosteroids for *Pneumocystis carinii* pneumonia in the acquired immunodeficiency syndrome. California Collaborative Treatment Group. N Engl J Med. 1990:323:1451-7. PMID: 2233917
2. **Bartlett JG**. Pneumonia in the patient with HIV infection. Infect Dis Clin North Am. 1998;12:807-20. PMID: 9779391

## HIV Disease Question 10
## Answer: B

**Educational Objective:**   *Recognize the manifestations of and manage HIV-related Kaposi's sarcoma.*

These diffuse pulmonary infiltrates are very likely due to Kaposi's sarcoma. The raised purple endobronchial lesion is most probably Kaposi's sarcoma. Kaposi's sarcoma can occur at any CD4 cell count, although its frequency increases as the CD4 cell count declines. Kaposi's sarcoma can cause diffuse pulmonary infiltrates. Patients typically have endobronchial lesions and a bloody pulmonary effusion at the time that they develop infiltrates, although many patients with endobronchial disease have no pulmonary parenchymal involvement. Diagnosis is difficult to establish by bronchoscopic biopsy because the sample may be obtained too superficially and the crush artifact may make the histologic findings difficult to interpret.

Disseminated Herpes simplex would not present with an isolated lesion, nor would leukocytoclastic vasculitis or immune thrombocytopenic purpura, which would present with purpuric skin lesions.

### Bibliography

1. **Gill PS, Akil B, Colletti P, Rarick M, Loureiro C, Bernstein-Singer M, et al**. Pulmonary Kaposi's sarcoma: clinical findings and results of therapy. Am J Med. 1989;87:57-61. PMID: 2472743
2. **Ognibene FP, Steis RG, Macher AM, Liotta L, Gelmann E, Pass HI, et al**. Kaposi's sarcoma causing pulmonary infiltrates and respiratory failure in the acquired immunodeficiency syndrome. Ann Intern Med. 1985;102:471-5. PMID: 3977195

## HIV Disease Question 11
## Answer: B

**Educational Objective:**   *Recognize the options for treatment of Pneumocystis carinii pneumonia (PCP).*

This patient has early signs of a severe cutaneous reaction to TMP-SMX, with fever and mucous membrane involvement, and the TMP-SMX should be discontinued. There are several alternatives for the treatment of *Pneumocystis carinii* pneumonia (PCP) for patients who cannot tolerate trimethoprim-sulfamethoxazole (TMP-SMX). The usual parenteral alternative to TMP-SMX for severe disease is intravenous pentamidine, although clindamycin, 600 mg intravenously every 8 hours, and primaquine also have been shown to be effective (but this regimen is not listed as one of the choices in the question). Aerosolized pentamidine can be used prophylactically but is not indicated for the treatment of PCP. Atovaquone is an option for oral treatment of PCP for patients with mild disease. However, this agent may not be as effective in patients with diarrhea. Prednisone alone would not be an appropriate therapy.

### Bibliography

1. **Safrin S, Finkelstein DM, Feinberg J, Frame P, Simpson G, Wu A, et al.** Comparison of three regimens for treatment of mild to moderate Pneumocystis carinii pneumonia in patients with AIDS. A double-blind, randomized, trial of oral trimethoprim-sulfamethoxazole, dapsone-trimethoprim, and clindamycin-primaquine. ACTG 108 Study Group. Ann Intern Med. 1996;124:792-802. PMID: 8610948

## HIV Disease Question 12
## Answer: B

**Educational Objective:**   *Recognize the clinical presentation of oral candidiasis, and determine the best test to establish the diagnosis.*

The presence of diffuse, pink-white plaques in the oral mucosae that can easily be scraped suggests oral candidiasis. This condition is common in various settings but is particularly prevalent in immunosuppressed persons such as in this 32-year-old man. But white lesions, even in the setting of HIV, do not always represent candidiasis.

The diffuse nature of the disease contrasts with the localized presentation of oral hairy leukoplakia, which is seen in HIV-infected patients and is secondary to infection with Epstein-Barr virus. In patients with candidiasis, the fragile nature of the lesions also distinguishes them from other white plaques in the oral mucosae, such as those seen in patients with oral hairy leukoplakia or oral lichen planus.

Although a biopsy and culture will establish the diagnosis of oral candidiasis, a potassium hydroxide preparation is done more easily and rapidly than are the biopsy and culture. Thus, the potassium hydroxide preparation can more readily confirm the diagnosis of candidiasis than can a biopsy and culture and should be the first test of any white plaque of the oral mucosae.

A Tzanck smear is a useful test for detecting immunobullous and herpetic infections but is generally not informative in candidiasis. Polymerase chain reaction for herpesviruses has been used as a research tool and has allowed investigators to determine the role of Epstein-Barr virus in oral hairy leukoplakia, but it is not useful in establishing the diagnosis of oral candidiasis.

**Bibliography**

1. **Priddy RW.** Inflammatory hyperplasias of the oral mucosa. J Can Dent Assoc. 1992;58:311-21. PMID: 1591647

## HIV Disease Question 13
## Answer: C

**Educational Objective:** *Recognize the clinical presentation of bacillary angiomatosis in a patient with HIV infection.*

This 27-year-old man with HIV infection has lesions most consistent with the diagnosis of bacillary angiomatosis. A distinct infection most commonly seen in patients infected with HIV, bacillary angiomatosis can present in the skin but also may involve the viscera and bones. It is most probably caused by *Rochalimaea (Bartonella) henselae.* In the skin, the morphology of the lesions varies, and the number of lesions ranges from one to many. Unlike Kaposi's sarcoma, these lesions commonly bleed.

Kaposi's sarcoma can present in the skin with lesions similar to those seen in patients with bacillary angiomatosis. It is therefore essential to biopsy any purple lesion that may arise in the skin of HIV-infected patients, because bacillary angiomatosis is treatable and, if undiagnosed, can be progressive and potentially fatal.

Histologically, the lesions of bacillary angiomatosis may resemble those of pyogenic granuloma, but silver stains often show organisms in the tissue of patients with bacillary angiomatosis. Although pyogenic granulomas may occur in any setting, the rapid onset of multiple pyogenic granulomas is rare.

Secondary syphilis is commonly seen in the setting of HIV. The lesions can vary, and a granulomatous form of this disease is recognized. Skin biopsies distinguish these two entities, and special silver stains show the presence of spirochetes in secondary syphilis.

Cutaneous cryptococcosis is an important manifestation of AIDS. The most common lesions in cutaneous cryptococcosis, however, are either scattered papules and nodules with central crusting resembling molluscum contagiosum or brown to purple nodules.

**Bibliography**

1. **Koehler JE, Quinn FD, Berger TG, Le Boit PE, Tappero JW.** Isolation of Rochalimaea species from cutaneous and osseous lesions of bacillary angiomatosis. N Engl J Med. 1992;327:1625-31. PMID: 1435899
2. **Tompkins DC, Steigbigel RT.** Rochalimaea's role in cat scratch disease and bacillary angiomatosis. Ann Intern Med. 1993;118:388-90. PMID: 8430985

## HIV Disease Question 14
## Answer: D

**Educational Objective:** *Recognize oral candidiasis and distinguish it from oral hairy leukoplakia, leukoplakia, and lichen planus.*

Oral candidiasis presents as solid white or yellow plaques that can occur anywhere on the oral mucosa. The plaque is a pseudomembrane, meaning that it can be partially scraped off, and bleeding will occur where the plaque is removed. The surrounding mucosa is bright red and swollen. On the palate, candidiasis appears as atrophic red erosions with a white or yellow pseudomembrane. Oral candidiasis is associated with burning and pain.

Lesions mimicking oral candidiasis include oral hairy leukoplakia, leukoplakia, and lichen planus. Oral hairy leukoplakia is an adherent, reticulate (lacy) white lesion that begins on the distal lateral tongue. Leukoplakia appears as adherent solid white patches on the buccal mucosa or tongue at sites of chronic irritation. As these lesions age, they become chalk-white and thick and can be palpated as a firm nodule. Lichen planus is a striated or reticulated white plaque that can have a serpiginous annular or linear configuration and can be associated with ulcers or erosions. If ulcers are present, they are painful. However, the lesions are usually asymptomatic. Lichen planus has a predilection for the buccal mucosa and tongue, but can occur anywhere inside the oral cavity.

**Bibliography**

1. **Priddy RW.** Inflammatory hyperplasias of the oral mucosa. J Can Dent Assoc. 1992;58:311-21. PMID: 1591647

## HIV Disease Question 15
## Answer: A

**Educational Objective:** *Recognize oral hairy leukoplakia and distinguish it from lichen planus, leukoplakia, and oral candidiasis.*

Oral hairy leukoplakia is characterized by painless, adherent, reticulate (lacy) white lesions that begin on the distal lateral tongue. The disorder is strongly associated with HIV infection.

Lesions mimicking oral hairy leukoplakia include lichen planus, leukoplakia, and oral candidiasis. Lichen planus is a striated or reticulated white plaque that can have a serpiginous annular or linear configuration and can be associated with ulcers or erosions. If ulcers are present, they are painful. However, the lesions are usually asymptomatic. Lichen planus has a predilection for the buccal mucosa and tongue, but can occur anywhere inside the oral cavity.

Leukoplakia is characterized by adherent, solid white patches on the buccal mucosa or tongue at sites of chronic irritation. As the lesions age, they become chalk-white and thick and can be palpatated as a firm nodule. In contrast to oral hairy leukoplakia, leukoplakia is a solid nodular plaque that can involve the dorsum of the tongue as well as the lateral margins. Oral candidiasis is a painful solid white or yellow plaque that can occur anywhere on the oral mucosa. The plaque is a pseudomembrane, meaning that it can be partially scraped off. Bleeding can occur where the plaque is removed. The mucosa surrounding the lesion is bright red and swollen.

### Bibliography

1. **Priddy RW.** Inflammatory hyperplasias of the oral mucosa. J Can Dent Assoc. 1992;58:311-21. PMID: 1591647

## HIV Disease Question 16
## Answer: B

**Educational Objective:** *Recognize the typical presentation of cerebral toxoplasmosis on MRI.*

The presentation here is a single, ring-enhancing lesion in a HIV-infected patient. The major differential diagnosis is between cerebral toxoplasmosis and lymphoma. While both are common in HIV-infected patients, the lack of central necrosis or mass effect makes CNS lymphoma less likely. HIV dementia will present with atrophy or progressive multifocal encephalopathy. Diffuse cerebral edema and thromboembolic strokes do not present with focal ring enhancing lesions.

### Bibliography

1. **Ammassari A, Murri R, Cingolani A, DeLuca A, Antinori A.** AIDS-associated cerebral toxoplasmosis: an update on diagnosis and treatment. Curr Top Microbiol Immunol. 1996;219:209-22. PMID: 8791702

## HIV Disease Question 17
## Answer: E

**Educational Objective:** *Recognize multifocal lesions consistent with a brain tumor on a contrast-enhanced CT scan of the brain.*

The main differential diagnosis for a patient with multiple, enhancing brain lesions on a CT scan includes metastases and primary central nervous system lymphoma. The five primary tumors that commonly metastasize to the brain are neoplasms of the lung, breast, kidney, and gastrointestinal tract and melanoma of the skin. Primary central nervous system lymphoma may also be multifocal and produce similar CT

findings. Other primary brain tumors, including astrocytomas and other gliomas, are typically unifocal.

The presentation here is multifocal, ring-enhancing lesions in an HIV-infected patient. The differential diagnosis is between cerebral toxoplasmosis and lymphoma. While both are common in HIV-infected patients the multifocal presentation makes toxoplasmosis less likely. HIV dementia will present with atrophy or progressive multifocal encphalopathy. Diffuse cerebral edema and thromboembolic strokes do not present with focal, ring-enhancing lesions.

### Bibliography

1. **Smirniotopoulos JG, Koeller KK, Nelson AM, Murphy FM.** Neuroimaging-autopsy correlations in AIDS. Neuroimaging Clin N Am. 1997;7:615-37. PMID: 9376971
2. **Provenzale JM, Jinkins JR.** Brain and spine imaging findings in AIDS patients. Radiol Clin North Am. 1997;35:1127-66. PMID: 9298090

## HIV Disease Question 18
## Answer: C

**Educational Objective:** *Select the most appropriate management for a patient with HIV infection and a central nervous system mass lesion.*

Central nervous system mass lesions in patients with HIV infection are caused most often by *Toxoplasma gondii* or lymphoma. *Mycobacteria,* endemic mycoses, *Nocardia,* and amebae can also cause mass lesions on occasion; glioblastoma multiforme, metastatic solid tumors, and conventional bacterial abscesses also occur. The computed tomographic (CT) scan is not highly specific for suggesting which diagnosis is most likely.

This patient is very unlikely to have cerebral toxoplasmosis for three reasons: his CD4 cell count is unusually high, he has a negative *Toxoplasma* serology, and he has been taking reasonably effective prophylaxis. Thus, another diagnosis must be sought.

There is urgency to establish a diagnosis in this patient because of the size of the two lesions and the presence of surrounding edema. Lymphomas can be readily diagnosed by CT-guided needle biopsies if the lesion can be visualized by CT scan and is anatomically accessible. An open brain biopsy is unnecessary if the lesion is accessible to needle biopsy.

### Bibliography

1. **Carr A, Tindall B, Brew BJ, Marriott DJ, Harkness JK, Penny R, et al.** Low-dose trimethoprim-sulfamethoxazole prophylaxis for toxoplasmic encephalitis in patients with AIDS. Ann Intern Med. 1992;117:106-11. PMID: 1351371
2. **Porter SB, Sande MA.** Toxoplasmosis of the central nervous system in the acquired immunodeficiency syndrome. N Engl J Med. 1992;327:1643-8. PMID: 1359410
3. **Luft BJ, Remington JS.** Toxoplasmic encephalitis in AIDS. Clin Infect Dis. 1992;15:211-22. PMID: 1520757

## HIV Disease Question 19
## Answer: A

**Educational Objective:** *Evaluate a patient with HIV infection and pulmonary disease.*

Establishing a microbiologic diagnosis in patients with HIV-related pulmonary disease is essential to guide therapy and assess response. In patients with symptoms and radiographic evidence of pneumonitis, specific tests to identify potential pathogens are required. In patients with induced sputum specimens that are unrevealing, bronchoscopy with bronchoalveolar lavage should be done and specimens sent for *Pneumocystis carinii* and acid-fast stains and bacterial, mycobacterial, and fungal cultures. Bronchoalveolar lavage is highly sensitive for diagnosing opportunistic pulmonary disease in patients with HIV disease, such as this 40-year-old man.

Nonspecific tests such as gallium lung scanning or CT scanning are of little use in identifying the specific cause of pneumonitis.

Empiric therapy for *P. carinii* is not an appropriate alternative to bronchoscopy, although presumptive anti-*Pneumocystis* therapy may be given while the evaluation proceeds. Because therapy for *P. carinii* pneumonia such as corticosteroids and high-dose trimethoprim-sulfamethoxazole is potentially toxic and differs greatly from therapy for bacterial pneumonia or tuberculosis, further evaluation of patients with normal induced sputum is warranted. Ventilation-perfusion lung scanning is not indicated, because there is no clinical evidence of pulmonary embolism.

### Bibliography

1. **Masur H**. Prevention and treatment of *Pneumocystis* pneumonia. N Engl J Med. 1992;327:1853-60. PMID: 1448123

2. **Broaddus C, Dake MD, Stulbarg MS, Blumfeld W, Hadley WK, Golden JA, et al.** Bronchoalveolar lavage and transbronchial biopsy for the diagnosis of pulmonary infections in the acquired immunodeficiency syndrome. Ann Intern Med. 1985;102:747-52. PMID: 2986505

## HIV Disease Question 20
## Answer: C

**Educational Objective:** *Diagnose Mycobacterium tuberculosis in HIV-infected patients.*

Although *Mycobacterium avium-intracellulare* complex (MAC) is an important cause of infection in HIV-infected persons, it almost never causes infections in patients with CD4 cell counts greater than $100/\mu L$. The most likely acid-fast organism causing infection in this particular patient is *Mycobacterium tuberculosis*. HIV seropositivity is clearly an important risk factor for the development of tuberculosis. One of the major reasons cited for the reversal of the trend of steady decline in the number of tuberculosis cases in the United States is increase in tuberculosis among HIV-infected persons. Those who are HIV-positive and use injected drugs are at a particular risk of developing infection with *M. tuberculosis*. Of particular concern is the increase in multidrug-resistant tuberculosis. Previously treated patients, those infected with HIV, and injected drug users are at increased risk for drug resistance. Spread of multidrug-resistant organisms from these patients to other patients and care providers in hospitals and institutions (prisons) has been reported.

Other organisms of clinical importance in HIV-infected patients, which may be completely or partially acid-fast, include *Rhodococcus equi* and *Nocardia* species. The protozoan parasites *Cryptosporidium* and *Isospora* may also stain with the acid-fast procedure. Although much less common than the mycobacteria, these organisms should be kept in mind when considering a report of "acid-fast organisms present" in an HIV-infected person. Notably in HIV-infected children, MAC is a frequent cause of pulmonary disease.

### Bibliography

1. **Frieden TR, Sterling T, Pablos-Mendez A, Kilburn JO, Cauthen GM, Dooley SW**. The emergence of drug-resistant tuberculosis in New York City. N Engl J Med. 1993;328:21-6. PMID: 8381207

2. **Selwyn PA, Hartel D, Lewis VA, Schoenbaum EE, Vermund SH, Klein RS, et al**. A prospective study of the risk of tuberculosis among intravenous drug users with human immunodeficiency virus infection. N Engl J Med. 1989;320:545-50. PMID: 2915665

## HIV Disease Question 21
## Answer: A

**Educational Objective:** *Determine the common causes of anal ulceration in HIV-infected men.*

There are many causes of a painful anal ulcer. The most common cause is reactivation of herpes simplex infection. The immunosuppression of HIV infection allows for an increased incidence of reactivation of latent infection to disease—even in people who are unaware of prior herpes infection. The diagnosis is easily made by the clinical appearance of the ulcers (vesicles or shallow ulcers in the anal/perianal area) and culture of the lesion for herpes simplex virus. The lesion usually responds well to acyclovir, but prolonged courses of therapy may be required for complete healing. For frequent recurrences, long-term suppressive therapy is recommended for both symptomatic relief as well as the observation that reactivation of herpes can result in increased HIV replication.

Primary syphilis typically presents as a painless mucosal lesion at the site of inoculation. This lesion is typically heaped up at the edge and has a clean center. For people who engage in anogenital sex, this lesion may appear at the anal verge or inside the anus or rectum. The VDRL and confirmatory test for syphilis are typically positive but may be negative or positive at very low titer at the time of initial clinical manifestation. If clinical suspicion is high and the VDRL is negative, the test should be repeated in a week or two. The lesions respond to intramuscular benzathine penicillin G.

Human papillomavirus is sexually transmitted and typically presents as painless, raised, warty-like structures on the anogenital mucosa. Certain strains are oncogenic and may be the precursors of carcinoma in situ and squamous cell carcinoma of the anus. The latter occurs more commonly in homosexual men than in the general population and may present as a painful or painless mucosal ulcer. Polymerase chain reaction (PCR) is a research tool used to determine the specific strain of human papillomavirus. Anal Pap smears can be used to determine the presence of dysplasia. Anal biopsy is required for the diagnosis of anal squamous cell carcinoma.

Gonorrhea can present as an anal or urethral discharge in homosexual men. The diagnosis is made by Gram's stain of the discharge demonstrating the characteristic intracellular diplococci that can be confirmed on culture. Ulcerated lesions are not typical.

### Bibliography

1.  **Melbye M, Cote TR, Kessler L, Gail M, Biggar RJ**. High incidence of anal cancer among AIDS patients. The AIDS/Cancer Working Group. Lancet. 1994;343:636-9. PMID: 7906812

2.  **Critchlow CW, Surawicz CM, Holmes KK, Kuypers J, Daling JR, Hawes SE, et al**. Prospective study of high grade anal squamous intraepithelial neoplasia in a cohort of homosexual men: influence of HIV infection, immunosuppression and human papillomavirus infection. AIDS. 1995;9:1255-62. PMID: 8561979

3.  **Schmitt SL, Wexner SD**. Treatment of anorectal manifestations of AIDS: past and present. Int J STD AIDS. 1994;5:8-10. PMID: 8142539

## HIV Disease Question 22
## Answer: D

**Educational Objective:** *Evaluate the cause of fever in an HIV-infected patient.*

The prophylactic agent of choice for *Pneumocystis carinii* pneumonia (PCP) is trimethoprim-sulfamethoxazole, given as one double-strength tablet daily or three times per week. For patients compliant with this therapy, the risk of PCP is less than 5%. PCP typically presents with fever, dry cough, and progressive dyspnea. The chest radiograph can be normal in the early stages. Decreases in oxygen saturation with exertion can be an early manifestation. For reasons that are not understood, patients with HIV infection have an increased rate of hypersensitivity reactions to trimethoprim-sulfamethoxazole relative to the general population. Rates of reaction have been reported in approximately 20% to 30% of patients on prophylactic doses and up to 50% of patients on treatment doses of the agent. The reaction is typically delayed, with mean onset approximately 2 weeks after the initiation of therapy. Reactions are characterized by a diffuse erythematous eruption, pruritus, general malaise, and fever. Internal organ involvement such as hepatitis, myocarditis, thyroiditis, arthritis, and nephritis occurs less frequently. Mild reactions can generally be treated with acetaminophen, antihistamines, low-dose prednisone, or dimenhydrate. More serious reactions require

discontinuation of the drug. Patients may subsequently be able to tolerate the drug after a course of desensitization.

As the CD4 count decreases below $200/\mu L$ the HIV-infected patient becomes increasingly at risk for opportunistic infections and malignancies that can present with fever. The earliest complications include bacterial pneumonia, lymphoma, and PCP. As the CD4 count decreases below $50/\mu L$, the HIV-infected patient is at increased risk for disseminated *Mycobacterium avium* (MAI) infection. The latter often presents with fever, night sweats, wasting, anemia, and increases in alkaline phosphatase. Disseminated MAI infection would be unlikely in a patient with a CD4 count of $150/\mu L$.

Bacterial pneumonia is usually caused by *Streptococcus pneumoniae*, *Haemophilus influenzae*, or *Mycoplasma pneumoniae*. Its presentation in the HIV-infected patient is similar to that in the HIV-negative patient, with cough, fever, shortness of breath, hypoxia, signs of consolidation on physical examination and an abnormal chest radiograph.

Fever without rash has been uncommonly described in patients receiving zidovudine. Fever typically occurs 5 to 7 days after initiation of therapy and recurs with rechallenge.

### Bibliography

1.  **Bayard PJ, Berger TG, Jacobson MA**. Drug hypersensitivity reactions and human immunodeficiency virus disease. J Acquir Immune Defic Syndr. 1992;5:1237-57. PMID: 1453334

2.  **Gordin FM, Simon GL, Wofsy CB, Mills J**. Adverse reactions to trimethoprim-sulfamethoxazole in patients with the acquired immunodeficiency syndrome. Ann Intern Med. 1984;100: 495-9. PMID: 6230976

3.  **Barat LM, Gunn JE, Steger KA, Perkins CJ, Craven DE**. Causes of fever in patients infected with human immunodeficiency virus who were admitted to Boston City Hospital. Clin Infect Dis. 1996;23:320-8. PMID: 8842271

# NORMAL LABORATORY VALUES
## MKSAP for Students 2

U.S. traditional units are followed in parentheses by equivalent values expressed in S.I. units.

## Blood, Plasma, and Serum Chemistries

**Acetoacetate,** plasma — Less than 1 mg/dL (0.1 mmol/L)
**Alpha-fetoprotein,** serum — 0-20 ng/mL (0-20 µg/L)
**Aminotransferase, alanine** (ALT, SGPT) — 0-35 U/L
**Aminotransferase, aspartate** (AST, SGOT) — 0-35 U/L
**Ammonia,** plasma — 40-80 µg/dL (23-47 µmol/L)
**Amylase,** serum — 0-130 U/L
**Antistreptolysin O titer** — Less than 150 units
**Ascorbic acid (vitamin C),** blood — 0.4-1.5 mg/dL (23-86 µmol/L); leukocyte — less than 20 mg/dL (< 3.5 µmol/L)
**Bicarbonate,** serum — 23-28 meq/L (23-28 mmol/L)
**Bilirubin,** serum
　Total — 0.3-1.2 mg/dL (5.1-20.5 µmol/L)
　Direct — 0-0.3 mg/dL (0-5.1 µmol/L)
**Blood gases,** arterial (room air)
　$P_{O_2}$ - 80-100 mm Hg
　$P_{CO_2}$ - 35-45 mm Hg
　pH - 7.38-7.44
**Calcium,** serum — 9-10.5 mg/dL (2.2-2.6 mmol/L)
**Carbon dioxide content,** serum — 23-28 meq/L (23-28 mmol/L)
**Carcinoembryonic antigen** — Less than 2 ng/mL (2 µg/L)
**Carotene,** serum — 75-300 µg/dL (1.4-5.6 µmol/L)
**Ceruloplasmin,** serum — 25-43 mg/dL (250-430 mg/L)
**Chloride,** serum — 98-106 meq/L (98-106 mmol/L)
**Cholesterol, total,** plasma — 150-199 mg/dL (3.88-5.15 mmol/L), desirable
**Cholesterol, low-density lipoprotein** (LDL), plasma — Less than or equal to 130 mg/dL (3.36 mmol/L), desirable
**Cholesterol, high-density lipoprotein** (HDL), plasma — Greater than or equal to 40 mg/dL (1.04 mmol/L), desirable
**Complement,** serum
　C3 - 55-120 mg/dL (550-1200 mg/L)
　Total - 37-55 U/mL (37-55 kU/L)
**Copper,** serum — 70-155 µg/dL (11-24.3 µmol/L)
**Creatine kinase,** serum — 30-170 U/L
**Creatinine,** serum — 0.7-1.3 mg/dL (61.9-115 µmol/L)
**Delta-aminolevulinic acid,** serum — 15-23 µg/dL (1.14-1.75 µmol/L)
**Ethanol,** blood — less than 50 mg/dL (11 nmol/L)
**Fibrinogen,** plasma — 150-350 mg/dL (1.5-3.5 g/L)
**Folate,** red cell — 160-855 ng/mL (362-1937 nmol/L)
**Folate,** serum — 2.5-20 ng/mL (5.7-45.3 nmol/L)
**Glucose,** plasma — Fasting, 70-105 mg/dL (3.9-5.8 mmol/L); 2 hours postprandial less than 140 mg/dL (7.8 mmol/L)
**Homocysteine,** plasma — Male: 4-16 µmol/L; female: 3-14 µmol/L
**Immunoglobulins**
　IgG - 640-1430 mg/dL (6.4-14.3 g/L)
　　$IgG_1$ - 280-1020 mg/dL (2.8-10.2 g/L)
　　$IgG_2$ - 60-790 mg/dL (0.6-7.9 g/L)
　　$IgG_3$ - 14-240 mg/dL (0.14-2.4 g/L)
　　$IgG_4$ - 11-330 mg/dL (0.11-3.3 g/L)
　IgA - 70-300 mg/dL (0.7-3.0 g/L)
　IgM - 20-140 mg/dL (0.2-1.4 g/L)
　IgD - Less than 8 mg/dL (80 mg/L)
　IgE - 0.01-0.04 mg/dL (0.1-0.4 mg/L)
**Iron,** serum — 60-160 µg/dL (11-29 µmol/L)
**Iron binding capacity,** serum — 250-460 µg/dL (45-82 µmol/L)
**Lactate dehydrogenase,** serum — 60-100 U/L
**Lactic acid,** venous blood — 6-16 mg/dL (0.67-1.8 mmol/L)
**Lead,** blood — Less than 40 µg/dL (1.9 µmol/L)
**Lipase,** serum — Less than 95 U/L
**Magnesium,** serum — 1.5-2.4 mg/dL (0.62-0.99 mmol/L)
**Manganese,** serum — 0.3-0.9 mg/mL (300-900 ng/L)
**Methylmalonic acid,** serum — 150-370 nmol/L
**Osmolality,** plasma — 275-295 mosm/kg $H_2O$
**Phosphatase, acid,** serum — 0.5-5.5 U/L
**Phosphatase, alkaline,** serum — 36-92 U/L
**Phosphorus, inorganic,** serum — 3-4.5 mg/dL (0.97-1.45 mmol/L)

**Potassium,** serum — 3.5-5 meq/L (3.5-5 mmol/L)
**Protein,** serum
　Total - 6.0-7.8 g/dL (60-78 g/L)
　Albumin - 3.5-5.5 g/dL (35-55 g/L)
　Globulins - 2.5-3.5 g/dL (25-35 g/L)
　　$Alpha_1$ - 0.2-0.4 g/dL (2-4 g/L)
　　$Alpha_2$ - 0.5-0.9 g/dL (5-9 g/L)
　　Beta - 0.6-1.1 g/dL (6-11 g/L)
　　Gamma - 0.7-1.7 g/dL (7-17 g/L)
**Rheumatoid factor** — less than 40 U/mL (less than 40 kU/L)
**Sodium,** serum — 136-145 meq/L (136-145 mmol/L)
**Triglycerides** — Less than 250 mg/dL (2.82 mmol/L), desirable
**Urea nitrogen,** serum — 8-20 mg/dL (2.9-7.1 mmol/L)
**Uric acid,** serum — 2.5-8 mg/dL (0.15-0.47 mmol/L)
**Vitamin $B_{12}$,** serum — 200-800 pg/mL (148-590 pmol/L)

## Cerebrospinal Fluid

**Cell count** — 0-5 cells/µL ($0-5 \times 10^6$ cells/L)
**Glucose** — 40-80 mg/dL (2.5-4.4 mmol/L); less than 40% of simultaneous plasma concentration is abnormal
**Protein** — 15-60 mg/dL (150-600 mg/L)
**Pressure (opening)** — 70-200 cm $H_2O$

## Endocrine

**Adrenocorticotropin (ACTH)** — 9-52 pg/mL (2-11 pmol/L)
**Aldosterone,** serum
　Supine - 2-5 ng/dL (55-138 pmol/L)
　Standing - 7-20 ng/dL (194-554 pmol/L)
**Aldosterone,** urine — 5-19 µg/24 h (13.9-52.6 nmol/24 h)
**Catecholamines** — Epinephrine (supine): less than 75 ng/L (410 pmol/L); norepinephrine (supine): 50-440 ng/L (296-2600 pmol/L)
**Catecholamines, 24-hour,** urine — Less than 100 µg/m² per 24 h (591 nmol/m² per 24 h)
**Cortisol**
　Serum - 8 am: 8-20 µg/dL (221-552 nmol/L); 5 pm: 3-13 µg/dL (83-359 nmol/L);
　1 h after cosyntropin; greater than 18 µg/dL (498 nmol/L); usually 8 µg/dL (221 nmol/L) or more above baseline
　overnight suppression test: less than 5 µg/dL (138 nmol/L)
　Urine free cortisol - less than 90 µg/24 h (248 nmol/24 h)
**Dehydroepiandrosterone sulfate,** plasma — Male: 1.3-5.5 mg/mL (3.5-14.9 µmol/L); female: 0.6-3.3 mg/mL (1.6-8.9 µmol/L)
**11-deoxycortisol,** plasma — Basal: less than 5 µg/dL (145 nmol/L); after metyrapone: greater than 7 µg/dL (203 nmol/L)
**Estradiol,** serum — Male: 10-30 pg/mL (37-110 pmol/L); female: day 1-10, 50-100 pmol/L; day 11-20, 50-200 pmol/L; day 21-30, 70-150 pmol/L
**Estriol,** urine — Greater than 12 mg/24 h (42 µmol/d)
**Follicle-stimulating hormone,** serum — Male (adult): 5-15 mU/mL (5-15 U/L); female: follicular or luteal phase, 5-20 mU/mL (5-20 U/L); midcycle peak, 30-50 mU/mL (30-50 U/L); postmenopausal, greater than 35 mU/mL (35 U/L)
**Growth hormone,** plasma — After oral glucose, less than 2 ng/mL (2 µg/L); response to provocative stimuli: greater than 7 ng/mL (7 µg/L)
**17-hydroxycorticosteroids,** urine (Porter-Silber) — Male: 3-10 mg/24 h (8.3-28 µmol/24 h); female: 2-8 mg/24 h (5.5-22.1 µmol/24 h)
**Insulin,** serum (fasting) — 5-20 mU/L (35-139 pmol/L)
**17-ketosteroids,** urine — Male: 8-22 mg/24 h (28-77 µmol/24 h); female: up to 15 µg/24 h (52 mmol/24 h)
**Luteinizing hormone,** serum — Male: 3-15 mU/mL (3-15 U/L); female: follicular or luteal phase, 5-22 mU/mL (5-22 U/L); midcycle peak, 30-250 mU/mL (30-250 U/L); postmenopausal, greater than 30 mU/mL (30 U/L)

**Metanephrine,** urine — Less than 1.2 mg/24 h (6.1 mmol/24 h)
**Parathyroid hormone,** serum — 10-65 pg/mL (10-65 ng/L)
**Progesterone**
  Luteal — 3-30 ng/mL (0.1-0.95 nmol/L)
  Follicular — less than 1 ng/mL (0.03-nmol/L)
**Prolactin,** serum — Male: less than 15 ng/mL (15 mg/L);
  female: less than 20 ng/mL (20 mg/L)
**Renin activity (angiotensin-I radioimmunoassay),** plasma
  Normal diet: supine, 0.3-1.9 ng/mL per h (0.3-1.9 µg/L per h);
  upright, 0.2-3.6 ng/mL per h (0.2-3.6 µg/L per h)
**Sperm concentration** — 20-150 million/mL (20-50 × 10^9/L)
**Sweat test for sodium and chloride** — Less than 60 meq/L
  (60 mmol/L)
**Testosterone,** serum — Adult male: 300-1200 ng/dL (10-42
  nmol/L); female: 20-75 ng/dL (0.7-2.6 nmol/L)
**Thyroid function tests** (normal ranges vary)
  Thyroid iodine ($^{131}$I) uptake - 10% to 30% of administered dose
  at 24 h
  Thyroid-stimulating hormone (TSH) - 0.5-5.0 µU/mL (0.5-5.0
  mU/mL)
  Thyroxine ($T_4$), serum
    Total - 5-12 µg/dL (64-155 nmol/L)
    Free - 0.9-2.4 ng/dL (12-31 pmol/L)
    Free $T_4$ index - 4-11
  Triiodothyronine, resin ($T_3$) - 25%-35%
  Triiodothyronine, serum ($T_3$) - 70-195 ng/dL (1.1-3.0 nmol/L)
**Vanillylmandelic acid,** urine — Less than 8 mg/24 h (40.4
  µmol/24 h)
**Vitamin D**
  1,25-dihydroxy, serum - 25-65 pg/mL (60-156 pmol/L)
  25-hydroxy, serum - 15-80 ng/mL (37-200 nmol/L)

## Gastrointestinal

**D-xylose absorption** (after ingestion of 25 g of D-xylose) — Urine
  excretion: 5-8 g at 5 h (33-53 mmol); serum D-xylose: greater
  than 20 mg/dL at 2 h (1.3 nmol/L)
**Fecal urobilinogen** — 40-280 mg/24 h (68-473 µmol/ 24 h)
**Gastric secretion** — Basal secretion: male: 4.0 ± 0.2 meq of HCl/h
  (4.0 ± 0.2 mmol/h); female: 2.1 ± 0.2 meq of HCl/h (2.1 ± 0.2
  mmol/h); peak acid secretion: male: 37.4 ± 0.8 meq/h (37.4 ±
  0.8 mmol/h); female: 24.9 ± 1.0 meq/h (24.9 ± 1.0 mmol/h)
**Gastrin,** serum — 0-180 pg/mL (0-180 ng/L)
**Lactose tolerance test** — Increase in plasma glucose: greater than
  15 mg/dL (0.83 mmol/L)
**Lipase,** ascitic fluid — Less than 200 U/L
**Secretin-cholecystokinin pancreatic function** — Greater than
  80 meq/L (80 mmol/L) of $HCO_3$ in at least 1 specimen
  collected over 1 h
**Stool fat** — Less than 5 g/d on a 100-g fat diet
**Stool nitrogen** — Less than 2 g/d
**Stool weight** — Less than 200 g/d

## Hematology

**Activated partial thromboplastin time** — 25-35 s
**Bleeding time** — Less than 10 min
**Coagulation factors,** plasma
  Factor I - 150-350 mg/dL (1.5-3.5 g/L)
  Factor II - 60%-150% of normal
  Factor V - 60%-150% of normal
  Factor VII - 60%-150% of normal
  Factor VIII - 60%-150% of normal
  Factor IX - 60%-150% of normal
  Factor X - 60%-150% of normal
  Factor XI - 60%-150% of normal
  Factor XII - 60%-150% of normal
**Erythrocyte count** — 4.2-5.9 million cells/µL (4.2-5.9 x 10^12 cells/L)
**Erythrocyte survival rate** ($^{51}$Cr) — T½ = 28 days
**Erythropoietin** — less than 30 mU/mL (30 U/L)
**D-dimer** — less than 0.5 µg/mL (500 mg/L)
**Ferritin,** serum — 15-200 ng/mL (15-200 mg/L)
**Glucose-6-phosphate dehydrogenase,** blood — 5-15 U/g Hgb
  (0.32-0.97 mU/mol Hgb)

**Haptoglobin,** serum — 50-150 mg/dL (500-1500 mg/L)
**Hematocrit** — Male: 41%-51%; female: 36%-47%
**Hemoglobin,** blood — Male: 14-17 g/dL (140-170 g/L);
  female: 12-16 g/dL (120-160 g/L)
**Hemoglobin,** plasma — 0.5-5 mg/dL (0.08-0.8 µmol/L)
**Leukocyte alkaline phosphatase** — 15-40 mg of phosphorus liber-
  ated/h per 10^10 cells; score = 13-130/100 polymorphonuclear
  neutrophils and band forms
**Leukocyte count** — Nonblacks: 4000-10,000/µL
  (4.0-10 × 10^9/L); Blacks: 3500-10,000/µL (3.5-10 x 10^9/L)
**Lymphocytes**
  CD4$^+$ cell count — 640-1175/µL (0.64-1.18 × 10^9/L)
  CD8$^+$ cell count — 335-875/µL (0.34-0.88 × 10^9/L)
  CD4: CD8 ratio — 1.0-4.0
**Mean corpuscular hemoglobin** (MCH) — 28-32 pg
**Mean corpuscular hemoglobin concentration** (MCHC) —
  32-36 g/dL (320-360 g/L)
**Mean corpuscular volume** (MCV) — 80-100 fL
**Osmotic fragility of erythrocytes** — Increased if hemolysis
  occurs in over 0.5% NaCl, decreased if hemolysis is incomplete
  in 0.3% NaCl
**Platelet count** — 150,000-350,000/µL (150-350 × 10^9/L)
**Platelet life span** ($^{51}$Cr) — 8-12 days
**Protein C activity,** plasma — 67%-131%
**Protein C resistance** — 2.2-2.6
**Protein S activity,** plasma — 82%-144%
**Prothrombin time** — 11-13 s
**Reticulocyte count** — 0.5%-1.5% of erythrocytes; absolute: 23,000-
  90,000 cells/µL (23-90 × 10^9/L)
**Schilling test** (oral administration of radioactive cobalamin-labeled
  vitamin B$_{12}$) — 8.5%-28% excreted in urine per 24-48 h
**Sedimentation rate,** erythrocyte (Westergren) — Male:
  0-15 mm/h; female: 0-20 mm/h
**Volume,** blood
  Plasma - Male: 25-44 mL/kg (0.025-0.044 L/kg) body weight;
    female: 28-43 mL/kg (0.028-0.043 L/kg) body weight
  Erythrocyte - Male: 25-35 mL/kg (0.025-0.044 L/kg) body
    weight; female: 20-30 mL/kg (0.020-0.030 L/kg) body
    weight

## Pulmonary

**Forced expiratory volume in 1 second (FEV$_1$)** — Greater than
  80% predicted
**Forced vital capacity (FVC)** — Greater than 80% predicted
**FEV$_1$/FVC** — Greater than 75% (0.75)

## Urine

**Amino acids** — 200-400 mg/24 h (14-29 nmol/24 h)
**Amylase** — 6.5-48.1 U/h
**Calcium** — 100-300 mg/d (2.5-7.5 mmol/d) on unrestricted diet
**Chloride** — 80-250 meq/d (80-250 mmol/d) (varies with intake)
**Copper** — 0-100 µg/24 h (0-1.6 µmol/d)
**Coproporphyrin** — 50-250 µg/24 h (76-382 nmol/d)
**Creatine** — Male: 4-40 mg/24 h (30-305 mmol/24 h);
  female: 0-100 mg/24 h (0-763 mmol/24 h)
**Creatinine** — 15-25 mg/kg per 24 h (133-221 mmol/kg per 24 h)
**Creatinine clearance** — 90-140 mL/min (0.09-0.14 l/min)
**5-hydroxyindoleacetic acid (5-HIAA)** — 2-9 mg/24 h
  (10.4-46.8 µmol/d)
**Osmolality** — 38-1400 mosm/kg $H_2O$
**Phosphate, tubular resorption** — 79%-94% (0.79-0.94) of filtered
  load
**Potassium** — 25-100 meq/24 h (25-100 mmol/24 h) (varies with
  intake)
**Protein** — Less than 100 mg/24 h
**Sodium** — 100-260 meq/24 h (100-260 mmol/24 h) (varies with
  intake)
**Uric acid** — 250-750 mg/24 h (1.48-4.43 mmol/24 h) (varies
  with diet)
**Urobilinogen** — 0.05-2.5 mg/24 h (0.08-4.22 µmol/24 h)

## American College of Physicians
190 N. Independence Mall West, Philadelphia, PA 19106-1572

# Notes

# Notes